Weight Loss - A Multidisciplinary Perspective

Edited by Hubertus Himmerich

Published in London, United Kingdom

Weight Loss - A Multidisciplinary Perspective
http://dx.doi.org/10.5772/intechopen.1001687
Edited by Hubertus Himmerich

Contributors
Alexandra Harvey, Amardeep Shrestha, Anayeli D.J. Patiño-Laguna, Andrew Kurt Thaw, Anıl Ergin, Bogdan Severus Gaspar, Camilla Day, Carla P. Barragán-Álvarez, Cihan Şahan, Citlalli E. Mora-Navarro, Elizabeth Contreras-López, Emmanuel Pérez-Escalante, Gemma Peachey, Georgia Faulkner, Hubertus Himmerich, Ines Green, Ivana Picek, Janet Treasure, Jessica Lizbeth Sebastián-Nicolás, Jessica McMahon, Jesús Guadalupe Pérez Flores, José Antonio Guerrero-Solano, José M. Mora-Martínez, Khang Jin Cheah, Laura García-Curiel, Lin Jia Cheah, Lizbeth Anahí Portillo-Torres, Luis Guillermo González-Olivares, Maija Huttunen-Lenz, Marek Soltes, Marie Hehl, Maryam Alkhatry, Matej Pekař, Michelle E. Gonzalez-Mora, Miriam A. Mora-Navarro, Monica Profir, Pavol Holéczy, Phoebe Saville, Prakriti Singh Shrestha, Sanda Maria Cretoiu, Susan Peirce Thompson, Titilope Omitogun

First published in London, United Kingdom, 2024 by IntechOpen
IntechOpen is the global imprint of INTECHOPEN LIMITED, registered in England and Wales, registration number: 11086078, 167-169 Great Portland Street, London, W1W 5PF, United Kingdom

British Library Cataloguing-in-Publication Data
A catalogue record for this book is available from the British Library

Additional hard and PDF copies can be obtained from orders@intechopen.com

Weight Loss - A Multidisciplinary Perspective
Edited by Hubertus Himmerich
p. cm.
Print ISBN 978-0-85466-692-8
Online ISBN 978-0-85466-691-1
eBook (PDF) ISBN 978-0-85466-693-5

For EU product safety concerns:
IN TECH d.o.o., Prolaz Marije Krucifikse Kozulić 3, 51000 Rijeka, Croatia,
info@intechopen.com or visit our website at intechopen.com.

Meet the editor

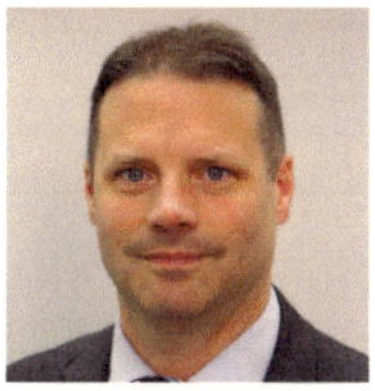

Professor Dr. Med. Hubertus Himmerich is a reader in eating disorders at King's College London and a consultant psychiatrist on an inpatient ward for patients with eating disorders at the Bethlem Royal Hospital in London, UK. Following medical school, Dr. Himmerich received his scientific and clinical training at the Max Planck Institute of Psychiatry, Germany, and the Universities of Mainz and Marburg, Germany. Afterward, he worked as a consultant psychiatrist at the RWTH Aachen University Hospital and as a professor of neurobiology of affective disorders at the University of Leipzig, Germany. He has led and performed national and international scientific projects with researchers from Africa, Asia, Australia, America, and Europe; and he has published more than 200 articles in peer-reviewed scientific journals, books, and book chapters.

Contents

Preface

The book *Weight Loss – A Multidisciplinary Perspective* depicts the relevance of weight loss as a clinical symptom or as a desired treatment outcome. It includes chapters on economic, pathophysiological, diagnostic, and therapeutic aspects of various eating, gut, and weight disorders. The book comprises contributions from scientists, clinicians, and an author with lived experience.

As the chapters cover timely research topics such as the microbiome–gut-brain axis, ultra-processed food, probiotics, bariatric and endoscopic surgery, lifestyle interventions, patient-centered communication, and shared decision-making, the book provides a comprehensive overview of current ideas about eating, gut, and weight disorders.

I am grateful to the team of diverse authors from Australia, the Czech Republic, Germany, Malaysia, Mexico, the Slovak Republic, Romania, Turkey, the United Arab Emirates, the United Kingdom, and the United States of America for their excellent contributions; and I would also like to thank IntechOpen and specifically Ms. Tea Jelaca for making this book project possible.

Hubertus Himmerich
Department of Psychological Medicine,
King's College London,
London, UK

Section 1

The Microbiome-Gut-Brain Axis and Probiotics

Chapter 1

Tryptophan Metabolites and the Microbiome-Gut-Brain Axis in Major Gut Disorders

Bogdan Severus Gaspar, Monica Profir and Sanda Maria Cretoiu

Abstract

Recently, the role of the gut microbiome has become more prominent in gut-brain interactions. The microbiota-gut-brain axis homeostasis is responsible for our emotional behavior, stress response, and brain neurotransmitter balance. This bidirectional communication axis between the gut and the brain is influenced by the effect of the microbiome on the metabolic pathways of the host. Intestinal bacteria intervene directly in Trp metabolism, generating signaling molecules and specific metabolites with physiological effects on both the brain and the intestine. Trp is also metabolized under the influence of the microbiome and suffers three major pathways in the organism: The serotonin (5-HT), kynurenine, and indole pathway resulting in the production of neuro-active metabolites. This current chapter aims to cover the most recent data referring to the Trp metabolites and the microbiome-gut-brain axis in major gut disorders, such as irritable bowel syndrome (IBS), inflammatory bowel disease (IBD), and celiac disease. These diseases are frequently associated with mood disorders.

Keywords: microbiome, indole, tryptophan, kynurenine pathway, serotonin

1. Introduction

Tryptophan (Trp) is an essential aromatic amino acid necessary for the normal growth and health of mammalian species [1]. The main source of Trp is the diet, however, small amounts can be produced by the gut microbiota, *Escherichia coli*, in particular [2]. Trp is found in foods with protein content, such as turkey, chicken, pork meat, fish, cheese, tofu, beans, nuts, and seeds [3]. Trp is absorbed at the intestinal level and its absorption and availability in the small intestine are limited by the simultaneous ingestion of carbohydrates and neutral amino acids because the release of insulin favors the absorption of the latter [4]. Free Trp can be incorporated into proteins, but it also serves as a precursor of serotonin and melatonin, the availability of Trp being dependent on vitamin B6 [5, 6]. A small part of Trp from food reaches the large intestine, where it is degraded under the action of the microbiota, following different metabolic routes (**Figure 1**). The resulting metabolites participate in the microbiota-gut-brain communication [7–9].

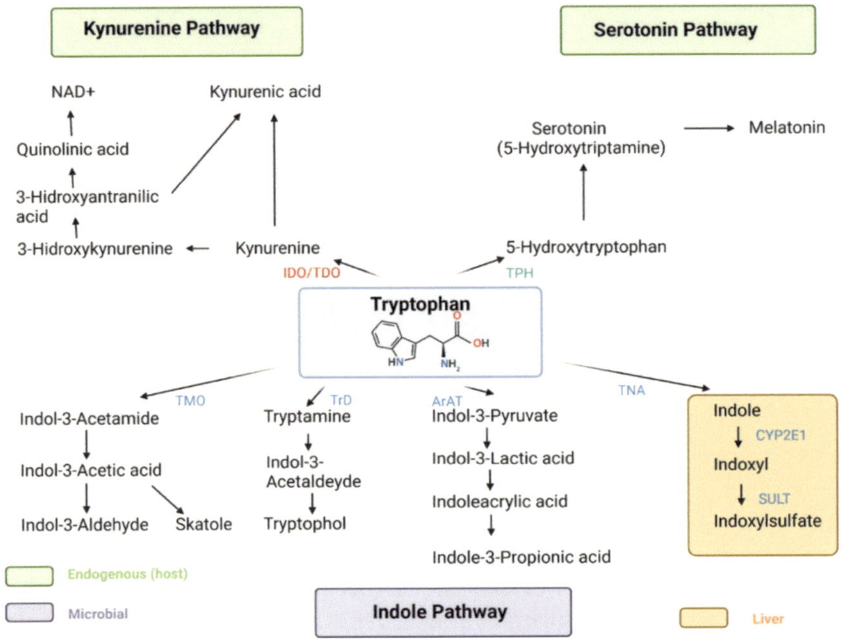

Figure 1.
The tryptophan metabolism. Tryptophan metabolism occurs via the kynurenine pathway or the serotonin pathway. Kynurenine is metabolized to kynurenic or quinolinic acid, which is then converted to nicotinamide adenine dinucleotide (NAD+). In the serotonin pathway, Trp is converted to 5-HTP in the enterochromaffin cells and enteric neurons and can be further metabolized to form melatonin. Microbiota metabolize Trp into indole and indole derivatives because they express different enzymes, resulting in end-products. Abbreviations: ArAT - aromatic amino acid aminotransferase; IDO - indoleamine 2,3-dioxygenase; NAD⁺- nicotinamide adenine dinucleotide; TDO - tryptophan 2,3-dioxygenase; TPH - tryptophan hydroxylase; TrD - tryptophan decarboxylase enzyme; TNA - tryptophanase; SULT - sulfotransferase. Created with BioRender.

Multiple studies demonstrated that the gut microbiota plays a key role in the gut-brain axis modulation by influencing the production of metabolites [10, 11].

Nowadays, microbiota located in the gut is regarded as a "virtual organ" outnumbering the human cells by a ratio of at least 10:1 [12]. However, this ratio was criticized by Sender et al. who suggested that the ratio is in fact 1:1 [13].

The intestinal microbiota is essential for normal brain development and for normal human behavior in adulthood, mainly based on the metabolism of Trp. This was demonstrated by studies on germ-free animals. These studies brought tremendous achievements in this regard, because it was demonstrated that the high Trp levels observed in germ-free mice decreased after colonization of their gut, indicating that microbiota plays a role in this decrease and also in the development of central serotonergic systems [14].

Some *in vitro* studies showed that there are specific bacterial strains such as *Lactococcus lactis subsp. cremoris* (MG 1363), *L. lactis subsp. lactis* (IL1403), *Lactobacillus plantarum* (FI8595), *Streptococcus thermophilus* (NCFB2392), *Escherichia coli* K-12, *Morganella morganii* (NCIMB, 10466), *Klebsiella pneumoniae* (NCIMB, 673), and *Hafnia alvei* (NCIMB, 11999) that can produce serotonin from Trp [15–17].

The brain-gut axis is a bidirectional communication network between the gastrointestinal tract, the (ENS), and the (CNS), mediated primarily by serotonin. Serotonin plays a major role in the normal functioning of the gut-brain axis, acting as a neurotransmitter in both the CNS and the ENS [18].

Numerous sensations and functions are under the bidirectional (sensory and motor) control of vagal system: Nausea, fullness, visceral pain, peristalsis, sphincter control, etc. During the development of the enteric vagal innervation, the microbiota might influence the developing axons of the ENS [19]. The gut microbiota is apparently responsible for the maturation of the adult ENS through the release of 5-HT and activation of 5-HT4 receptors, indicating its involvement in the normal peristaltic function of the gut [20].

Trp metabolites, either of endogenous origin (kynurenine, kynurenic acid, and NAD+) or resulting from bacterial degradation (indole, indole propionic acid, indole acetic acid, skatole, and tryptamine), are involved in gut immune homeostasis and mucosal homeostasis, and in serotonergic signaling [21].

Trp metabolites produced by microbes play an important role in gut physiology. The Trp metabolite indole has anti-inflammatory activities and *in vitro* studies have demonstrated that indole promotes health by inducing the expression of tight junction proteins and anti-inflammatory cytokines along with decreasing the level of pro-inflammatory interleukin-8 (IL-8) [22]. Other studies have demonstrated that indole-3-lactic acid (ILA) is able to reduce inflammation in immature epithelial cells [23, 24].

Therefore, it is considered that dysbiosis is implicated in many functional disorders of the gut-brain axis, such as (IBS), irritable bowel disease (IBD), and certain neuropsychiatric disorders like autism or depression [25–28].

In this chapter, we summarize the Trp metabolic pathways and we provide an in-depth description of their interrelation with the gut microbiota and their impact on the gut-brain axis in major gut disorders, such as IBS, IBD, and celiac disease (CeD).

2. Trp metabolic pathways

2.1 The serotonin pathway

The serotonin synthesis occurs primarily in the gastrointestinal tract (90%) and partially in the CNS (10%) starting from its precursor Trp [5]. The initial step in the serotonin pathway is represented by the Trp hydrolysis to 5-hydroxy Trp (5-HTP) via Trp hydroxylase 1 and 2 (TPH1/2). TPH1 is found in the periphery, while TPH2 is found in the CNS. 5-HTP is then rapidly decarboxylated by the aromatic L-amino decarboxylase (ALAAD) to 5-hydroxytryptamine (5-HT) known as serotonin [29].

5-HT is finally converted to melatonin in the pineal gland and the periphery or it is metabolized by monoamine oxidase (MAO) to 5-hydroxyindole acetaldehyde, which aldehyde dehydrogenase (ALDH) further oxidizes to 5-hydroxyindoleacetic acid (5-HIAA). The serotonin metabolite 5-HIAA is eliminated via urinary excretion [30].

2.2 The kynurenine pathway

Only 5% of the Trp is utilized as a substrate for the production of 5-HT. The remaining fraction of Trp enters the kynurenic pathway [31]. The Trp degradation arises primarily in the liver via the Trp 2,3-dioxygenase (TDO) and partially extrahepatic in the brain and the gastrointestinal tract via the indoleamine 2,3-dioxygenase (IDO). TDO and IDO are enzymes induced by glucocorticoids and pro-inflammatory cytokines and convert Trp to kynurenine as a first step in the kynurenine pathway [32]. Therefore, infections and chronic stress can reduce the amount of Trp that is converted to serotonin having a negative effect on mental health and the neuroendocrine stress axis [33–35].

After this initial step, kynurenine can be catabolized by three different enzymes. Kynurenine aminotransferase (KAT) converts kynurenine into kynurenic acid (KA). KA is an N-methyl-D-aspartate (NMDA) receptor antagonist and α7 nicotinic acetylcholine receptor and it exhibits immunosuppressive, anti-oxidative, and neuroprotective roles [31].

Part of kynurenine can also be converted to 3-hydroxykynurenine (3-HK) by the kynurenine-3-monooxygenase (KMO). 3-HK is further converted to 3-hydroxyanthranilic (3-HAA) via the enzyme kynureninase. Both 3-HK and 3-HAA are neurotoxic and oxidative mediators [31]. 3-HK has been shown to induce endogenous oxidative stress and neuronal cell apoptosis and has been linked to a series of neurodegenerative disorders [36]. 3-HK can further be converted to xanthurenic acid (XA). 3-HAA can be converted to quinolinic acid (QA), which is further catabolized into nicotinamide adenine dinucleotide (NAD^+) and niacin. KA and QA are both neuroactive inflammatory mediators [5]. Studies have found a link between high levels of QA and numerous neurological disorders such as anxiety, depression, Huntington's disease, and Alzheimer's disease [37–39]. In addition, kynureninase converts kynurenine to anthranilic acid (AA), a metabolite generally accepted as biologically inactive [40].

2.3 The indole pyruvate pathway

Most of the available Trp comes from dietary intake via foods such as nuts, seeds, milk, cheese, or tuna, and the majority of Trp is absorbed in the small intestine. However, the fraction that remains unabsorbed serves as a substrate for the gut microbes [5]. Through microbial degradation, Trp is metabolized into indole and indole derivatives via the indole pathway.

Several microbes in the gut express enzymes that use Trp to generate indole and other indole catabolites [5]. The microbial species involved in the indole pathway have been summarized in recent reviews [41, 42]. Trp is converted to indole via the enzyme Trp identified in gut bacteria such as *Escherichia coli* (*E. coli*), *Clostridium* spp., and *Bacteroides* spp. [41]. The Trp decarboxylase that converts Trp to tryptamine is expressed in *Clostridium*, *Ruminococcus*, *Blautia,* and *Lactobacillus* bacteria [43].

The first step in the degradation of Trp to indole-3-propionic acid (IPA) is the conversion to indole-3-pyruvic acid (IPYA) via the aromatic amino acid decarboxylase, followed by the conversion to ILA and anholocyclic acid (IA), and finally IPA. In addition, through different enzymes gut microbes degrade Trp to indole-3-aldehyde (IAld) and indole-3-acetaldehyde (IAAld) [5].

3. Trp metabolites and gastrointestinal disorders

3.1 Irritable bowel syndrome

IBS is a functional gastrointestinal disorder characterized by chronic abdominal pain associated with altered bowel habits [44]. It is the most commonly diagnosed gastrointestinal disorder, representing a significant social problem [45]. Visceral hypersensitivity accounts for the symptoms of chronic pain that patients with IBS report to their physicians. Pain perception might be influenced by the gut microbiota, which participates in pain signaling [46]. Species like *Streptococcus*, *Escherichia*, and *Enterococcus*, which are known to produce 5-HT may influence visceral pain perception [47].

The stimulation of receptors in the gut wall sends signals via the spinal cord to the brain [48]. Specific mediators such as serotonin and kinins have been associated with the visceral pain observed in IBS patients along with the increased spinal cord excitability as a result of the NMDA receptor [49–51].

The role of Trp metabolites in IBS has been demonstrated by Fitzgerald et al. when comparing patients with IBS to healthy controls. They found that IBS patients' blood had more kynurenine than the control group, and that there was a positive link between the severity of IBS symptoms and the kynurenine/tryptophan (Kyn/Trp) ratio [52]. A shift in Trp metabolism toward kynurenine production has also been observed by Han et al. along with a link between a Trp dysregulated metabolism and the severity of IBS depression [53].

Several other authors have observed increased levels of serotonin in patients with IBS compared to healthy controls. By comparing serum 5-HT levels under fasting conditions in patients with IBS and healthy controls Moskwa et al. demonstrated that serotonin levels are increased in both patients with diarrhea predominant and constipation predominant IBS [54]. However, Atkinson et al. reported increased levels of 5-HT in patients with diarrhea predominant IBS in both fasting and fed conditions, whereas patients with constipation predominant IBS did not show increased levels of 5-HT after meal ingestion. The results of this study suggest that reduced serotonin reuptake characterizes patients with diarrhea predominant IBS [55]. Other studies have demonstrated that serotonin levels are not significantly different in patients with IBS compared to controls. However, an altered serotonin metabolism appears to be implicated, with decreased 5-HIAA levels significantly lower 5-HIAA/5-HT ratio [56].

The mechanisms underlying altered plasma serotonin levels in IBS remain incompletely understood. However, in addition to modulating psychological and behavioral processes through the CNS, serotonin, and its metabolites are also known to play important modulatory roles in the ENS, co-regulating intestinal secretion, motility, and visceral perception [57]. One study demonstrated an association between increased plasma 5-HT levels in patients with IBS and the presence of *Bifidobacteriaceae*, *Bacteroidaceae*, *Oscillospiraceae,* and the bacteriophages *Podoviridae* in the gut microbiota. The authors have observed a pattern of altered serotonin metabolism associated with identified fecal microbiome-metabolome signatures and an exaggerated stress response in patients with IBS. These findings support the microbiota-gut-brain link in the IBS pathogenesis [58].

The 5-HT mucosal levels also play an important role. Existing studies demonstrated that the 5-HT levels are lower in IBS patients compared to the healthy controls and it is associated with a low expression of the re-uptake transporters for TPH1 and serotonin [59]. According to the studies, there might be differences in the 5-HT levels between IBS subtypes, since in IBS-C the levels are low in the colonic mucosa, and increased for IBS-D, respectively [60].

3.2 Inflammatory bowel diseases

Inflammatory bowel diseases (IBDs) are a group of chronic inflammatory disorders of the gastrointestinal tract, represented by Crohn's disease (CD) and ulcerative colitis (UC). IBDs represent a healthcare problem globally, with increasing incidence and prevalence in the Western civilization [61]. Although diarrhea and abdominal pain dominate the clinical presentation of patients with CD and UC, there are major differences between the two disorders. In UC the inflammation is limited to the colonic mucosal layer, it involves the rectum in almost all of the cases and it is extended to the proximal part of the colon in a continuous fashion [62]. On the other hand, in CD the inflammation occurs in all the layers of the gut wall and it can involve any part of the gastrointestinal tract. The CD is typically characterized by segments of normal appearing bowel interrupted by areas of disease [63].

The pathogenesis of IBDs is not yet completely understood, however, genetic, environmental, and immunologic factors and an altered gut microbiota have been demonstrated to play key roles in the development of IBDs [63, 64]. Recent studies suggest that IBD is possibly caused by the improper functionality of the immune system, but also by a pronounced dysbiosis accompanied by modifications in its metabolome [65, 66]. Adult patients with CD showed decreased amounts of *Faecalibacterium prausnitzii* and high amounts of *E. coli*, while *Clostridium clusters* XIVa and IV are shown to be decreased in patients showing CD recurrence after surgery [67, 68].

When comparing healthy volunteers to patients with IBD, researchers have observed that IBD patients had lower Trp levels in both serum and fecal samples [69, 70].

Experimental animal studies demonstrated that Trp is responsible for the expression of secretory immunoglobulin A (sIgA) and β-defensins [71]. A decreased level of Trp is followed by a production of inflammatory interleukins in the immune cells, such as IL-10 and transforming growth factor-β (TGF-β) [72]. It was demonstrated that IBD has an early onset if a functional deficient mutation in the IL-10 gene is present [73].

IBDs are known to be characterized by a pro-inflammatory state with increased levels of pro-inflammatory cytokines, such as tumor necrosis factor-α (TNF-α), interleukin-12 (IL-12), interleukin-17 (IL-17), and IFN-gamma [74]. These cytokines can enhance the kynurenine pathway by inducing IDO expression, thus leading to higher levels of Trp metabolites [31]. A meta-analysis of the transcriptome and a systematic review of the metabolome demonstrated that patients with IBD exhibit decreased Trp absorption, enhanced kynurenine pathway, altered indole pathway along, and altered indole pathway with decreased Trp plasma levels. In addition, the authors identified increased expression levels of aryl hydrocarbon receptor (AhR), which is a ligand-activated transcription factor [75]. AhR plays a key role in maintaining gut homeostasis (**Figure 2**). The activated Trp-AhR pathway modulates cell renewal and turnover, induces expression of IL-10 receptors and tight junctions in intestinal epithelial cells, thus promoting intestinal barrier integrity and helping to regulate tissue regeneration [76].

Several Trp metabolites, such as kynurenine, 5-HT, XA, and KA have the capacity to bind to AhR and activate it leading to expression of cytokines such as interleukin-22 (IL-22) and IL-17 [22].

One study showed that the Trp metabolites XA and KA have been negatively correlated to inflammation not only in colitis mice models but also in humans with IBD. Lower XA and KA levels have been linked to clinical, biological, and endoscopic markers of disease activity and to a higher expression of pro-inflammatory cytokines. The authors demonstrated that XA and KA have an anti-inflammatory role and that increasing XA and KA levels could represent a promising new therapeutic approach for IBD patients [77].

Moreover, the gut microbiota plays a key role in the kynurenine pathway metabolism and IBD pathophysiology due to its ability to metabolize Trp via the indole pathway. In other words, dysbiosis can alter the kynurenine pathway and promote

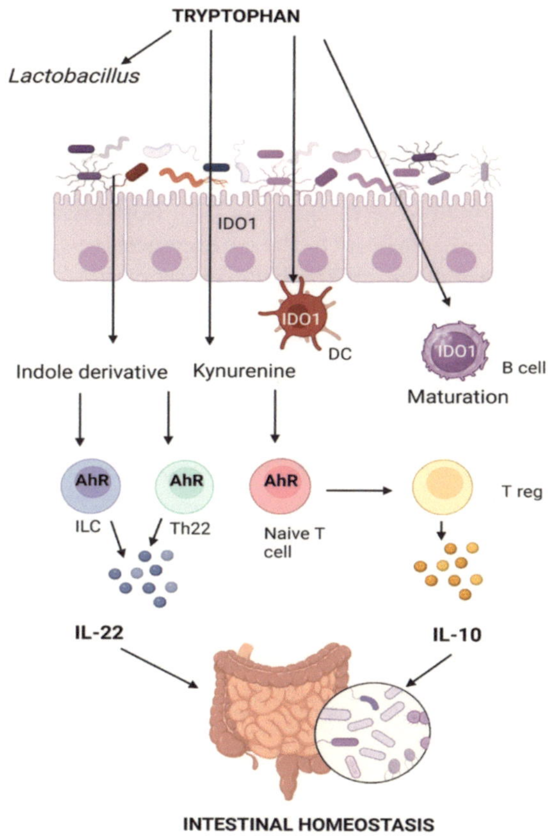

Figure 2.
The role of tryptophan in intestinal homeostasis. Kynurenine and indole derivatives (indole-3-aldehyde, and indole-3-acetic acid) bind to AhR on immune cells and stimulate the production of Il-10 and IL-22. AhR- aryl hydrocarbon receptor; DC - dendritic cell; IDO1 - Indoleamine 2,3 dioxygenase-1; ILC - innate lymphoid cells. Created with BioRender.

inflammation in IBD [78]. Recent studies have identified a number of substances that could regulate Trp metabolism. Ginsenoside Rg1, a natural compound, showed promising results in colitis model mice, alleviating inflammation by regulating several microbiota metabolic pathways, including reducing the levels of Trp metabolites [79]. Fucose administration increased the levels of Trp-producing *E. coli* and thus normalized Trp serum levels [80]. Fructooligosaccharides have been shown to modulate the gut microbial composition, by decreasing the abundance of *Akkermansiaceae* (family level) and *Verrucomicrobia* (phylum level) and increasing the abundance of *Ruminococcaceae* (phylum level), and to increase the levels of Trp and 5-HT in mice models [81]. The Fuzhuan brick tea polysaccharide administration increased the abundance of beneficial microbes such as *Lactobacillus* and *Akkermansia*, altered the Trp metabolism and led to higher IA1d and IAA levels [82].

The involvement of the kynurenine pathway in inflammation has been linked to the development and severity of IBD. Thus, targeting different parts of this metabolic pathway could represent a new treatment strategy for treating IBD. Diets rich in foods that contain Trp and dietary supplements containing Trp can be beneficial since there are studies demonstrating Trp rich diets are associated with a decrease in inflammation, while Trp deficient diets have been linked to exacerbation of colitis [83, 84].

3.3 Celiac disease

CeD is an immune-mediated inflammatory disease of the small intestine caused by sensitivity to dietary gluten affecting genetically predisposed individuals. The global prevalence of CeD is estimated to be around 1% based on serologic testing [85, 86]. Epidemiological studies have reported a prevalence of around 1:70 to 1:300 when biopsy verification was added to serologic tests [87]. Both environmental (dietary gluten) and genetic factors contribute to the pathogenesis of CeD. The high frequency of intrafamilial incidence and the strikingly close association with the human leukocyte antigen (HLA) DR3-DQ2 and/or DR4-DQ8 gene locus provide evidence for the genetic basis of CeD [88, 89]. As early as 1964, the association between CeD and altered Trp metabolism was demonstrated by measuring the urinary levels of several Trp metabolites. The authors reported increased urinary levels of Trp metabolites and low vitamin B6 levels [90]. The role of the gut microbiota was also demonstrated in both earlier and more recent studies and increased abundance of some bacterial strains such as *Pseudomonas aeruginosa*, *Neisseria flavescens,* and *E. coli* have been associated with CeD [91–96]. Some Gram-negative genra such as *Bacteroides, Prevotella*, and *Escherichia*, were found in increased amounts while *Bifidobacteria* and *Lactobacilli* were found to be decreased [97].

Dysbiosis is apparently responsible for CeD with the onset in adult life and for the cases that do not respond well to a gluten-free diet [98, 99].

Recent studies have demonstrated that the gut microbiota of CeD patients has a reduced capacity of converting Trp into metabolites capable of activating the AhR, leading to intestinal inflammation [97, 98]. The correlation between decreased AhR activity and CeD is supported by several authors [99–103]. One of the mechanisms by which beneficial bacteria could alleviate CeD is by modulating the AhR pathway. Studies on rodent models demonstrated that treating mice with lactobacilli strains known to produce AhR ligands such as *Lactobacillus reuteri*, led to increased AhR activity in the small intestine and ameliorated intestinal inflammation [69, 97]. In addition, a Trp rich diet was able to shift the gut microbial composition of mice toward the increased abundance of bacteria able to produce AhR ligands such as *Lactobacillus* and *Ruminococcus gnavus*, thus reducing gluten immunopathology [98]. Further studies should focus on identifying strain-specific probiotic treatments and dietary approaches that could modulate the AhR pathway and improve CeD symptoms.

4. The relationship between Trp metabolites, related gastrointestinal disease, and weight loss

Serotonin, a neurotransmitter derived from Trp, plays a role in regulating mood and appetite. However, the relationship between serotonin levels and weight loss is complex and not fully understood. While serotonin itself is not directly linked to weight loss, its influence on appetite and mood can indirectly impact weight management [18].

The relationship between serotonin and weight is complex and can involve various factors. Serotonin is known to contribute to feelings of satiety and fullness [104, 105]. Low serotonin levels have been associated with an increased appetite and cravings for carbohydrate-rich foods [106]. Some individuals may engage in emotional eating to boost serotonin levels, especially during periods of stress or low mood [107].

Changes in serotonin levels can influence mood, and mood disturbances may affect eating habits. For example, people with depression may experience changes in appetite, leading to weight gain or loss [108]. Certain medications, such as selective serotonin reuptake inhibitors (SSRIs), which are commonly prescribed for the treatment of depression and anxiety, can affect serotonin levels. Some individuals may experience weight changes as a side effect of these medications [108].

The link between gastrointestinal diseases and weight loss has been studied from several points of view and will be detailed in the following paragraphs as stated in the literature.

IBD can affect the absorption of nutrients in the intestines [109]. Chronic inflammation and damage to the intestinal lining can impair the body's ability to absorb essential nutrients, leading to malabsorption. This malabsorption can result in weight loss and nutritional deficiencies [110].

Symptoms of IBD, such as abdominal pain, diarrhea, and nausea, can contribute to a reduced appetite. Individuals with IBD may experience discomfort or pain during or after eating, leading to a decrease in food intake and subsequent weight loss [110].

The chronic inflammation associated with IBD can increase the body's metabolic rate. This increased demand for energy, coupled with malabsorption, can contribute to weight loss, even when individuals are not intentionally restricting their calorie intake [111].

The inflammation and other factors associated with IBD can lead to changes in body composition, including muscle wasting and loss of fat tissue. This can contribute to overall weight loss and weakness [111]. The severity of IBD symptoms can vary, and individuals may experience periods of flare-ups with more intense symptoms. During flare-ups, the impact on weight loss may be more pronounced [112]. It's important to note that weight loss in IBD is often unintentional and can be a sign of underlying disease activity [113]. Managing IBD involves a multidisciplinary approach, including medical treatment, nutritional support, and lifestyle modifications.

IBS is different from IBD, and it is essential to distinguish between the two conditions. Unlike IBD (Crohn's disease and ulcerative colitis), IBS is a functional gastrointestinal disorder characterized by symptoms such as abdominal pain, bloating, and changes in bowel habits without evidence of inflammation or damage to the digestive tract [60]. In general, IBS is not typically associated with significant weight loss. Weight loss is usually not a primary symptom of IBS, and any changes in body weight are more likely to be subtle or unintentional. However, there are a few indirect ways in which IBS might be linked to changes in weight [114].

Individuals with IBS may make changes to their diet to manage symptoms, such as avoiding certain trigger foods. This modification in dietary habits could potentially impact calorie intake and, in some cases, lead to weight changes [115].

Some people with IBS may experience symptoms such as diarrhea or abdominal pain that can affect their appetite or eating patterns. While this might not necessarily lead to significant weight loss, it can contribute to fluctuations in body weight [116]. IBS symptoms are known to be influenced by stress and psychological factors. Stress-related changes in eating patterns or behaviors may indirectly impact weight [117, 118]. It's important to emphasize that IBS is a chronic condition, and its symptoms can vary widely among individuals. While weight loss is not a primary characteristic of IBS, other gastrointestinal conditions or non-gastrointestinal factors could contribute to changes in body weight.

CeD is an autoimmune disorder characterized by an intolerance to gluten, a protein found in wheat, barley, and rye [119]. The ingestion of gluten triggers an immune response in individuals with CeD, leading to inflammation and damage to the lining of the small intestine. This damage can result in malabsorption of nutrients, affecting various aspects of health, including body weight [119].

The relationship between CeD and weight loss is often observed due to a number of factors. The damage to the small intestine in CeD impairs the absorption of essential nutrients, including proteins, fats, carbohydrates, vitamins, and minerals. This malabsorption can lead to nutrient deficiencies, contributing to weight loss [110].

Individuals with CeD may experience symptoms such as abdominal pain, bloating, diarrhea, and nausea. These symptoms can affect appetite and food intake, leading to reduced caloric consumption and subsequent weight loss. Chronic diarrhea is a common symptom of CeD. Frequent bowel movements can result in fluid loss and contribute to weight loss [120]. The inflammation in the small intestine associated with CeD can increase the body's metabolic rate, causing an elevated demand for energy. This increased metabolic activity, combined with malabsorption, can lead to weight loss [119]. In severe cases of untreated CeD, the body may start to break down muscle tissue for energy, contributing to muscle wasting and additional weight loss [121].

It's important to note that while weight loss is a common symptom of CeD, not everyone with the condition experiences this. Some individuals with CeD may have atypical or minimal symptoms, making diagnosis challenging.

The treatment for CeD involves strict adherence to a gluten-free diet, which typically leads to the resolution of symptoms and the restoration of a healthy body weight. Early detection and adherence to a gluten-free diet can help manage symptoms and prevent complications associated with CeD [122].

5. Future perspectives

To date, several studies focused on the importance of the gut microbiota, this "virtual symbiotic organ" that clearly interferes with many metabolic and immune functions in our organism. The human health and disease state are depending on the microbial metabolites resulted by host-microorganism or microorganism – microorganism interactions at gut level [107]. The complete understanding of the gut microbiota complexity and the possibility to manipulate the microbes as future therapeutic strategy will open new perspectives regarding our understanding of gastrointestinal and psychiatric pathologies. An appealing approach for the patients associating depression or anxiety that usually accompany IBS, IBD, or CeD is provided by the administration of probiotics and/or prebiotics [108]. Some other diseases involving the gut-microbiota-brain axis, such as anorexia nervosa apparently produced by changes in dietary intake and pre-morbid gut microbiota changes might benefit of the use of probiotics [109]. We mentioned here anorexia nervosa because there are many similarities between this eating disorder and the above-mentioned gastrointestinal diseases and mental health disorders [110].

The probiotics rich in *Lactobacillus* and *Bifidobacteria* species, nowadays known under the term "psychobiotics" may be capable of modulating the brain-gut-microbiota axis improving mood, anxiety, and cognition [111]. The advance in microbiome and psychiatric research is still at the beginning and hold promise for the future.

Acronyms and abbreviations

AA	anthranilic acid
ALAAD	aromatic L-amino decarboxylase,
ALDH	aldehyde dehydrogenase
AhR	aryl hydrocarbon receptor
CD	Crohn's disease
CeD	celiac disease
CNS	central nervous system
ENS	enteric nervous system
IA	anholocyclic acid
IAAld	indole-3-acetaldehyde
IAld	indole-3-aldehyde
IBD	inflammatory bowel disease
IBS	irritable bowel syndrome
IDO	indoleamine 2,3-dioxygenase
IL-8	interleukin-8
IL-12	interleukin-12
IL-17	interleukin-17
ILA	indole-3-lactic acid
IPA	indole-3-propionic acid
IPYA	indole-3-pyruvic acid
KA	kynurenic acid
KMO	kynurenine-3-monooxygenase
MAO	monoamine oxidase
NAD^+	nicotinamide adenine dinucleotide
NMDA	N-methyl-D-aspartate
QA	quinolinic acid
sIgA	immunoglobulin A
TDO	tryptophan 2,3-dioxygenase
TGF-β	transforming growth factor-β
TNF-α	necrosis factor-α
TPH	tryptophan hydroxylase
UC	ulcerative colitis
XA	xanthurenic acid
3-HAA	3-hydroxyanthranilic acid
3-HK	3-hydroxykynurenine
5-HIAA	5-hydroxyindoleacetic acid
5-HT	5-hydroxytryptamine
5-HTP	5-hydroxytryptophan

Author details

Bogdan Severus Gaspar[1,2], Monica Profir[3] and Sanda Maria Cretoiu[4*]

1 Surgery Clinic, Emergency Clinical Hospital of Bucharest, Bucharest, Romania

2 Department of Surgery, Carol Davila University of Medicine and Pharmacy, Bucharest, Romania

3 Department of Oncology, Elias University Emergency Hospital, Bucharest, Romania

4 Department of Morphological Sciences, Cell and Molecular Biology and Histology, "Carol Davila" University of Medicine and Pharmacy, Bucharest, Romania

*Address all correspondence to: sanda@cretoiu.ro

References

[1] Xue C et al. Tryptophan metabolism in health and disease. Cell Metabolism. 2023;**35**(8):1304-1326

[2] Li G, Young KD. Indole production by the tryptophanase TnaA in *Escherichia coli* is determined by the amount of exogenous tryptophan. Microbiology (Reading). 2013;**159**(Pt 2):402-410

[3] Friedman M. Analysis, nutrition, and health benefits of tryptophan. International Journal of Tryptophan Research. 2018;**11**:1178646918802282

[4] Liu M et al. Microbial tryptophan metabolism tunes host immunity, metabolism, and extraintestinal disorders. Metabolites. 2022;**12**(9):834

[5] Roth W et al. Tryptophan metabolism and gut-brain homeostasis. International Journal of Molecular Sciences. 2021;**22**(6):2973

[6] Ciorba MA. Kynurenine pathway metabolites: Relevant to vitamin B-6 deficiency and beyond. The American Journal of Clinical Nutrition. 2013;**98**:863-864

[7] Li S. Modulation of immunity by tryptophan microbial metabolites. Frontiers in Nutrition. 2023;**10**:1209613

[8] Gao K et al. Increasing carbohydrate availability in the hindgut promotes hypothalamic neurotransmitter synthesis: Aromatic amino acids linking the microbiota-brain axis. Journal of Neurochemistry. 2019;**149**(5):641-659

[9] Sherwin E, Dinan TG, Cryan JF. Recent developments in understanding the role of the gut microbiota in brain health and disease. Annals of the New York Academy of Sciences. 2018;**1420**(1):5-25

[10] Fröhlich EE et al. Cognitive impairment by antibiotic-induced gut dysbiosis: Analysis of gut microbiota-brain communication. Brain, Behavior, and Immunity. 2016;**56**:140-155

[11] De Vadder F et al. Microbiota-generated metabolites promote metabolic benefits via gut-brain neural circuits. Cell. 2014;**156**(1-2):84-96

[12] Bianconi E et al. An estimation of the number of cells in the human body. Annals of Human Biology. 2013;**40**(6):463-471

[13] Sender R, Fuchs S, Milo R. Are we really vastly outnumbered? Revisiting the ratio of bacterial to host cells in humans. Cell. 2016;**164**(3):337-340

[14] Clarke G et al. The microbiome-gut-brain axis during early life regulates the hippocampal serotonergic system in a sex-dependent manner. Molecular Psychiatry. 2013;**18**(6):666-673

[15] Ozogul F, Kuley E, Ozogul Y, Ozogul I. The function of lactic acid bacteria on biogenic amines production by food-borne pathogens in arginine decarboxylase broth. Food Science and Technology Research. 2012;**18**(6):795-804

[16] Ma J, Kobayashi DY, Yee N. Role of menaquinone biosynthesis genes in selenate reduction by enterobacter cloacae SLD1a-1 and *Escherichia coli* K12. Environmental Microbiology. 2009;**11**(1):149-158

[17] Clark A, Mach N. Exercise-induced stress behavior, gut-microbiota-brain axis and diet: A systematic review for athletes. Journal of the International Society of Sports Nutrition. 2016;**13**:43

[18] Jenkins TA et al. Influence of tryptophan and serotonin on mood and cognition with a possible role of the gut-brain Axis. Nutrients. 2016;**8**(1):56

[19] Ratcliffe EM, Farrar NR, Fox EA. Development of the vagal innervation of the gut: Steering the wandering nerve. Neurogastroenterology and Motility. 2011;**23**(10):898-911

[20] De Vadder F et al. Gut microbiota regulates maturation of the adult enteric nervous system via enteric serotonin networks. Proceedings of the National Academy of Sciences of the United States of America. 2018;**115**(25):6458-6463

[21] Rhee SH, Pothoulakis C, Mayer EA. Principles and clinical implications of the brain-gut-enteric microbiota axis. Nature Reviews. Gastroenterology & Hepatology. 2009;**6**(5):306-314

[22] Sun M et al. Tryptophan (Trp) modulates gut homeostasis via aryl hydrocarbon receptor (AhR). Critical Reviews in Food Science and Nutrition. 2020;**60**(10):1760-1768

[23] Ehrlich AM et al. Indole-3-lactic acid associated with bifidobacterium-dominated microbiota significantly decreases inflammation in intestinal epithelial cells. BMC Microbiology. 2020;**20**(1):357

[24] Meng D et al. Indole-3-lactic acid, a metabolite of tryptophan, secreted by *Bifidobacterium longum* subspecies infantis is anti-inflammatory in the immature intestine. Pediatric Research. 2020;**88**(2):209-217

[25] Labus JS et al. Differences in gut microbial composition correlate with regional brain volumes in irritable bowel syndrome. Microbiome. 2017;**5**(1):49

[26] Pinto-Sanchez MI et al. Probiotic *Bifidobacterium longum* NCC3001 reduces depression scores and alters brain activity: A pilot study in patients with irritable bowel syndrome. Gastroenterology. 2017;**153**(2):448-459.e8

[27] Strati F et al. New evidences on the altered gut microbiota in autism spectrum disorders. Microbiome. 2017;**5**(1):24

[28] Jiang H et al. Altered fecal microbiota composition in patients with major depressive disorder. Brain, Behavior, and Immunity. 2015;**48**:186-194

[29] Höglund E, Øverli Ø, Winberg S. Tryptophan metabolic pathways and brain serotonergic activity: A comparative review. Frontiers in Endocrinology (Lausanne). 2019;**10**:158

[30] Badawy AA. Tryptophan metabolism: A versatile area providing multiple targets for pharmacological intervention. Egyptian Journal of Basic and Clinical Pharmacology. 2019;**9**

[31] Sheibani M et al. Kynurenine pathway and its role in neurologic, psychiatric, and inflammatory bowel diseases. Molecular Biology Reports. 2023;**50**(12):10409-10425

[32] Takikawa O. Biochemical and medical aspects of the indoleamine 2,3-dioxygenase-initiated L-tryptophan metabolism. Biochemical and Biophysical Research Communications. 2005;**338**(1):12-19

[33] O'Farrell K, Harkin A. Stress-related regulation of the kynurenine pathway: Relevance to neuropsychiatric and degenerative disorders. Neuropharmacology. 2017;**112**(Pt B):307-323

[34] Dantzer R et al. From inflammation to sickness and depression: When the immune system subjugates the brain. Nature Reviews. Neuroscience. 2008;**9**(1):46-56

[35] Maes M et al. The inflammatory & neurodegenerative (I & ND) hypothesis of depression: Leads for future research and new drug developments in depression. Metabolic Brain Disease. 2009;**24**(1):27-53

[36] Okuda S et al. 3-hydroxykynurenine, an endogenous oxidative stress generator, causes neuronal cell death with apoptotic features and region selectivity. Journal of Neurochemistry. 1998;**70**(1):299-307

[37] Stone TW, Darlington LG. Endogenous kynurenines as targets for drug discovery and development. Nature Reviews. Drug Discovery. 2002;**1**(8):609-620

[38] Irwin MR, Miller AH. Depressive disorders and immunity: 20 years of progress and discovery. Brain, Behavior, and Immunity. 2007;**21**(4):374-383

[39] Schwarcz R. The kynurenine pathway of tryptophan degradation as a drug target. Current Opinion in Pharmacology. 2004;**4**(1):12-17

[40] Reyes Ocampo J et al. Kynurenines with neuroactive and redox properties: Relevance to aging and brain diseases. Oxidative Medicine and Cellular Longevity. 2014;**2014**:646909

[41] Roager HM, Licht TR. Microbial tryptophan catabolites in health and disease. Nature Communications. 2018;**9**(1):3294

[42] Su X, Gao Y, Yang R. Gut microbiota-derived tryptophan metabolites maintain gut and systemic homeostasis. Cells. 2022;**11**(15):2296

[43] Williams BB et al. Discovery and characterization of gut microbiota decarboxylases that can produce the neurotransmitter tryptamine. Cell Host & Microbe. 2014;**16**(4):495-503

[44] Gaspar B et al. The intestinal microbiome in humans: It's role for a healthy life and in the onset of disease. In: MIcrobiome - the Key for Human Health. London, UK: IntechOpen; 2024

[45] Drossman DA et al. AGA technical review on irritable bowel syndrome. Gastroenterology. 2002;**123**(6):2108-2131

[46] Cryan JF et al. The microbiota-gut-brain axis. Physiological Reviews. 2019;**99**(4):1877-2013

[47] Agus A, Planchais J, Sokol H. Gut microbiota regulation of tryptophan metabolism in health and disease. Cell Host & Microbe. 2018;**23**(6):716-724

[48] Arnold W. Pathophysiology of irritable bowel syndrome. 2023. Available from: https://www.uptodate.com/contents/pathophysiology-of-irritable-bowel-syndrome?search=irritable%20bowel%20syndrome&source=search_result&selectedTitle=3~150&usage_type=default&display_rank=3#H1

[49] Buéno L, Fioramonti J, Garcia-Villar R. Pathobiology of visceral pain: Molecular mechanisms and therapeutic implications. III. Visceral afferent pathways: A source of new therapeutic targets for abdominal pain. American Journal of Physiology. Gastrointestinal and Liver Physiology. 2000;**278**(5):G670-G676

[50] Faure C et al. Serotonin signaling is altered in irritable bowel syndrome with diarrhea but not in functional dyspepsia in pediatric age patients. Gastroenterology. 2010;**139**(1):249-258

[51] Willert RP et al. The development and maintenance of human visceral pain hypersensitivity is dependent on the N-methyl-D-aspartate receptor. Gastroenterology. 2004;**126**(3):683-692

[52] Fitzgerald P et al. Tryptophan catabolism in females with irritable bowel syndrome: Relationship to interferon-gamma, severity of symptoms and psychiatric co-morbidity. Neurogastroenterology and Motility. 2008;**20**(12):1291-1297

[53] Han L et al. Altered metabolome and microbiome features provide clues in understanding irritable bowel syndrome and depression comorbidity. The ISME Journal. 2022;**16**(4):983-996

[54] Moskwa A et al. Serum serotonin concentration and urine 5-hydroxyindole acetic acid excretion in patients with irritable bowel syndrome. Polski Merkuriusz Lekarski. 2007;**22**(131):366-368

[55] Atkinson W et al. Altered 5-hydroxytryptamine signaling in patients with constipation- and diarrhea-predominant irritable bowel syndrome. Gastroenterology. 2006;**130**(1):34-43

[56] Thijssen AY et al. Alterations in serotonin metabolism in the irritable bowel syndrome. Alimentary Pharmacology & Therapeutics. 2016;**43**(2):272-282

[57] Gershon MD, Tack J. The serotonin signaling system: From basic understanding to drug development for functional GI disorders. Gastroenterology. 2007;**132**(1):397-414

[58] Mujagic Z et al. Integrated fecal microbiome-metabolome signatures reflect stress and serotonin metabolism in irritable bowel syndrome. Gut Microbes. 2022;**14**(1):2063016

[59] Foley S et al. Impaired uptake of serotonin by platelets from patients with irritable bowel syndrome correlates with duodenal immune activation. Gastroenterology. 2011;**140**(5):1434-43.e1

[60] Saha L. Irritable bowel syndrome: Pathogenesis, diagnosis, treatment, and evidence-based medicine. World Journal of Gastroenterology. 2014;**20**(22):6759-6773

[61] M'Koma AE. Inflammatory bowel disease: An expanding global health problem. Clinical Medicine Insights. Gastroenterology. 2013;**6**:33-47

[62] Iancu MA et al. Revisiting the intestinal microbiome and its role in diarrhea and constipation. Microorganisms. 2023;**11**(9):2177

[63] Ruxandra Florentina I et al. Intestinal Microbiomics in physiological and pathological conditions. In: Vasudeo Z et al., editors. Advances in Probiotics for Health and Nutrition. London, UK, Rijeka: IntechOpen; 2023. p. Ch. 6

[64] Zhang YZ, Li YY. Inflammatory bowel disease: Pathogenesis. World Journal of Gastroenterology. 2014;**20**(1):91-99

[65] Ni J et al. Gut microbiota and IBD: Causation or correlation? Nature Reviews. Gastroenterology & Hepatology. 2017;**14**(10):573-584

[66] Imhann F et al. Interplay of host genetics and gut microbiota underlying the onset and clinical presentation of inflammatory bowel disease. Gut. 2018;**67**(1):108-119

[67] Barnich N, Denizot J, Darfeuille-Michaud A. *E. coli*-mediated gut inflammation in genetically predisposed Crohn's disease patients. Pathologie Biologie (Paris). 2013;**61**(5):e65-e69

[68] Walker AW et al. High-throughput clone library analysis of the mucosa-associated microbiota reveals dysbiosis and differences between inflamed and non-inflamed regions of the intestine in inflammatory bowel disease. BMC Microbiology. 2011;**11**:7

[69] Lamas B et al. CARD9 impacts colitis by altering gut microbiota metabolism of tryptophan into aryl hydrocarbon receptor ligands. Nature Medicine. 2016;**22**(6):598-605

[70] Shiomi Y et al. GCMS-based metabolomic study in mice with colitis induced by dextran sulfate sodium. Inflammatory Bowel Diseases. 2011;**17**(11):2261-2274

[71] Liang H et al. Dietary l-tryptophan supplementation enhances the intestinal mucosal barrier function in weaned piglets: Implication of tryptophan-metabolizing microbiota. International Journal of Molecular Sciences. 2018;**20**(1):20

[72] Sorgdrager FJH et al. Tryptophan metabolism in inflammaging: From biomarker to therapeutic target. Frontiers in Immunology. 2019;**10**:2565

[73] Neurath MF. Cytokines in inflammatory bowel disease. Nature Reviews. Immunology. 2014;**14**(5):329-342

[74] Sanchez-Munoz F, Dominguez-Lopez A, Yamamoto-Furusho JK. Role of cytokines in inflammatory bowel disease. World Journal of Gastroenterology. 2008;**14**(27):4280-4288

[75] Wang S et al. The involvement of intestinal tryptophan metabolism in inflammatory bowel disease identified by a meta-analysis of the transcriptome and a systematic review of the metabolome. Nutrients. 2023;**15**(13):2886

[76] Rothhammer V, Quintana FJ. The aryl hydrocarbon receptor: An environmental sensor integrating immune responses in health and disease. Nature Reviews. Immunology. 2019;**19**(3):184-197

[77] Michaudel C et al. Rewiring the altered tryptophan metabolism as a novel therapeutic strategy in inflammatory bowel diseases. Gut. 2023;**72**(7):1296-1307

[78] O'Mahony SM et al. Serotonin, tryptophan metabolism and the brain-gut-microbiome axis. Behavioural Brain Research. 2015;**277**:32-48

[79] Cheng H et al. Ginsenoside Rg1 alleviates acute ulcerative colitis by modulating gut microbiota and microbial tryptophan metabolism. Frontiers in Immunology. 2022;**13**:817600

[80] Borisova MA et al. Fucose ameliorates tryptophan metabolism and behavioral abnormalities in a mouse model of chronic colitis. Nutrients. 2020;**12**(2):445

[81] Yan X et al. Fructooligosaccharides protect against OVA-induced food allergy in mice by regulating the Th17/Treg cell balance using tryptophan metabolites. Food & Function. 2021;**12**(7):3191-3205

[82] Yang W et al. Fuzhuan brick tea polysaccharide improved ulcerative colitis in association with gut microbiota-derived tryptophan metabolism. Journal of Agricultural and Food Chemistry. 2021;**69**(30):8448-8459

[83] Islam J et al. Dietary tryptophan alleviates dextran sodium sulfate-induced colitis through aryl hydrocarbon receptor in mice. The Journal of Nutritional Biochemistry. 2017;**42**:43-50

[84] Lanis JM et al. Tryptophan metabolite activation of the aryl hydrocarbon receptor regulates IL-10 receptor expression on intestinal epithelia. Mucosal Immunology. 2017;**10**(5):1133-1144

[85] Rubio-Tapia A et al. The prevalence of celiac disease in the United States. The American Journal of Gastroenterology. 2012;**107**(10):1538-1544; quiz 1537, 1545

[86] Choung RS et al. Prevalence and morbidity of undiagnosed celiac disease from a community-based study. Gastroenterology. 2017;**152**(4):830-839.e5

[87] Gujral N, Freeman HJ, Thomson AB. Celiac disease: Prevalence, diagnosis, pathogenesis and treatment. World Journal of Gastroenterology. 2012;**18**(42):6036-6059

[88] Liu E et al. Risk of pediatric celiac disease according to HLA haplotype and country. The New England Journal of Medicine. 2014;**371**(1):42-49

[89] Pietzak MM et al. Stratifying risk for celiac disease in a large at-risk United States population by using HLA alleles. Clinical Gastroenterology and Hepatology. 2009;7(9):966-971

[90] Kowlessar OD, Haeffner LJ, Benson GD. Abnormal tryptophan metabolism in patients with adult celiac disease, with evidence for deficiency of vitamin B6. The Journal of Clinical Investigation. 1964;**43**(5):894-903

[91] Stěpánková R et al. Changes in jejunal mucosa after long-term feeding of germfree rats with gluten. Scandinavian Journal of Gastroenterology. 1996;**31**(6):551-557

[92] Galipeau HJ et al. Intestinal microbiota modulates gluten-induced immunopathology in humanized mice. The American Journal of Pathology. 2015;**185**(11):2969-2982

[93] Ashorn S et al. Elevated serum anti-Saccharomyces cerevisiae, anti-I2 and anti-OmpW antibody levels in patients with suspicion of celiac disease. Journal of Clinical Immunology. 2008;**28**(5):486-494

[94] D'Argenio V et al. Metagenomics reveals dysbiosis and a potentially pathogenic *N. flavescens* strain in duodenum of adult celiac patients. The American Journal of Gastroenterology. 2016;**111**(6):879-890

[95] Galipeau HJ, Verdu EF. The double-edged sword of gut bacteria in celiac disease and implications for therapeutic potential. Mucosal Immunology. 2022;**15**(2):235-243

[96] Nadal I et al. Imbalance in the composition of the duodenal microbiota of children with coeliac disease. Journal of Medical Microbiology. 2007;**56**(Pt 12): 1669-1674

[97] Natividad JM et al. Impaired aryl hydrocarbon receptor ligand production by the gut microbiota is a key factor in metabolic syndrome. Cell Metabolism. 2018;**28**(5):737-749.e4

[98] Lamas B et al. Aryl hydrocarbon receptor ligand production by the gut microbiota is decreased in celiac disease leading to intestinal inflammation. Science Translational Medicine. 2020;**12**(566):eaba0624

[99] Dinallo V et al. Protective effects of aryl hydrocarbon receptor signaling in celiac disease mucosa and in poly I:C-induced small intestinal atrophy mouse model. Frontiers in Immunology. 2019;**10**:91

[100] Xu H et al. Gluten-sensitive enteropathy coincides with decreased capability of intestinal T cells to secrete IL-17 and IL-22 in a macaque model for celiac disease. Clinical Immunology. 2013;**147**(1):40-49

[101] Bodd M et al. HLA-DQ2-restricted gluten-reactive T cells produce IL-21 but not IL-17 or IL-22. Mucosal Immunology. 2010;**3**(6):594-601

[102] Li Y et al. Exogenous stimuli maintain intraepithelial lymphocytes via aryl hydrocarbon receptor activation. Cell. 2011;**147**(3):629-640

[103] Suwanai H et al. A defective Il15 allele underlies the deficiency in natural killer cell activity in nonobese diabetic mice. Proceedings of the National Academy of Sciences of the United States of America. 2010;**107**(20):9305-9310

[104] van Galen KA, Ter Horst KW, Serlie MJ. Serotonin, food intake, and obesity. Obesity Reviews. 2021;**22**(7):e13210

[105] Voigt JP, Fink H. Serotonin controlling feeding and satiety. Behavioural Brain Research. 2015;**277**:14-31

[106] Wurtman RJ, Wurtman JJ. Brain serotonin, carbohydrate-craving, obesity and depression. Obesity Research. 1995;**3**(Suppl 4):477s-480s

[107] Grajek M et al. Prevalence of emotional eating in groups of students with varied diets and physical activity in Poland. Nutrients. 2022;**14**(16):3289

[108] Felton J et al. The relation of weight change to depressive symptoms in adolescence. Development and Psychopathology. 2010;**22**(1):205-216

[109] Balestrieri P et al. Nutritional aspects in inflammatory bowel diseases. Nutrients. 2020;**12**(2):372

[110] Montoro-Huguet MA, Belloc B, Domínguez-Cajal M. Small and large intestine (I): Malabsorption of nutrients. Nutrients. 2021;**13**(4):1254

[111] Roncoroni L et al. Nutrition in patients with inflammatory bowel diseases: A narrative review. Nutrients. 2022;**14**(4):751

[112] Sun Y et al. Stress triggers flare of inflammatory bowel disease in children and adults. Frontiers in Pediatrics. 2019;**7**:432

[113] Elsherif Y, Alexakis C, Mendall M. Determinants of weight loss prior to diagnosis in inflammatory bowel disease: A retrospective observational study. Gastroenterology Research and Practice. 2014;**2014**:762191

[114] Pickett-Blakely O. Obesity and irritable bowel syndrome: A comprehensive review. Journal of Gastroenterology and Hepatology (N Y). 2014;**10**(7):411-416

[115] Guo YB et al. Association between diet and lifestyle habits and irritable bowel syndrome: A case-control study. Gut Liver. 2015;**9**(5):649-656

[116] Harer KN. Irritable bowel syndrome, disordered eating, and eating disorders. Journal of Gastroenterology and Hepatology (N Y). 2019;**15**(5):280-282

[117] Hayes PA, Fraher MH, Quigley EM. Irritable bowel syndrome: The role of food in pathogenesis and management. Journal of Gastroenterology and Hepatology (N Y). 2014;**10**(3):164-174

[118] Qin HY et al. Impact of psychological stress on irritable bowel syndrome. World Journal of Gastroenterology. 2014;**20**(39):14126-14131

[119] Sharma N et al. Pathogenesis of celiac disease and other gluten related disorders in wheat and strategies for mitigating them. Frontiers in Nutrition. 2020;7:6

[120] Sabença C et al. Wheat/gluten-related disorders and gluten-free diet misconceptions: A review. Food. 2021;**10**(8):1765

[121] De Risi LL. Starving in the midst of plenty: Adult celiac disease. The American Journal of Nursing. 1970;**70**(5):1048-1053

[122] Simón E et al. The gluten-free diet for celiac disease: Critical insights to better understand clinical outcomes. Nutrients. 2023;**15**(18):4013

Chapter 2

The Microbiota-Gut-Brain Axis: Tryptophan Metabolism and Potential Therapeutic Strategies

Miriam A. Mora-Navarro, José M. Mora-Martínez, Anayeli D.J. Patiño-Laguna, Carla P. Barragán-Álvarez, Michelle E. Gonzalez-Mora and Citlalli E. Mora-Navarro

Abstract

Tryptophan is an essential amino acid. It is metabolized through two main pathways: the kynurenine pathway and the methoxyidol pathway. The intestinal microbiota has been identified as a modifier of the metabolism of tryptophan and its derived metabolites. The resulting metabolites can trigger immune, metabolic, and neuronal effects, at the systemic and distant levels, as well as therapeutic specific and nonspecific targets. The reader reviewing this content will learn the importance of tryptophan biotransformation through metabolism and the host-microbiome complex, the formation of serotonin and kynurenine, the pathways of unwinding and the physiological effects of metabolites within the intestinal part, energy metabolism and neurotransmitters. The effects and pathologies that dysregulation may have with this metabolism will be reviewed, as well as the therapeutic targets and related drugs.

Keywords: gut microbiome, tryptophan metabolism, therapeutic strategies, microbiota-gut-brain axis, probiotics

1. Introduction

The intestine is an ecosystem harboring a dense and diverse microbial community called "gut microbiota" considered an endocrine organ. Many of the effects are mediated by metabolites that are either produced by microbes from the transformation of environmental or host molecules.

L-tryptophan is an amino acid that has emerged as a critical player in the microbiota-gut-brain axis. It is the only precursor for the neurotransmitter serotonin, contributes to the normal grown and health of both animals and humans.

The intestinal microbiota influences the metabolism of tryptophan, specific to microbial control over the kynurenine pathway and the indole pathway, which are important for host physiology. These metabolites participate in processes such as immune system regulations, regulations of metabolism, gastrointestinal motility, inflammation, and oxidative and anti-oxidative effects. Deciphering the complex equilibrium between intestinal microbiota and tryptophan metabolism will facilitate the understanding of the diversity of pathogenesis of human diseases and new therapeutic opportunities.

2. Microbiota-gut-brain axis: tryptophan metabolism

The human gut microbiota plays an essential role in host health and physiology. Its colonization begins in the earliest moments of life after birth. It is composed of microorganisms such as bacteria, viruses, fungi, yeasts, and bacteriophages [1, 2]. Throughout one's lifespan, the composition of the microbiota can be influenced by various factors, starting with the type of birth delivery, nutrition, antibiotic exposure, inflammation, aging, psychological stress, and lifestyle [1, 3].

As mentioned earlier, the gut microbiota influences multiple physiological processes, including digestion, metabolism, the balance between host defense and immune tolerance, pathogen resistance, epithelial cell proliferation and differentiation, insulin resistance, as well as the behavioral and neurological functions of the host [4, 5]. This last effect is particularly associated with bidirectional gut-brain interactions, better known as the gut-brain axis (GBA). The GBA facilitates communication between the central nervous system (CNS), the enteric nervous system (ENS), and the gastrointestinal (GI) tract (**Figure 1**) [6, 7]. Given the significance of GBA, numerous studies have been conducted to characterize the molecular and functional connections between the gut and the brain. Currently, the most extensively documented network is between the CNS, ENS, and the hypothalamic-pituitary-adrenal

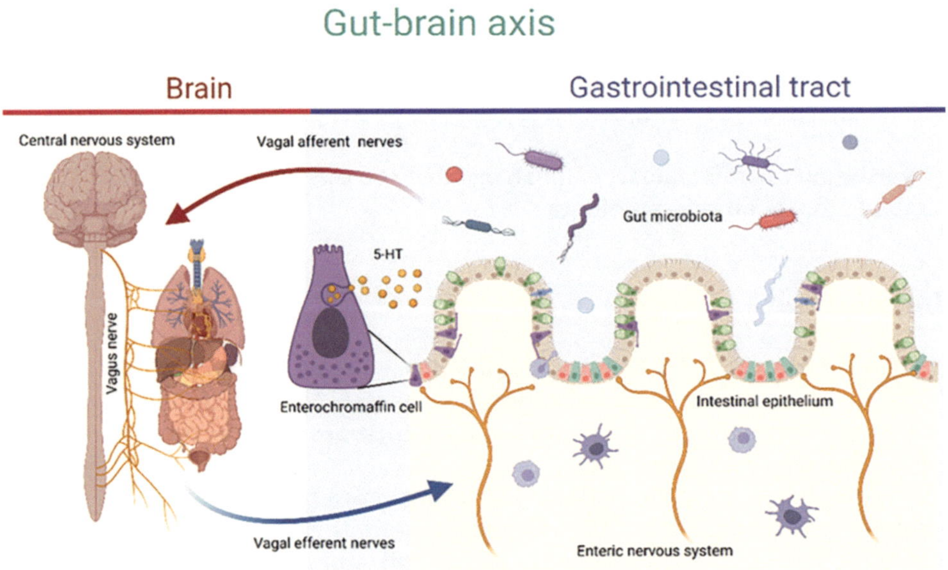

Figure 1.
The gut-brain axis (GBA). Schematic representation of the bidirectional crosstalk between the central nervous system (CNS), the enteric nervous system (ENS), and the gastrointestinal (GI) tract. Vagal efferent and afferent nerves send signals reciprocally between the brain and the gut. Enterochromaffin cells produce and release serotonin (5-HT- 5-hydroxytryptamine) into the gut. Created with BioRender.com.

axis. The ENS resides in the intestinal wall, and its communication with the CNS occurs through neuroimmune and neuroendocrine signaling, mediated by the vagus nerve [8, 9].

The vagus nerve is the longest cranial nerve and is considered the main component of the parasympathetic nervous system; it sends information about the state of the inner organs to the brain and is involved in the control of multiple functions such as immune response, digestion, heart rate, endocrine functions, the mood, among others. The vagus nerve is crucial to the brain-gut axis since establishes the connections between the brain and the gastrointestinal tract; vagal efferents send the signals from the brain to the gut and the vagal afferents from the intestinal wall to the brain. The vagal afferent pathways are involved in the regulation of the hypothalamic-pituitaryadrenal (HPA) axis, and in conjunction allow the brain to influence the activities of intestinal functional effector cells (immune cells, epithelial cells, enteric neurons, smooth muscle cells, interstitial cells of Cajal, and enterochromaffin cells) [9–11]. Enterochromaffin cells (ECs) are the most abundant enteroendocrine cell type in the intestinal epithelium, their arrangement in the colon lets them be in direct contact with gut microbiota, as well as with the afferent and efferent nerve endings (**Figure 1**). Its importance resides in its ability to produce, store, and release serotonin in the gut. They produce 90% of the serotonin in the body, which is essential for intestinal motility, platelet function, immune response, and bone development [11–13]. Recently, Dodds et al. [13] developed an *in vivo* anterograde tracing technique to study the spatial relationship between nerve endings and their proximity to specific cell types in the inner surface of the gastrointestinal tract. Their findings suggest that colonic 5-HT-containing EC cells release neurochemical substances to activate afferent nerves likely *via* diffusion, which then relay this sensory information to the spinal cord and brain [13].

2.1 Tryptophan

Tryptophan (Trp) is an aromatic amino acid that in humans is obtained exclusively by the diet since its biosynthesis is performed in bacteria and plant cells. Although Trp can be metabolized in mammals, microorganisms, and plants, they use different metabolic pathways and produce a vast diversity of metabolites. In mammals, the kynurenine pathway is the most used to degrade it, and only a small proportion is metabolized into serotonin (5-HT, 5-hydroxytryptamine); as the precursor of these metabolites, Trp is considered a key player in the microbiota-gut-brain axis since these neuroactive compounds are involved in depression and other neuropsychiatric disorders [14, 15].

2.2 Kynurenine pathway

Almost 90% of total tryptophan is oxidized to kynurenine across the kynurenine pathway. The initial enzymes of this pathway are the indoleamine-2,3-dioxygenase (IDO) and tryptophan 2,3-dioxygenase (TDO) both of which are responsible for converting tryptophan into kynurenine (**Figure 2**). IDO is present in various organs (brain, GI tract, and liver), and it is typically activated in response to immune stimuli. In contrast, TDO is predominantly expressed in the liver, and its activity depends on tryptophan's availability. Inflammation plays a central role in IDO and TDO activation since IDO is stimulated by proinflammatory cytokines, particularly interferon gamma, and TDO is stimulated by glucocorticoids. On the other hand, kynurenine can be transformed into two different precursors: kynurenic acid and quinolinic acid.

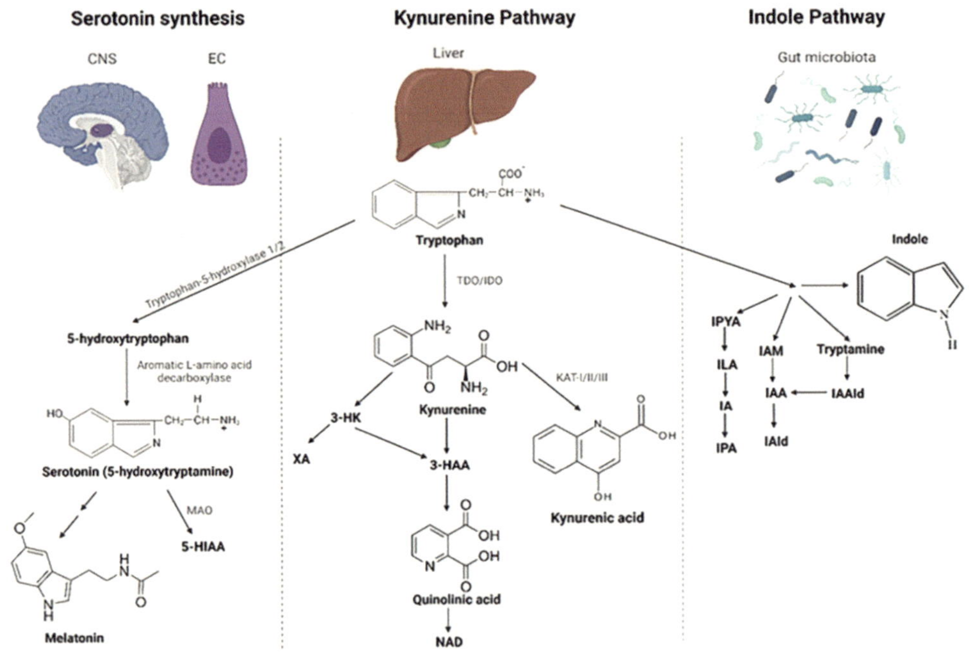

Figure 2.
Tryptophan metabolism host and microbial tryptophan catabolites. Modified from Roth et al. [14]. Overview of the different tryptophan pathways. Microbes degrade tryptophan in the human gut. CNS, central nervous system; EC, Enterochromaffin cells; 5HIAA, 5-Hydroxyindolacetic acid; MAO, monoamine oxidase; IDO, indoleamine 2,3-dioxygenase; TDO, tryptophan 2,3-dioxygenase; 3HAA, 3-Hydroxyanthranilic acid; 3HK, 3-Hydroxykynurenine; XA, Xanthurenic acid; NAD, nicotinamide adenine dinucleotide; IPYA, indole-3-pyurvic acid; ILA, indole-3-lactic acid; IA, indole acrylic acid; IPA, indolic-3-propionic acid; IAM, indole-3-acetamide; IAA, indole-3-acetic acid; IAld, indole-3-aldehyde; IAAld, indole-3-acetaldehyde. Created with BioRender.com.

These metabolites are neuroactive and stimulate N-methyl D-aspartate (NMDA) and alpha-7 nicotinic receptors. Its effects are contrasting, whereas kynurenic acid may act as an anti-inflammatory molecule with neuroprotective features, quinolinic acid is excitotoxic [6, 16].

2.3 Serotonin pathway (CNS and enterochromaffin cells)

The serotonin or 5-HT pathway is also crucial to human physiology as this neurotransmitter influences physiological and behavioral functions such as cognitive and emotional processes, autonomic control, and circadian rhythm. 5-HT acts not only in the CNS but also has various effects externally. For example, it regulates GI and heart rate regulation and mammary gland development, and more recently, potential roles beyond being a neurotransmitter have been reported. The latest studies have revealed that 5-HT can regulate neuronal growth and differentiation during early brain development. Additionally, it has been reported that 5-HT can undergo serotonylation, a mechanism in which covalent bonds are formed with certain substrate proteins, such as histones, giving rise to a class of histone posttranslational modifications that play important roles in regulating neuronal transcriptional programs [15, 17].

5-HT is a monoamine that can be synthesized in the brain and gut by two isoforms of Trp hydroxylase (TPH). In the brain, TPH2 catalyzes 5-HT conversion in monoaminergic neurons (central 5-HT); it represents only a small proportion of the body's total 5-HT. In contrast, peripheral 5-HT (the most abundant) is produced by ECs across TPH1. After 5-HT synthesis, it can be metabolized to form melatonin or 5-hydroxyindoleacetic acid (5-HIAA) and the major 5-HT metabolite (**Figure 2**). Normally, 5-HT cannot cross the blood-brain barrier, so there are differences in the availability of serotonin along the GBA [6, 17].

2.4 Indole pathway and microbial tryptophan catabolites

Most proteins are digested and absorbed in the small intestine; however, increased protein intake lets a significant amount of these proteins and amino acids reach the colon, where a wide range of commensal bacteria triggers their catabolism. Trp is metabolized into indole and indole derivatives (indole-3-aldehyde (IAld), indole3-acetic-acid (IAA), and indole-3-propionic acid (IPA)) (**Figure 2**). Gram-negative and Gram-positive bacterial species, such as *Escherichia coli*, Clostridium sp., and Bacteroides sp., can activate the enzyme tryptophanase (TnaA) to form indole. In the case of its derivates, some species such as Clostridium sp., Bacteroides sp., and Bifidobacterium sp. can form IAA from indole-acetamide. The intermediate indole3-lactic acid (ILA) is produced by Lactobacillus sp. and Bifidobacterium sp., which is transformed into IPA by bacteria, such as Clostridium sp. and Peptostreptococcus sp. [6, 18].

Recent advances have suggested that microbiota-derived tryptophan catabolites are crucial for maintaining intestinal homeostasis, and several mechanisms have been described (**Figure 3**). Indole, IPA, and IA can influence gut cells, reducing intestinal permeability and thus affecting mucosal homeostasis. On the other hand, indole induces enteroendocrine L-cells to release glucagon-like peptide 1 (GLP-1), which triggers effects such as appetite suppression and insulin secretion, and slowed gastric emptying.

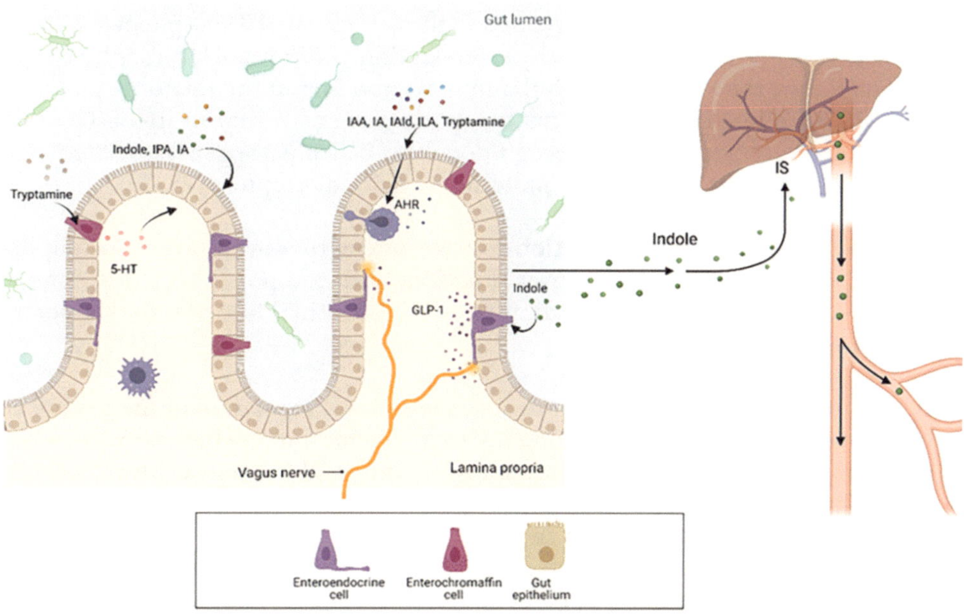

Figure 3.
Microbial tryptophan catabolites host effects. Modified from Roager and Licht [19]. IA, indole acrylic acid; IPA, indolic-3-propionic acid; IAA, indole-3-acetic acid; IAld, indole-3-aldehyde; 5-HT, 5-hydroxytryptamine; GLP-1, glucagon-like peptide 1; AHR, aryl hydrocarbon receptor; IS, indoxyl sulfate. Created with BioRender.com.

Additionally, some catabolites stimulate intestinal immune cells *via* the aryl hydrocarbon receptor (AHR), leading to increased production of interleukin-22 (IL-22). Furthermore, enterochromaffin cells can release 5-HT through tryptamine induction, consequently stimulating enteric neurons and enhancing gastrointestinal motility. In the bloodstream, certain tryptophan catabolites, such as IPA and IA, have anti-oxidative and anti-inflammatory effects. In addition, IPA and its precursors help the proliferation, differentiation, and barrier function of human intestinal epithelial cells. In contrast, indoxyl sulfate (IS), an indole metabolite, can have cytotoxic effects [19–21].

3. Physiological effects (hunger and satiety, intestinal health, mental health, and insulin sensitivity)

The gut-brain axis is a bidirectional complex that maintains communication between the central nervous system and the digestive tract. The brain integrates it, the spinal cord, the autonomic nervous system (sympathetic, parasympathetic, and enteric nervous systems), and the neuroendocrine and neurohumoral systems [19, 22].

The intestinal microbiota is composed of 1013–1014 microbial cells. Its distribution is 90% bacteria, predominantly Firmicutes and Bacteroidetes; the other 10% between Actinobacteria and Proteobacteria and in smaller proportion between Verrucomicrobes, Fusobacteria, Cyanobacteria, and nonbacterial microorganisms, such as archaea and yeasts [23, 24].

The microbiota has four main functions:

- Metabolic function is related to the production of short-chain fatty acids (SCFA), the balance between fatty acid oxidation and lipogenesis, and vitamin synthesis [25].

- The immunological function is related to the activation of T lymphocytes, the production of immunoglobulins by B production of immunoglobulins by B lymphocytes, the release of proinflammatory and immunoregulatory cytokines, and the secretion of hormones, neuropeptides, and neurotransmitters. These processes are triggered by the recognition of so-called pathogen-associated molecular patterns (PMAPs) by pattern recognition receptors [25, 26].

- Physiological and barrier function consists of cell turnover, linked to apoptosis and maintenance of the barrier function, with components of the immune system, hormones, and metabolites from the intestinal lumen into the bloodstream [26, 27].

These functions are important for the production and regulation of the passage of proinflammatory cytokines, toxins, and microorganisms into the bloodstream, which stimulates the release of hormones, immunoglobulins, and the activation of systems, such as the hypothalamic-pituitary-adrenal (HPA) axis with the consequent production of cortisol and the activation of the vagal system [25, 28].

The small intestine has a layer called mucosa, which is the first line of defense, and digests, and absorbs nutrients, electrolytes, and water. The mucosa-associated lymphoid tissue (MALT) and the intestine-associated lymphoid tissue (GALT) are in charge of the immune response, which is formed by lymphoid nodules and isolated lymphocytes that generate their own response and originate innate and adaptive (humoral) immune response and production of inflammatory cytokines, among them tumor necrosis factor-alpha (TNF-α) and interleukin I and 6 regulatory and cooperator T lymphocytes [28, 29].

The large intestine acts as a selective barrier to microorganisms and participates in conjunction with the epithelium, lymphoid tissue, and calciform cells [29].

The microbiome is formed by signaling from the microorganisms themselves and their postbiotics called "quorum sensing," which participate in physiological processes. This microbiota-brain axis has been related to several homeostatic physiological processes such as digestion, hunger-satiety axis, metabolism, eating behaviors, and neural problems. The three main related axes are immune, neuronal, and metabolic, as seen in **Figure 4** [28, 30, 31].

3.1 Metabolic effects

Signals following ingestion are transmitted to the central nervous system (CNS) where the hypothalamus integrates signals emitted from the neuroendocrine cells of the intestinal epithelium that sense the luminal milieu and release glucagon-like peptide and cholecystokinin (CCK), gastric intestinal polypeptide (GIP), and pancreatic polypeptide (PYY) acting in a paracrine manner, which is directed to peripheral organs. These peptides are released near afferent neurons, these send signals to the solitary nucleus and the arcuate nucleus, and this signal is also activated by the enteric nervous system, which is activated by the production of serotonin at the intestinal level, by tryptophan metabolism and intraganglionic laminar endings, also the peptides can go directly to the circulation and arrive directly to the solitary tract [31–33].

In the arcuate nucleus, the signals emitted by these intestinal peptides can regulate glucose and energy homeostasis, where the orexigenic (hunger) and anoxygenic (satiety) neurons intervene [31, 33].

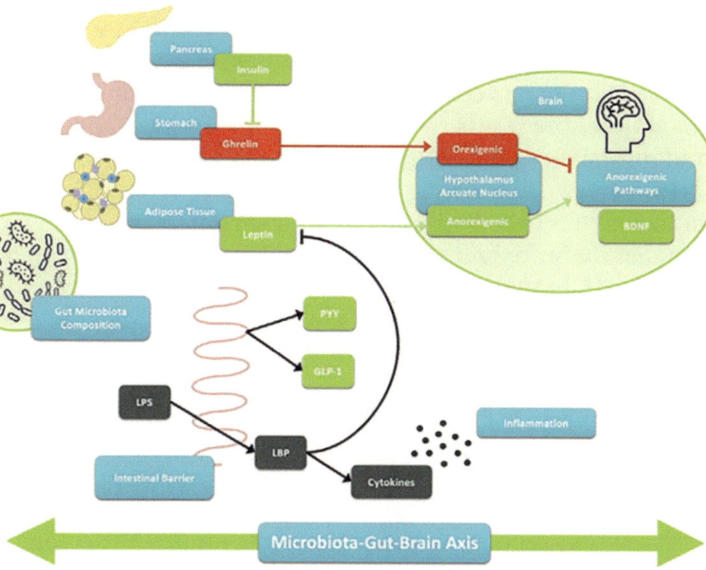

Figure 4.
Effects of the microbiota-gut-axis.

On the other hand, the vagus nerve transmits information to regulate energy homeostasis and glucose levels. Chronic stimulation of vagal afferent pathways is known to reduce energy intake. Glucose consumption increases this vagal signaling [34].

3.2 Effects on blood glucose

In the intestine, glucose is also formed by gluconeogenesis, which improves insulin sensitivity. Other peptides increase glucose-6-phosphatase. Changes in the microbiota contribute to vagal afferent desensitization. It is known that the consumption of fat in food may also play a role in this desensitization [34, 35].

The enteroendocrine cells of the small and large intestine secrete GLP-1 and GIP, although it is greater in the large intestine and to a greater extent GLP-1 through the action of metabolites secreted from microorganisms (**Figure 1**). On the other hand, the release of SCFA, which is a product of intestinal microbiota metabolism, induces the release of GLP-1 by G protein-bound receptors in enterocytes [36, 37].

Additionally, GLP-1 release reduces food intake by the aforementioned mechanisms. GIP acts in the pancreas by stimulating the release of insulin and neurons found in the paraventricular nucleus so that an impairment in the production and intestinal permeability or reduction in SCFA has been related to increased body weight, dyslipidemia, and increased appetite signaling as well as leptin resistance [37, 38].

More recent studies have described that tryptophan metabolism *via* the kineturin pathway (quinurenine, quinurenate, xanthurenic, and quinolinate) and indolactate is associated with the risk of developing type 2 diabetes; however, it has also been found that the combination with indolpropionate has an inverse, that is, protective and relationship. This metabolite is formed by the intestinal microorganism Bifidobacterium intestinal in the consumption of foods rich in tryptophan and protein of high biological value [39].

3.3 Brain function

The microbiome can influence brain function by pathways that include the release of neurotransmitters and neurotransmitter metabolites that modulate the immune system and the regulation of the hypothalamic-pituitary-adrenal axis. The enteric nervous system is connected to the central nervous system, and the vagal nerve modulates the release of neurotransmitters such as acetylcholine, dopamine, and norepinephrine, which additionally also affects hormone production [40].

The gut-brain axis has been implicated in brain aging, plasticity, and cognition, and it is known that there are four messengers involved in this brain operation: short-chain fatty acids, branched amino acids, peptides, gut hormones, cytokines and sensory neurons. There are four messengers involved in this brain function: short-chain fatty acids, branched amino acids, peptidoglycans, gut hormones, cytokines and sensory neurons [41].

Short-chain fatty acids are produced by the fermentation of gastrointestinal microorganisms, and these act by regulating neuroplasticity, epigenetic expression, and the immune system. Sodium butyrate improves serotonin production and behavior, for example, in mice, it has decreased depression and intestinal hormones, such as GLP-1, and GIP, not only regulate appetite but also stimulate the colonic vagal system. Amines (such as tryptophan, and tyramine), travel through the blood system and also affect local neurons and cells of the central nervous system and afferent pathways of the vagus nerve [42].

Within the production of neurotransmitters, it is known that Bacteroides, Bifidobacterium, Parabacteroides, and Escherichia spp. produce γ-aminobutyric acid (GABA) and are important in the production of serotonin (5-hydroxytryptamine 5-HT); most of this component is produced in the intestine, and although it does not affect the amount of serotonin in the brain and does not cross the blood-brain barrier, it has been shown that it does have a modulatory role in the 5HT signaling pathways in the brain. The mechanism is not yet fully elucidated; however, it is known that cells of the innate immune system such as dendritic cells, monocytes, and mast cells express serotonin receptors and transporters. Something similar occurs in the adaptive system and any blood cell except erythrocytes. Therefore, 5HT regulates inflammation and chemotaxis, in addition to the fact that practically all organs and cells have one or more serotonin receptors [42, 43].

The microorganisms that can lead to the production of metabolites that interact with the nervous system are:

Lactobacillus reuteri regulates oxytocin levels, and *Lactobacillus rhamnosus* regulates and produces GABA, which in mice regulates anxiety. Bifidobacteria longum has been linked to increased neuronal neuroplasticity. Bifidobacteria fragilis by its reduction of 4-ethylphenylsulfate modulates anxiety [43, 44].

As mentioned above, this relationship is bidirectional and there are factors such as stress that activate the HPA system, which releases corticotropin-releasing hormone into the bloodstream, or the brain, which releases adrenocorticotropic hormone and cortisol, which affects the intestinal barrier. There are also immunomodulators and neurotransmitters that activate neurons in the intestinal system and the vagus nerve, which in turn changes the composition of the microbiota [43, 45].

4. The intestinal microbiota as a modifier of tryptophan metabolism: dysregulation and associated pathologies

As mentioned earlier, the composition of the microbiota can be influenced by age, sex, genetics, geography, probiotics, race, stress, smoking, diet, medication (especially antibiotics), or gastrointestinal infections. These differences can alter availability and tryptophan metabolism and be associated with various pathologies [14, 46].

The luminal tryptophan availability is influenced by microbial tryptophan metabolism. Restrictive diets, low in protein or essential amino acids, in addition to causing anorexia and weight loss [10, 47, 48], can reduce microbial proliferation (Lactobacillus) and through dietary intake improve microbial metabolism and increase Indol 3-aldehyde (IAld). In animal models, high-fat diets deplete microbial metabolites of indole-3-acetic (IAA) acid and tryptamine, indicating that microbial degradation is diminished. Formula milk alters serotonin to tryptamine metabolism. A diet rich in carbohydrates the microbial metabolism of tryptophan is affected, indigestible carbohydrates (starch) facilitate the production of (SCFAs), and reduce the degradation of tryptophan and Indole compounds, in addition to the increase in tryptophan levels in the large intestine and serum [6].

Oral antibiotics modify the composition and metabolism of the IM, in case of depletion, serotonin levels are reduced, the colon motility is delated, the kynurenine pathway is affected, and the availability of Trp is increased [6, 49]. In addition to the administration antibiotics increase the levels of indol and compounds in the large intestine [49].

4.1 Inflammatory bowel disease and irritable bowel syndrome

Among the diseases mort linked to the IM inflammatory bowel disease, patients with ulcerative colitis and Crohn's disease, and tryptophan levels in serum are lower than healthy controls, this suggests that changes in metabolism are involved in the etiology of inflammatory bowel disease. Metagenomic analysis of tool samples a reduction of intestinal microorganisms involved in Trp in addition to a lower production of ligands AHR observed [14]. The increase in the catabolism of Typ in intestinal immune cells is associated with impaired ability to degrade Typ limiting the bioavailability of beneficial indole derivatives and contributing to the severity of the disease [50].

Irritable bowel syndrome is characterized by abdominal pain and changes in bowel habits. Kynurenine to Trp levels have been shown to be increased in plasma. The composition of the gut microbiota may play an important role in pathogenesis since bacterial abundance and brain connectivity are different in healthy controls [6].

4.2 Alzheimer disease

There is evidence of the influence of Trp metabolites, the IM, and the neuroinflammatory process associated with Alzheimer's disease (AD) [51]. In patients with AD, a significant difference has been found in the taxonomy of the intestinal microbiota with a predominance in the decrease of Fermicutes and Actinobacteria in addition to an increase in Bacteroidetes species, compared to agematch control patients. Another study reported that patients with AD had reduced circulating Trp levels and elevated kynurenine/TPH ratios, it is also associated with greater cognitive impairment and elevated proinflammatory cytokines [51].

4.3 Parkinson disease

Current evidence suggests that the microbiota is involved in the pathogenesis through inflammatory neurotoxicity. The abundance of Bacteroidetes in this type of patient correlates with the clinical severity of motor symptoms and high levels of proinflammatory TNFα and INFγ. Verrucomicrobia is associated with higher levels of INFγ and possible interaction with metabolites of IDO and Trp. Parkinson's disease patients have elevated proportions of kynurenine/TPH in plasma, as well as reduced KAT activity relative to control patients [14].

4.4 Multiple sclerosis

Analysis of stool from multiple sclerosis patients showed an increase in Methanobrevibacter and Akkermansia, as well as a decrease in Butyricimones compared to control patients. Patients have reduced circulation of the aryl hydrocarbon receptor of tryptophan hydrolase metabolites, indicating a metabolic dysregulation in pathogenesis [14].

4.5 Migraine

Clinical studies focusing on intestinal microbial changes in migraine patients have shown that intestinal dysbiosis worsens migraine pain in a TNFa-dependent process. The analysis of fecal samples of elderly women showed elevation of Firmicutes, especially of the Clostridium species, compared to the control group of the same age. In addition, Kynurenine metabolites have also been found to be elevated in this same group of patients [14].

4.6 Anxiety and depression

Serotonin is widely studied in anxiety and depression. In susceptible populations, such as older adults, a decrease in plasma tryptophan concentration may cause mood changes. It has been observed that decreased Trp levels and a higher ratio of kynurenine to Trp in plasma are associated with depression [6]. There is evidence of the role of the intestinal microbiota in the onset and clinical phenotype of this type of disorder. It has been observed that depression affects the HPA axis, neurotransmitter levels, and the inflammatory process are affected [52]. A study in mice revealed that in chronic sleep restriction stress, and these animals had depressive behavior, strong activation of the Kyn pathway, and IDO in the brain and gut. In germ-free mice, more anxious behavior has been observed in contrast to conventionally bred mice. Even with microbial repopulation after weaning, the behavior was not easily reversible, which is why it is described as a critical period during which the gut microbiota can aid psychological development [6]. In addition, children born overweight and overweight mothers have been observed to show higher scores of anxiety, shyness, and depression, correlated with the abundance of Actinobacteria and Fusobacteria [53].

4.7 Autism spectrum disorder

Autism spectrum disorder (ASD) is a disorder characterized by social and behavioral impairment. In addition to neurological symptoms, the patient often suffers from gastrointestinal abnormalities. Some microbial species have been linked to the pathogenesis of this disease; symptoms have been linked to a reduction of *Pretovella, Coprococcus, Veillonellaceae*, and *Bracteroides fragilis* and a reduction in the availability of TPH [6, 14].

4.8 Cerebrovascular disease

Tryptophan metabolites may influence the development and severity of cerebrovascular disease. It has been observed that in stroke patients, there is a positive correlation between the kyn/Trp ratio and the severity of stroke. Patients with acute ischemic stroke metabolic profiles showed elevated levels of serum lactate, carbonate, and glutamate, in addition to lower levels of Try and other amino acids [14].

The IM has been studied in animal models, such as stroke patients, and the microbial diversity has been observed to collapse after ischemic stroke metabolic in the days after stroke onset. Gut dysbiosis contributes additionally to the pathogenesis of stroke risk factors such as diabetes mellitus, hypertension, obesity, and metabolic syndrome [14].

4.9 Metabolic disorder

The IM plays a fundamental role in the metabolic balance of the host. It is now known that the intestinal IM is involved in the pathogenesis of metabolic disorders [50]. Metabolic disorders represent a group of interrelated pathological conditions that combine obesity, dyslipidemia, glucose intolerance, insulin resistance, hypertension, and diabetes mellitus, which, as mentioned above, increase the incidence of cardiovascular disease and increase mortality [54].

Specific classes where IM-derived metabolites, such as bile acids, branched-chain amino acids, Trp metabolites, and indole derivatives, have been implicated in metabolic disorders [50].

Cross-sectional studies have shown that tryptophan catabolism is altered in individuals with obesity and metabolic syndrome, and kynurenine/tryptophan ratios of blood concentrations are elevated in obese, metabolic syndrome, or hyperuricemia patients compared to healthy controls. In addition, kynurenine/tryptophan ratios correlate positively with BMI, triglyceride, and uric acid levels [50].

In a cohort study of diabetic patients, kynurenine levels were found to be positively associated with BMI and a higher HOMA2 insulin resistance index. Another study focused on alterations in plasma and fecal levels of Trp catabolites found that plasma levels of kynurenine were higher in obese or type 2 diabetic subjects than in control patients. In addition, in feces, a change in Trp catabolism toward kynurenine and lower production of indole-3-acetic acid were observed in obese and diabetic patients without treatment. Rationale suggests increased intestinal IDO1 activity and inhibition of the microbial indole pathway [50, 54].

Alterations in Tpy levels have also been observed in older adults with diabetes mellitus with aging, and the composition and function of adipose tissue changes, leading to insulin resistance. There are also cellular changes such as mitochondrial dysfunction, antioxidant deficiency, inflammation, and decreased immune response, changes that affect the Kyn pathway. It has also been observed that adults over 65 years of age have lower Tpy levels than younger groups [55].

Carcinogenesis is related to immune status and environmental factors, among them the intestinal microbiota and its metabolites, the bacterial metabolites of Trp play a role in the development of several types of cancer [54]. Under physiological conditions and as a defense mechanism, local inflammation depletes Tpy, which limits the growth of microbes and the proliferation of malignant cells. Under tumor conditions, the degradation of Trp and the accumulation of its metabolites increases, suppressing the tumor's immune response as a defense mechanism [56].

Between 16 and 20% of cancers are the result of pathogenic infections. Patients with Crohn's disease harbor pathogenic *Escherichia coli* that contributes to a proinflammatory state, changes in IDO1 expression, and cell proliferation. In some types of cancer (breast and colon), a significant increase in Kyn has been observed compared to healthy controls [57].

Trp catabolism exerts immunosuppressive actions in many types of cancer. Aryl hydrocarbon receptor activation in myeloid cells promotes an immunosuppressive tumor microenvironment and facilitates pancreatic ductal adenocarcinoma growth. In gastrointestinal, lung, melanoma, prostate, and pancreatic cancers, over-activation of the Kyn pathway, particularly IDO, predicts a bad prognosis [54].

4.10 Dermatological disorders

The skin and the intestine have similar characteristics with microorganisms that regulate their function and use of metabolites. Of the main related reactions, it has been demonstrated that the immune inflammation is caused by leukocytes, keratinocytes, macrophages, neutrophils, and T cells that increase inflammation and psoriasis by releasing proinflammatory cytokines. The gut axis and gut microbiota are the key elements of the gut-brain-skin axis and play an important role in the association between psoriasis and depression.

It has also been found that abnormal induction of the Kyn pathway is associated with dermal fibroblast infiltration and the release of inflammatory interleukins. Physiologically the skin microbiota degrades host tryptophan to regulate inflammation *via* the indole pathway; however, with dysbiosis, this activity is impaired [58].

5. Therapeutic strategies

The intestinal microbiota IM develops numerous metabolic processes. It needs to maintain an adequate state in its composition and functions (eubiosis) to maintain its state of health [8]. The genetic diversity of microbial communities determines a large number of enzymes and biochemical pathways, which are modified according to the conditions of the host, even in severe pathological states, such as cancer [59]. Its metabolic function makes it a therapeutic target when it is altered (dysbiosis). The advances achieved in the sequencing 16S rRNA, metagenomics, proteomics, and transcriptomics, allow to know its composition and functions, providing criteria with therapies according to the existing pathology [31, 60].

The intestinal microbiota, in our gut, plays a critical role in maintaining our overall health. It is responsible for various metabolic processes and must remain in a healthy state to ensure that we stay healthy. The diversity of microbial communities in our gut determines the many enzymes and biochemical pathways that are present, and these can be altered in response to the host's condition, even in severe cases such as cancer. When the microbiota is altered, it can become a therapeutic target, and advances in sequencing and analysis have allowed us to better understand its composition and functions. With this knowledge, we can develop targeted therapies that are tailored to the patient's specific needs [31].

5.1 Intestinal microbiota as a therapeutic target

The therapeutic targets at this level are numerous due to the complexity of existing microorganisms, whose influence and role within MI are increasingly found. This forces us to search for the best possible scenario to acquire knowledge of its importance and role played in health (eubiosis) and an alternative in disease management (dysbiosis), as well as an adequate perspective of its disease preventive capacity [61]. Because the modifications of microorganisms and their genes and enzymes affect the metabolism of the nutrients and substances that enter, they give rise to metabolites in an inappropriate way that leads to multiple pathologies. The relationship between metabolites/products is known as the microbiome since it implies genetic participation [31]. The study of dysbiosis is so important that specific databases have been developed since 2018, where every time new microorganisms, related diseases, or metabolites are registered; they are automatically added to these data [62]. It is expected that the use of microbes in genetic form will achieve disease preventive effects. In studies carried out, some metabolites exhibit the ability to potentiate other drugs by enhancing their beneficial effect, for example, for chemotherapeutic agents in the pancreas and ovary. Every day advances in the knowledge of therapeutic targets to restore not only the alteration of the beneficial and commensal species specific to the individual but also their capacity for participatory microbiome [61, 63].

In dysbiosis, strategies have been applied to restore the native microbiome. These range from fecal microbiota transplantation (FMT), and the use of pre, pro, and synbiotics to the use of new biotechnological drugs with inhibition of enzymes involved in the metabolism of such essential substances as tryptophan [19]. Other alternatives, both natural, traditional, and pharmacological medicines with synthetic biology are also studied [61, 64].

Genetic engineering offers the possibility of generating molecules, antitoxins, bacteriophages, peptides, and microbial metabolites, but most studies have been carried out in rodents. At the moment, the pharmaceutical industry is conducting studies at different phases of research with encouraging results based on well-established knowledge [65]. So, certain bacterial types are found to improve diseases, where *Christensenella sp*. has been used and defined to reduce anxiety and depression, *Akkermansia muciniphila* in metabolic disorders, *Lactobacillus johnsonii*, which protects against cancer, and *Bifidobacterium longum* reduces the severity in Crohn's disease and restores the mucus layer [61]. In the management of the MI – microbiome, three things are intended: increase its quantity, decrease it, or modulate it [66].

5.2 Increase the amount of gut microbiota

It involves directing the benefits of the host-microbiome interaction by adding strains of microbes that are diminished. They can be individual strains or a group of them. The microbes used can be natural or genetically modified to produce therapeutic molecules. It can be with probiotics or fecal microbiota transplantation (FMT).

FMT, in general, involves the therapeutic administration of healthy microbial populations to replace disease-causing ones. There are different types of selection, preparation, and management for FMT found in the literature. The main diseases that have responded adequately to FMT are listed: *Clostridium difficile* infection; recurrent *Clostridium difficile* infection; irritable bowel syndrome; insulin resistance; recurrent urinary tract infection; alcoholic liver disease; autism; multiple sclerosis; Parkinson's disease; cancer; pseudomembranous colitis, ulcerative colitis; Crohn's disease; hepatic encephalopathy; alcoholic hepatitis, diarrhea; adulthood; Stroke; Alzheimer's disease and sepsis. The use of probiotics is a method of additive therapy, which is based on administering microbes as monotherapy, whether natural or genetically modified. They are conceptualized as live microorganisms that when administered in adequate quantities provide a beneficial effect to the host [64].

The most used are Lactobacilli, bifidobacteria, and *E. Coli*, which act by producing bacteriocins among other effects and work is being done to improve their microbiome composition (gene processing). The use of FMT can be considered as a super probiotic.

The main probiotics, both native and modified, make up such an extensive list for the purposes of the book that it is suggested to go to the review done by Yadav and Chauhan [61].

5.3 Reduce gut microbiota

It is intended to reduce the number of pathogenic microbes through bacteriocins and bacteriophages. It is intended to achieve the desired effect without significantly affecting the other members of the IM. Bacteriocins are peptides synthesized in ribosomal form that show antimicrobial activity. Two classes have been identified and the bacteria that produce bacteriocins are Firmicutes, Bacteroidetes, Proteobacteria, and Actinobacteria. There is a long list of bacteriocins that are very helpful in various fields, both medicine and other areas. Resistance to bacteriocins can also be found.

Bacteriophages are viruses that have specificity for a bacterium. It inserts itself into the genome and causes bacterial membrane disintegration. They are considered a suitable alternative to antibiotic-resistant germs. Engineered phages use a CRISPR-cas system to destroy pathogens. Unlike IM and probiotics, their specific targets are pathogenic bacteria [61].

5.4 Modulatory therapy

Includes the modulation of IM or its interactions with the host for therapeutic purposes. It considers the restoration of diminished MI and the transformation of existing flora to achieve a healthier MI. It can be through diet, exercise, and antibiotics. Diet plays a critical role in the use of vitamin D.

Other types of therapeutic targets and beneficial germs that can help have been added to the literature such as psychobiotics (help in improving mental health in mental illness), postbiotics (inanimate microbes or their products that provide benefits), and synbiotics (mixtures of pre- and probiotics).

An important model for understanding therapies for MI is inflammatory bowel disease (IBD), which includes Crohn's disease and ulcerative colitis. The disorder of the intestinal flora of this disease is considered to offer the greatest number, both in pharmacological strategies and the use of natural remedies and traditional medicines, and some tested with adequate results. In IBD, the participation of the intestinal microbiota (IM) stands out. Significant growth of proinflammatory microorganisms is found, including *Ruminococcus gnavus* and *Escherichia Coli,* and reduction of anti-inflammatory microorganisms such as *Bacteroidetes, Lachnospiracea*, and *Faecalibacterium prasnitzi*. The presence of abundant mucus can aggravate the invasion of pathogens and commensal flora inducing inflammation. In addition, bacterial enterotoxins can damage the epithelial structure of the host. Most studies indicate that the presence of bacteria, such as adherent *E. coli, proteobacteria*, and *E. coli,* are possible causative agents, and the release of colibactin by *E. coli* may influence the presence of colorectal cancer. Host immunology can be altered and produce both inflammation and anti-inflammation according to local factors. Changes in bacterial structure, as well as in its metabolites stand out for the development of new therapies, including 5-ASA, immunosuppressants, glucocorticoids, polyphenols, polysaccharides, and herbal combinations [67].

5.5 Pharmacological interventions and possible therapeutic targets on tryptophan metabolism

At the level of the brain, the amino acid tryptophan plays a vital role in the synthesis of important biological molecules. Its metabolites are involved in a large number of processes; many beneficial types, depending on the metabolic pathways it follows, can give rise to malignant types, such as proteins in cancer cells. It also produces the activation of immunity and antitumor effects, which makes it a very complex component to achieve therapeutic interventions, due to the complex management within the host. One component is the administration of D tryptophan as a supplement, but within the body, its therapeutic targets are found in its metabolites and enzymes that intervene according to metabolic pathways. An important marker is the Kyn: Trp ratio, which increases with age causing frailty in adults. The KYNU enzyme is one of the most gene expressed. The main enzymes are tryptophan-2,3-dioxygenase (TDO), indolamine2,3-dioxygenase 1 (IDO1), indolamine-2,3-dioxygenase (IDO2), and KMO. All can be managed with inhibitors, modulators, agonists, and antagonists primarily [68].

6. Conclusions

The knowledge about the interaction between tryptophan metabolism and the gut microbiota has expanded greatly in recent years. Tryptophan and its metabolites modulated through the gut microbiota are involved in several host physiological and pathological processes. Degradation of tryptophan and its metabolites is an important target from a therapeutic perspective; however further. Research is required to refine effective dose ranges and gut microbial species to modulate host physiology.

Conflict of interest

The authors declare that there is no conflict of interest for the publication of this work; no financial or material assistance was received from any company.

Author details

Miriam A. Mora-Navarro[1*], José M. Mora-Martínez[1], Anayeli D.J. Patiño-Laguna[2], Carla P. Barragán-Álvarez[3], Michelle E. Gonzalez-Mora[1] and Citlalli E. Mora-Navarro[4]

1 Department of Philosophical and Methodological Discipline, University Center of Health Sciences, University of Guadalajara, Mexico

2 Institute of Experimental and Clinical Therapeutics, University Center of Health Sciences, University of Guadalajara, Mexico

3 Center for Research and Assistance in Technology and Design of the State of Jalisco, Mexico

4 Regional Hospital Dr. Valentin Gómez Farías, The Institute of Security and Social Services of State Workers, Mexico

*Address all correspondence to: miriam.mora@live.com.mx

References

[1] Ratsika A, Codagnone MC, O'mahony S, Stanton C, Cryan JF. Priming for life: Early life nutrition and the microbiota-gut-brain Axis. Nutrients. 2021;**13**(2):1-33. DOI: 10.3390/NU13020423

[2] Chen Y, Zhou J, Wang L. Role and mechanism of gut microbiota in human disease. Frontiers in Cellular and Infection Microbiology. 2021;**11**(625913):1-12. DOI: 10.3389/FCIMB.2021.625913/PDF

[3] Milani C et al. The first microbial colonizers of the human gut: Composition, activities, and health implications of the infant gut microbiota. Microbiology and Molecular Biology Reviews. 2017;**81**(4):e00036-17. DOI: 10.1128/MMBR.00036-17

[4] Rowland I et al. Gut microbiota functions: Metabolism of nutrients and other food components. European Journal of Nutrition. 2018;**57**(1):1-24. DOI: 10.1007/S00394-017-1445-8

[5] Hasan N, Yang H. Factors affecting the composition of the gut microbiota, and its modulation. PeerJ. 2019;7(8):1-31. DOI: 10.7717/PEERJ.7502

[6] Gao K, Mu CL, Farzi A, Zhu WY. Tryptophan metabolism: A link between the gut microbiota and brain. Advances in Nutrition. 2020;**11**(3):709-723. DOI: 10.1093/ADVANCES/NMZ127

[7] Mayer EA, Nance K, Chen S. The gut-brain Axis. Annual Review of Medicine. 2022;**73**:439-453. DOI: 10.1146/ANNUREV-MED-042320-014032

[8] Carloni S, Rescigno M. Unveiling the gut-brain axis: Structural and functional analogies between the gut and the choroid plexus vascular and immune barriers. Seminars in Immunopathology. 2022;**44**(6):869-882. DOI: 10.1007/S00281-022-00955-3

[9] Breit S, Kupferberg A, Rogler G, Hasler G. Vagus nerve as modulator of the brain-gut axis in psychiatric and inflammatory disorders. Frontiers in Psychiatry. 2018;**9**(44):1-15. DOI: 10.3389/FPSYT.2018.00044/PDF

[10] Browning KN, Verheijden S, Boeckxstaens GE. The Vagus nerve in appetite regulation, mood, and intestinal inflammation. Gastroenterology. 2017;**152**(4):730-744. DOI: 10.1053/J.GASTRO.2016.10.046

[11] Qin HY, Wong HLX, Zang KH, Li X, Bian ZX. Enterochromaffin cell hyperplasia in the gut: Factors, mechanism and therapeutic clues. Life Sciences. 2019;**239**:116886. DOI: 10.1016/J.LFS.2019.116886

[12] Xu X, Chen R, Zhan G, Wang D, Tan X, Xu H. Enterochromaffin cells: Sentinels to gut microbiota in hyperalgesia? Frontiers in Cellular and Infection Microbiology. 2021;**11**(760076):1-14. DOI: 10.3389/FCIMB.2021.760076/PDF

[13] Dodds KN, Travis L, Kyloh MA, Jones LA, Keating DJ, Spencer NJ. The gut-brain axis: Spatial relationship between spinal afferent nerves and 5-HT-containing enterochromaffin cells in mucosa of mouse colon. American Journal of Physiology. Gastrointestinal and Liver Physiology. 2022;**322**(5):G523-G533. DOI: 10.1152/AJPGI.00019.2022

[14] Roth W, Zadeh K, Vekariya R, Ge Y, Mohamadzadeh M. Tryptophan metabolism and gut-brain homeostasis. International Journal of Molecular

Sciences. 2021;**22**(6):1-23. DOI: 10.3390/IJMS22062973

[15] Correia AS, Vale N. Tryptophan metabolism in depression: A narrative review with a focus on serotonin and kynurenine pathways. International Journal of Molecular Sciences. 2022;**23**(15):8493. DOI: 10.3390/IJMS23158493

[16] Kim YK. Anxiety disorders: Rethinking and understanding recent discoveries. 2020;p. 566

[17] Al-Kachak A et al. Histone H3 serotonylation dynamics in dorsal raphe nucleus contribute to stress- and antidepressant-mediated gene expression and behavior. bioRxiv. 2023;**05**(04):539464, 1-71. DOI: 10.1101/2023.05.04.539464

[18] Höglund E, Øverli Ø, Winberg S. Tryptophan metabolic pathways and brain serotonergic activity: A comparative review. Frontiers in Endocrinology (Lausanne). 2019;**10**(158):1-11. DOI: 10.3389/FENDO.2019.00158

[19] Roager HM, Licht TR. Microbial tryptophan catabolites in health and disease. Nature Communications. 2018;**9**(1):1-10. DOI: 10.1038/S41467-018-05470-4

[20] Ismael S et al. IPA and its precursors differently modulate the proliferation, differentiation, and integrity of intestinal epithelial cells. Nutrition Research and Practice. 2023;**17**(4):616-630. DOI: 10.4162/NRP.2023.17.4.616

[21] Tan YQ et al. Host/microbiota interactions-derived tryptophan metabolites modulate oxidative stress and inflammation via aryl hydrocarbon receptor signaling. Free Radical Biology & Medicine. 2022;**184**:30-41. DOI: 10.1016/J.FREERADBIOMED.2022.03.025

[22] Carlos Pineda-Cortes J, Carlos Pineda J. El Microbioma y las enfermedades neurodegenerativas del Sistema Nervioso Central Autor para correspondencia. Revista biomédica. 2017;**1**:28

[23] Rodriguez-Valera F et al. Explaining microbial population genomics through phage predation. Nature Precedings. 2009;**07**(11):828-836. DOI: 10.1038/npre.2009.3489.1

[24] Rooks MG et al. Gut microbiome composition and function in experimental colitis during active disease and treatment-induced remission. The ISME Journal. 2014;**8**(7):1403. DOI: 10.1038/ISMEJ.2014.3

[25] Cryan JF et al. The microbiota-gut-brain Axis. Physiological Reviews. 2019;**99**(4):1877-2013. DOI: 10.1152/PHYSREV.00018.2018

[26] Fernandez-Real JM et al. Gut microbiota interacts with brain microstructure and function. The Journal of Clinical Endocrinology and Metabolism. 2015;**100**(12):4505-4513. DOI: 10.1210/JC.2015-3076

[27] Zhou H, Wang L, Liu F. Immunological impact of intestinal T cells on metabolic diseases. Frontiers in Immunology. 2021;**12**(639902):1-13. DOI: 10.3389/FIMMU.2021.639902

[28] Taleb S. Tryptophan dietary impacts gut barrier and metabolic diseases. Frontiers in Immunology. 2019;**10**(2113):1-7. DOI: 10.3389/FIMMU.2019.02113

[29] Valle-Noguera A, Ochoa-Ramos A, Gomez-Sánchez MJ, Cruz-Adalia A. Type 3 innate lymphoid cells as regulators of

the host-pathogen interaction. Frontiers in Immunology. 2021;**12**(748851):1-19. DOI: 10.3389/FIMMU.2021.748851

[30] Jostins L et al. Host-microbe interactions have shaped the genetic architecture of inflammatory bowel disease. Nature. 2012;**491**(7422):119-124. DOI: 10.1038/NATURE11582

[31] Falà AK, Álvarez-Ordóñez A, Filloux A, Gahan CGM, Cotter PD. Quorum sensing in human gut and food microbiomes: Significance and potential for therapeutic targeting. Frontiers in Microbiology. 2022;**13**:1002185. DOI: 10.3389/FMICB.2022.1002185/BIBTEX

[32] Moser B, Milligan MA, Dao MC. The microbiota-gut-brain Axis: Clinical applications in obesity and type 2 diabetes. Revista de Investigación Clínica. 2022;**74**(6):302-313. DOI: 10.24875/RIC.22000197

[33] Wachsmuth HR, Weninger SN, Duca FA. Role of the gut–brain axis in energy and glucose metabolism. Experimental & Molecular Medicine. 2022;**54**(4):377-392. DOI: 10.1038/s12276-021-00677-w

[34] Christensen LW, Kuhre RE, Janus C, Svendsen B, Holst JJ. Vascular, but not luminal, activation of FFAR1 (GPR40) stimulates GLP-1 secretion from isolated perfused rat small intestine. Physiological Reports. 2015;**3**(9):e12551, 1-13. DOI: 10.14814/PHY2.12551

[35] Müller M et al. Circulating but not faecal short-chain fatty acids are related to insulin sensitivity, lipolysis and GLP-1 concentrations in humans. Scientific Reports. 2019;**9**(1):1-9. DOI: 10.1038/s41598-019-48775-0

[36] Palmnäs-Bedard MSA et al. The human gut microbiota and glucose metabolism: A scoping review of key bacteria and the potential role of SCFAs. The American Journal of Clinical Nutrition. 2022;**116**(4):862-874. DOI: 10.1093/AJCN/NQAC217

[37] Müller TD et al. Glucagon-like peptide 1 (GLP-1). Molecular Metabolism. 2019;**30**:72-130. DOI: 10.1016/J.MOLMET.2019.09.010

[38] He J et al. Short-chain fatty acids and their association with Signalling pathways in inflammation, glucose and lipid metabolism. International Journal of Molecular Sciences. 2020;**21**(17):1-16. DOI: 10.3390/IJMS21176356

[39] Qi Q et al. Host and gut microbial tryptophan metabolism and type 2 diabetes: An integrative analysis of host genetics, diet, gut microbiome and circulating metabolites in cohort studies. Gut. 2022;**71**(6):1095. DOI: 10.1136/GUTJNL-2021-324053

[40] Muller PA et al. Microbiota modulate sympathetic neurons via a gut–brain circuit. Nature. 2020;**583**(7816):441-446. DOI: 10.1038/s41586-020-2474-7

[41] Pang S, Wen-Yi J, Zi W. The interplay between the gut microbiome and neurological disorders: Exploring the gut-brain Axis. Neurology Letters. 2023;**2**(1):25-29. DOI: 10.52547/NL.2.1.25

[42] Smith PA. The tantalizing links between gut microbes and the brain. Nature. 2015;**526**(7573):312-314. DOI: 10.1038/526312A

[43] Sarubbo F, Moranta D, Tejada S, Jiménez M, Esteban S. Impact of gut microbiota in brain ageing: Polyphenols as beneficial modulators. Antioxidants. 2023;**12**(4):1-19. DOI: 10.3390/ANTIOX12040812

[44] Morais LH, Schreiber HL, Mazmanian SK. The gut microbiota-brain axis in behaviour and brain

disorders. Nature Reviews. Microbiology. 2021;**19**(4):241-255. DOI: 10.1038/S41579-020-00460-0

[45] Blacher E et al. Potential roles of gut microbiome and metabolites in modulating ALS in mice. Nature. 2019;**572**(7770):474-480. DOI: 10.1038/S41586-019-1443-5

[46] Ortiz GG et al. Gut-brain Axis: Role of microbiota in Parkinson's disease and multiple sclerosis. Eat, Learn, Remember. 2019:11-30. DOI: 10.5772/INTECHOPEN.79493

[47] Zapata RC, Singh A, Ajdari NM, Chelikani PK. Dietary tryptophan restriction dose-dependently modulates energy balance, gut hormones, and microbiota in obesity-prone rats. Obesity. 2018;**26**(4):730-739. DOI: 10.1002/OBY.22136

[48] Strasser B, Fuchs D. Diet versus exercise in weight loss and maintenance: Focus on tryptophan. International Journal of Tryptophan Research. 2016;**9**(1):9-16. DOI: 10.4137/IJTR.S33385/ASSET/IMAGES/LARGE/10.4137_IJTR.S33385-FIG2.JPEG

[49] Zhang C, Yu M, Yang Y, Mu C, Su Y, Zhu W. Differential effect of early antibiotic intervention on bacterial fermentation patterns and mucosal gene expression in the colon of pigs under diets with different protein levels. Applied Microbiology and Biotechnology. 2017;**101**(6):2493-2505. DOI: 10.1007/S00253-016-7985-7

[50] Liu M, Nieuwdorp M, de Vos WM, Rampanelli E. Microbial tryptophan metabolism tunes host immunity, metabolism, and Extraintestinal disorders. Metabolites. 2022;**12**(9):1-24. DOI: 10.3390/METABO12090834

[51] Savonije K, Weaver DF. The role of tryptophan metabolism in Alzheimer's disease. Brain Sciences. 2023;**13**(2):1-12. DOI: 10.3390/BRAINSCI13020292

[52] Klimova B, Novotny M, Valis M. The impact of nutrition and intestinal microbiome on elderly depression-a systematic review. Nutrients. 2020;**12**(3):1-12. DOI: 10.3390/NU12030710

[53] Nieto-Ruiz A et al. Maternal weight, gut microbiota, and the association with early childhood behavior: The PREOBE follow-up study. Child and Adolescent Psychiatry and Mental Health. 2023;**17**(1):2-18. DOI: 10.1186/S13034-023-00589-9

[54] Su X, Gao Y, Yang R. Gut microbiota-derived tryptophan metabolites maintain gut and systemic homeostasis. Cells. 2022;**11**(15):2296, 1-20. DOI: 10.3390/CELLS11152296

[55] Khoshnevisan K, Chehrehgosha M, Sajjadi-Jazi SM, Meftah AM. Tryptophan and serotonin levels as potent biomarkers in diabetes mellitus complications: A new approach of diagnostic role. Journal of Diabetes and Metabolic Disorders. 2022;**21**(2):1923-1934. DOI: 10.1007/S40200-022-01096-Y

[56] Ghiboub M, Verburgt CM, Sovran B, Benninga MA, de Jonge WJ, Van Limbergen JE. Nutritional therapy to modulate tryptophan metabolism and aryl hydrocarbon-receptor signaling activation in human diseases. Nutrients. 2020;**12**(9):1-21. DOI: 10.3390/NU12092846

[57] Wyatt M, Greathouse KL. Targeting dietary and microbial tryptophan-indole metabolism as therapeutic approaches to colon cancer. Nutrients. 2021;**13**(4):1-23. DOI: 10.3390/NU13041189

[58] Guenin-Macé L et al. Dysregulation of tryptophan catabolism at the

host-skin microbiota interface in hidradenitis suppurativa. JCI Insight. 2020;**5**(20):e140598, 1-15. DOI: 10.1172/JCI.INSIGHT.140598

[59] Tintelnot J et al. Microbiota-derived 3-IAA influences chemotherapy efficacy in pancreatic cancer. Nature. 2023;**615**(7950):168-174. DOI: 10.1038/S41586-023-05728-Y

[60] Guillot CC. Microbiota intestinal y salud infantil intestinal microbiota and child health. Revista Cubana de Pediatría. 2018;**90**(1):94-110. Available from: http://scielo.sld.cu [Accessed: August 19, 2023]

[61] Yadav M, Chauhan NS. Microbiome therapeutics: Exploring the present scenario and challenges. 2021;**15**(10):1-19. DOI: 10.1093/gastro/goab046

[62] Janssens Y et al. Disbiome database: Linking the microbiome to disease. BMC Microbiology. 2018;**18**(1):1-6. DOI: 10.1186/S12866-018-1197-5

[63] Agus A, Clément K, Sokol H. Gut microbiota-derived metabolites as central regulators in metabolic disorders. Gut. 2021;**70**(6):1174-1182. DOI: 10.1136/GUTJNL-2020-323071

[64] Zhu HZ et al. Xiaoyaosan improves depressive-like behavior in rats with chronic immobilization stress through modulation of the gut microbiota. Biomedicine & Pharmacotherapy. 2019;**112**:108621, 1-13. DOI: 10.1016/J.BIOPHA.2019.108621

[65] Charbonneau MR, Isabella VM, Li N, Kurtz CB. Developing a new class of engineered live bacterial therapeutics to treat human diseases. 2020;**11**(1):1-11 DOI: 10.1038/s41467-020-15508-1

[66] Mimee M, Citorik RJ, Lu TK. Microbiome therapeutics – Advances and challenges. Advanced Drug Delivery Reviews. 2016;**105**(Pt A):44. DOI: 10.1016/J.ADDR.2016.04.032

[67] Zhu M, Song Y, Xu Y, Xu H. Manipulating microbiota in inflammatory bowel disease treatment: Clinical and natural product interventions explored. International Journal of Molecular Sciences. 2023;**24**(13):11004. DOI: 10.3390/IJMS241311004

[68] Platten M, Nollen EAA, Röhrig UF, Fallarino F, Opitz CA. Tryptophan metabolism as a common therapeutic target in cancer, neurodegeneration and beyond. Nature Reviews Drug Discovery. 2019;**18**(5):379-401. DOI: 10.1038/s41573-019-0016-5

Chapter 3

Probiotics and Metabolic Syndrome: A Bibliometric Analysis and Overview of Dietary Interventions

Laura García-Curiel, Jesús Guadalupe Pérez Flores,
Luis Guillermo González-Olivares, José Antonio Guerrero-Solano,
Elizabeth Contreras-López, Emmanuel Pérez-Escalante,
Lizbeth Anahí Portillo-Torres
and Jessica Lizbeth Sebastián-Nicolás

Abstract

This chapter addressed the problem of understanding the role of probiotics in managing metabolic syndrome. Therefore, the objective was to analyze the clinical evidence surrounding using probiotics and prebiotics for metabolic syndrome through a bibliometric analysis and to evaluate the impact of dietary interventions on the microbiota. The most significant results from the data analysis reveal that probiotics have a beneficial effect on various aspects of metabolic syndrome, including blood pressure, glucose metabolism, blood lipid profiles, and inflammatory biomarkers. Visualization techniques such as word clouds and scientometric mapping illustrate the thematic landscape and distribution of research articles, highlighting the emphasis on cardiovascular and metabolic health and the modulation of women's health and gut microbiota. Despite the substantial evidence supporting the beneficial effects of probiotics, discrepancies across studies were found, indicating variability in outcomes, potentially due to differences in the specific probiotic strains used and their dosages. In conclusion, the study provides a comprehensive overview of the favorable effects of probiotics on metabolic syndrome. It suggests that dietary modulation through probiotics could be a viable strategy for managing metabolic health. Moreover, this book chapter emphasizes the importance of standardization in improving the reliability and comparability of results across different studies.

Keywords: metabolic syndrome, dysbiosis, microbiota, dietary fiber, probiotics

1. Introduction

The composition of the microbiota is highly variable among individuals and can fluctuate significantly within an individual due to various environmental factors such as antibiotic use, lifestyle, hygiene, and diet, all of which have a direct impact on the host's health [1].

Probiotics and prebiotics are the primary modulators of the intestinal microbiota, and together, they are known as synbiotics [2]. This synergy has been shown to benefit the immune system and gut microbiota, offering potential strategies for preventing and treating dietary component-induced intestinal inflammation and inflammatory diseases [3].

Prebiotics, as defined by the Food and Agriculture Organization of the United Nations (FAO), are non-digestible food ingredients that reach the colon in an unaltered form and are fermented by saccharolytic bacteria [2]. These compounds predominantly include complex carbohydrates such as resistant starch, inulin, cellulose, pectin, hemicellulose, and gum, as well as substances like lactulose, fructooligosaccharides, and galactooligosaccharides [4]. Upon fermentation, prebiotics enhance the size and activity of beneficial bacteria in the colon, promoting the growth of a healthy gut microbiota [5].

The effects of prebiotics on the gut microbiota and their potential health benefits have been extensively studied. Research has shown that prebiotics can modulate the intestinal microbiota and benefit the host's health [6]. Furthermore, prebiotics have been associated with producing short-chain fatty acids with immunomodulatory properties, which can contribute to regulating gut permeability and reducing inflammation [7]. Additionally, prebiotics have been investigated for their potential to improve metabolic health, with studies revealing their influence on the production of glucagon-like peptide 1 and peptide YY and their ability to decrease ghrelin levels [8].

Probiotics defined by FAO/OMS are "live microorganisms which, when administered in adequate amounts, confer a health benefit on the host" [9]. These microorganisms primarily consist of lactic acid bacteria and yeasts, and their beneficial effects are attributed to various mechanisms, including the generation of short-chain fatty acids by specific beneficial bacteria, which play a crucial role in regulating glucose homeostasis [10].

The effects of probiotic supplementation on metabolic issues such as hyperglycemia, hypertension, and hyperlipidemia have been extensively studied. Clinical studies, systematic reviews, meta-analyses, and umbrella reviews have been conducted to assess the quality of the information in these reviews, providing a comprehensive understanding of the impact of probiotics on metabolic health [11–17]. These studies have investigated the potential of probiotics to ameliorate various metabolic parameters, including glucose metabolism, lipid profiles, and insulin resistance, among others. While some studies have reported positive effects of probiotics on metabolic parameters, others have failed to find significant benefits, leading to a lack of consensus in the field [18–20].

The variability in the results may be attributed to differences in study designs, participant characteristics, probiotic strains, and dosages used, highlighting the complexity of evaluating the overall impact of probiotics on metabolic health. Despite the challenges in reaching a consensus, evidence from several randomized controlled trials and meta-analyses indicates that probiotics can have a beneficial effect on aspects of metabolic syndrome, including blood pressure, glucose metabolism, and blood lipid profiles, as well as improving inflammatory biomarkers [21–23].

This book chapter aims to analyze the clinical evidence surrounding the use of probiotics for metabolic syndrome. It includes a bibliometric analysis of clinical studies, systematic reviews, meta-analyses, and umbrella reviews, thoroughly evaluating the existing literature on probiotics and their impact on metabolic syndrome. Additionally, the chapter reviews the principal dietary interventions for metabolic syndrome and their reported effects on the microbiota, exposing the potential mechanisms underlying the observed outcomes.

2. Bibliometric and authors' keywords analysis

Data gathering relied on scientific articles on Web of Science© (WoS) published and indexed. On January 23, 2024, a search was conducted on WoS using the "advanced search" section, employing the following logical operation: (TI = ('probiotic*' AND 'metabolic syndrome') OR AB = ('probiotic*' AND 'metabolic syndrome')) AND (TI = ('systematic review' OR 'meta-analysis' OR 'umbrella review' OR 'controlled trial*' OR 'overview') OR AB = ('systematic review' OR 'meta-analysis' OR 'umbrella review' OR 'controlled trial*' OR 'overview')) NOT KP = ('probiotic*' AND 'metabolic syndrome' AND 'systematic review' AND 'meta-analysis' AND 'umbrella review' AND 'controlled trial*' AND 'overview'). This function allowed search articles containing the terms probiotic or probiotics ("probiotic*") and metabolic syndrome in the title (TI) and abstract (AB). Also, it included at least one of the terms "systematic review", "meta-analysis", or "umbrella review" rather than relying on the keywords-plus associated with each document (NOT KP). The logical operators combined the conditions. The search excluded Book Chapters, Proceeding Papers, Early Access Articles, and Retracted Publications.

An analysis was conducted on publications spanning from 2014 to 2023, encompassing all records available in WoS. This examination yielded a total of 92 documents. Data were exported as BibTeX (savedrecs.bib) and Research Information Systems (savedrecs.ris) files using the "Record Content: Full Record" option. Analysis was performed with the software VOSviewer version 1.6.20 and with software R-package bibliometrix version 4.1.4 [24] for the scientific mapping analysis, using R version 4.1.2 as the programming language (2021-11-01) [25], and R-studio version 2023.12.0 as integrated development environment [26]. The analysis was conducted utilizing the biblioshiny() function.

The outcome of data analysis is presented in **Table 1**, which comprehensively analyzes research data spanning the timespan study (2014–2023). It highlights significant trends in document content, authorship, collaboration, and document types. Notably, the research landscape witnessed a robust annual growth rate of 31.8%, with 69 sources contributing to 92 documents. The absence of single-authored documents suggests a prevalent culture of collaboration among 475 authors. The 23.91% international co-authorships emphasize the study's global dimension. Document content is rich, featuring 413 Keywords Plus (ID) and 275 Author's Keywords (DE). The average document age of 3.52 years indicates the timeliness of the research, while the citation rate of 26.36 reflects its impact. Categorically, the documents include 51 articles and 41 reviews, showcasing a balanced mix of original research and critical assessments. The analysis provided valuable insights into research activities' dynamic and collaborative nature during the specified period.

Additionally, **Figure 1** serves as a multifaceted tool for understanding the intricacies of scientific production from 2014 to 2023. Each sub-figure provides a unique perspective, collectively contributing to a nuanced and comprehensive portrayal of the research landscape during the specified timespan. Researchers and stakeholders can leverage this information to identify trends, assess global contributions, and gain valuable insights into the evolving dynamics of scientific output.

Figure 1a outlines the annual scientific production from 2014 to 2023, revealing distinctive trends. Initial years (2014–2015) show sparse output, with two articles annually, followed by a notable absence in 2016. From 2017 to 2020, a gradual increase occurred, peaking at 15 articles in 2021 but experiencing fluctuations in 2020 and 2022. Notably, 2023 sees a significant surge with 24 articles, suggesting a particularly

Description	Results
Main information about data	
Timespan	2014:2023
Sources (Journals, Books, etc)	69
Documents	92
Annual growth rate %	31.8
Document average age	3.52
Average citations per doc	26.36
References	0
Document contents	
Keywords plus (ID)	413
Author's keywords (DE)	275
Authors	
Authors	475
Authors of single-authored docs	0
Authors collaboration	
Single-authored docs	0
Co-authors per doc	5.89
International co-authorships %	23.91
Document types	
article	51
review	41

Table 1.
Analysis of research data: 2014–2023—Document trends, authorship patterns, and collaboration insights.

productive year. The data underscores dynamic shifts in research output, potentially influenced by evolving research priorities, external events, and varying funding scenarios. This analysis provides valuable insights for researchers and stakeholders, identifying influential periods and informing strategic planning for future research endeavors.

Figure 1b presents a frequency distribution in research output across different regions, indicating the number of occurrences for each area. Iran leads with 171 instances, followed by Spain with 72 and China with 64. The United States, often a prominent contributor to scientific research, ranks fourth with 56 occurrences. Germany, India, Italy, Australia, Canada, and Brazil follow in descending order, contributing 34 to 14 instances each. This distribution suggests a varied global landscape of research contributions, with Iran demonstrating a notable presence in the dataset. **Figure 1b** provides valuable insights into regional research activity, aiding in understanding the geographical distribution of scientific output in the analyzed context.

Figure 1c provides an overview of the leading journals where articles were published, detailing the frequency of publications for each source. "Nutrients" emerges as the primary source with six articles, suggesting a significant focus on this avenue within the analyzed dataset. Following closely are "Gut Microbes", "Journal of Functional Foods", and "Trials", each with four articles indicating substantial research

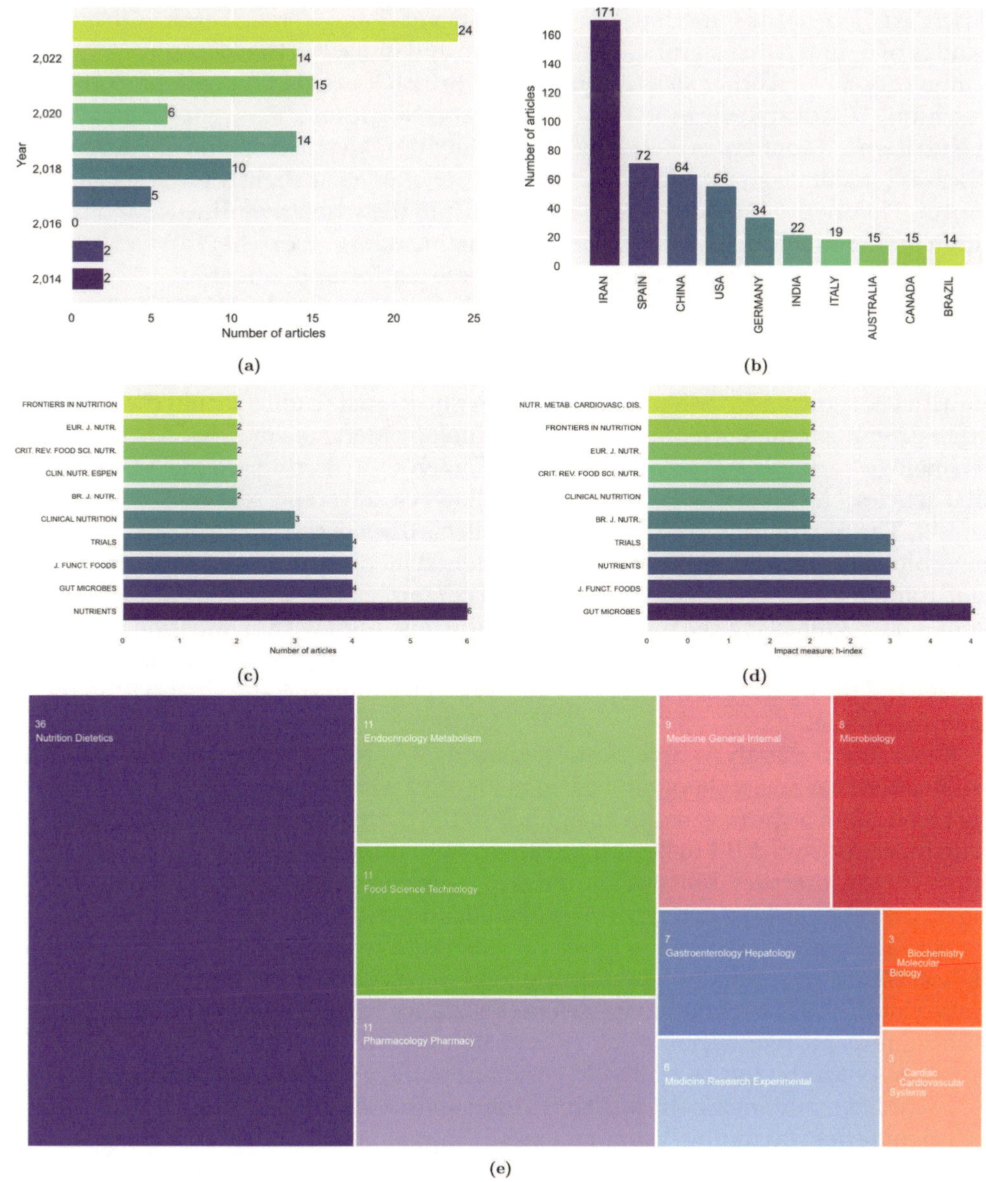

Figure 1.
Overview of scientific production from 2014 to 2023 timespan. (a) Annual scientific production. (b) Country scientific production. (c) Main journals where articles were published. (d) Treemap chart of the number of publications in different disciplines according to the classification of Web of Science©.

output from these platforms. Several other journals, such as "Clinical Nutrition", "British Journal of Nutrition", and "Critical Reviews in Food Science and Nutrition", contribute two to three articles each. Researchers and stakeholders can leverage this information to identify critical platforms driving discussions and insights within the realm of nutrition.

Figure 1d highlights the local impact of various sources in the field, as measured by their h-index. "Gut Microbes" leads with an h-index of 4, signifying its substantial influence and broad citation impact within the analyzed dataset. Following closely are "Journal of Functional Foods", "Nutrients", and "Trials", each with an h-index of 3, indicating significant recognition and impact in the local scholarly community. Several other sources, including "British Journal of Nutrition", "Clinical Nutrition", "Critical Reviews in Food Science and Nutrition", "European Journal of Nutrition", "Frontiers in Nutrition", and "Nutrition Metabolism and Cardiovascular Diseases", maintain an h-index of 2, reflecting a notable but slightly lower local impact. This metric provides valuable insights into the scholarly influence and recognition of these sources within the specific domain, aiding researchers and stakeholders in gauging the significance and reach of these platforms in nutrition.

Finally, **Figure 1e** categorizes the research articles into various Web of Science categories, indicating the record count and the corresponding percentage of 92 articles. "Nutrition Dietetics" is the predominant category, encompassing 39.13% of the articles, showcasing a significant focus on nutritional studies within the dataset. Other prominent categories include "Endocrinology Metabolism", "Food Science Technology", and "Pharmacology Pharmacy", each contributing around 12% of the total articles. "Medicine General Internal" follows closely, representing 9.78% of the dataset. The distribution across categories reflects diverse research interests, with microbiology, gastroenterology, and experimental medicine also making notable contributions. This categorization provides a comprehensive overview of the research landscape, highlighting the multifaceted nature of studies within nutrition and related disciplines. Researchers and stakeholders can leverage this information to understand the distribution of topics and the emphasis on specific areas within the analyzed dataset.

Regarding the analysis of authors' keywords, **Figure 2** provides a comprehensive exploration that researchers can utilize to identify patterns, recognize emerging trends, and acquire valuable insights into the thematic landscape of research contributions from 2014 to 2023. The integration of these visualization techniques improves the interpretability of the dataset, enabling a more nuanced understanding of the relationships and dynamics embedded within the usage of authors' keywords. **Figure 2a** shows a word cloud generated from the top 50 words with the highest frequency, visually representing vital thematic elements in the dataset. "Gut microbiota", "double-blind", and "insulin resistance" emerge as central terms, each with significant frequencies of 28, 25, and 18, respectively. These terms suggest a strong emphasis on topics related to gut microbiota, experimental design (double-blind studies), and metabolic health (insulin resistance) within the corpus. Other prevalent terms, including "meta-analysis", "supplementation", "inflammation", "obesity", "health", "lipid profile", and "probiotics", contribute to a rich thematic landscape. The prominence of these terms in the word cloud indicates their recurrent presence in the dataset, offering researchers valuable insights into the focal points of research contributions and potential areas of emphasis within the analyzed period.

Figure 2b–d depict the scientometric mapping conducted using VOSviewer v. 1.6.18 software, following the first two steps reported in a prior study [27]. The next steps followed the methodology reported in a previous investigation (3). The counting method was configured to utilize full counting. (4) A threshold of five occurrences was established to ensure the inclusion of numerous concepts in the map. Of the 2208 terms, 72 meet the threshold. (5) The software calculated a relevance score for each of the 72 terms [28]. Using this score, the terms deemed most relevant were chosen. The default setting, which comprised 60% of the most relevant terms, was selected, resulting in 43 terms. However, the terms "mg/dL", "baseline", "individual",

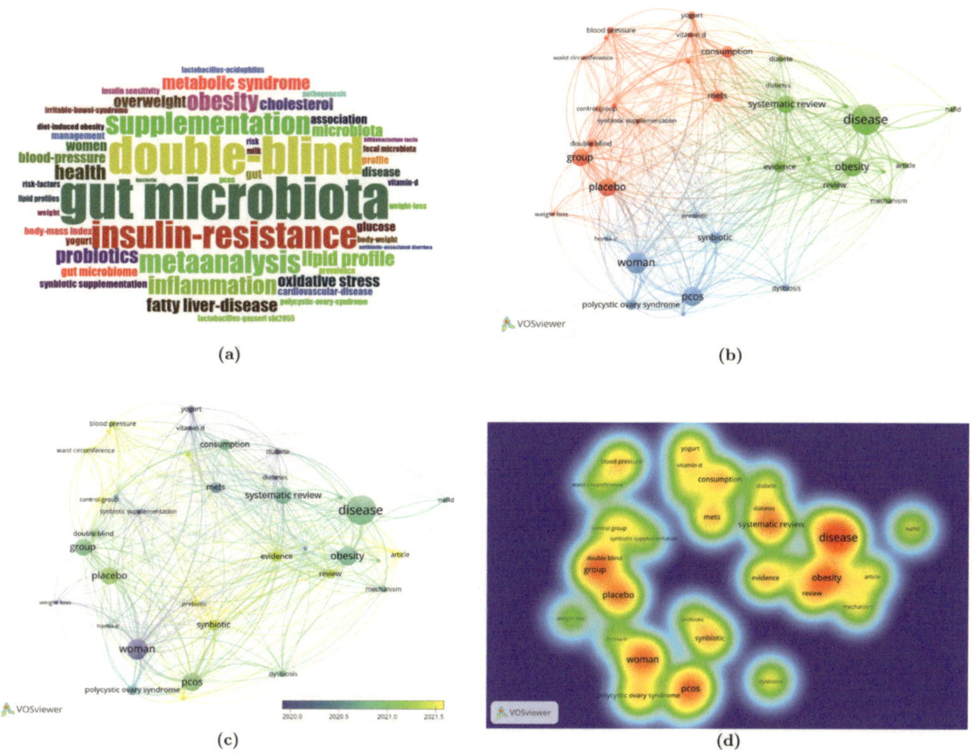

Figure 2.
Authors' keywords analysis from the period 2014–2023. (a) Word cloud containing the 50 principal authors' keywords. Scientometric mapping with the occurrence of the 42 principal authors' keywords: (b) network visualization, (c) overlay visualization, and (d) density visualization.

"type", "patient", "participant", and "week" were excluded because they are common terms related to clinical studies, leaving a final count of 36 terms. Although certain words may appear in different nodes, they refer to the same term. That is the case of "polycystic ovary syndrome, pco and pcos" "diabetes and diabete" and "synbiotic supplementation and symbiotic". (6) The maps were created. The normalization method chosen was the association strength. The cluster size was maintained at least one term per cluster, adhering to the default setting. The resolution parameter was set to one (default value). Finally, the maps were exported as PNG image files.

Figure 2b displays 36 items, 3 clusters, and 471 links, with a total link strength of 4944. The sizes of the letters and circles correspond to the frequency of occurrences, highlighting significant points within the chosen research domain. The proximity of keywords in the visualization reflects their connectedness through occurrence links, with closer keywords indicating a stronger relationship. The distances between keywords can serve as indicators of knowledge gaps within specific areas.

The dataset analysis with VOSviewer has revealed three distinct clusters, each highlighting specific areas of health research. The first cluster explores cardiovascular and metabolic health, emphasizing factors like blood pressure and weight loss. The second cluster focuses on evidence-based research into metabolic disorders such as diabetes and obesity. The third cluster delves into women's health and gut microbiota modulation, particularly hormonal aspects. Collectively, these clusters offer valuable insights into diverse aspects of metabolic health research:

The first cluster with 15 items, "Cardiovascular and Metabolic Health", red (R: 214, G: 39, B: 40), comprises terms closely associated with cardiovascular health, metabolic disorders, and related interventions. The presence of terms such as "blood pressure", "lipid profile", "waist circumference", and "weight loss" suggests a focus on factors related to cardiovascular risk assessment and management. Additionally, "vitamin D" and "yogurt" indicate potential dietary and lifestyle interventions that may influence cardiovascular and metabolic health outcomes. Including terms like "double-blind" and "placebo" underscores the importance of rigorous experimental design and control groups in studies investigating interventions targeting cardiovascular and metabolic parameters. Overall, this cluster reflects a comprehensive exploration of factors and interventions relevant to cardiovascular and metabolic health, highlighting the interdisciplinary nature of research in this domain.

The second cluster with 13 items, "Metabolic Disorders and Evidence-Based Research", green (R: 44, G: 160, B:44), encompasses terms indicative of in-depth investigations into metabolic disorders, particularly diabetes, obesity, and non-alcoholic fatty liver disease (NAFLD). The inclusion of terms like "evidence", "mechanisms", and "systematic review" suggests a strong emphasis on rigorous and evidence-based research methodologies within the cluster. The term "overview" implies a holistic approach, possibly involving comprehensive reviews or analyses of the current state of knowledge in the field of metabolic disorders. The presence of terms related to prevention underscores the proactive exploration of strategies to mitigate or manage metabolic disorders. Thus, Cluster 2 signifies a research focus on metabolic conditions, supported by evidence-based approaches, with an overarching goal of understanding mechanisms and prevention and offering comprehensive overviews through systematic reviews and articles.

The third cluster with 8 items, "Women's Health and Gut Microbiota Modulation", blue (R: 31, G: 119, B: 180), centers around terms related to women's health and the modulation of gut microbiota. The inclusion of terms like "PCOS" (Polycystic Ovary Syndrome), "woman", and "insulin resistance" (indicated by "homa ir") points toward a specific focus on women's health concerns, particularly those related to hormonal and reproductive aspects. Additionally, terms such as "dysbiosis", "prebiotic", "probiotic", and "synbiotic" highlight an interest in understanding and potentially modulating the gut microbiota as it relates to women's health. This cluster suggests a nuanced exploration of the interplay between gut health, hormonal imbalances, and conditions like PCOS, indicating a comprehensive investigation into the potential role of microbiota modulation in women's health and associated disorders.

On the other hand, **Figure 2c** displays an "overlay visualization" graph, employing a score range from 2020 to 2021.5, with the color scheme set to Viridis default. This visualization effectively represents the distribution and relationships among elements in the dataset over time. The "overlay visualization" offers a dynamic and detailed representation of data evolution, enabling a quick and precise interpretation of variations from 2020 to 2021.5.

Finally, **Figure 2d** displays the "density visualization", representing item density within the dataset. The "item density" option from VOSviewer software shows the graph's spatial concentration or distribution of elements. In a density visualization, areas with higher color intensity indicate a greater density of components, potentially suggesting the presence of denser thematic clusters or groups in those regions. Conversely, lighter-colored areas denote lower density, indicating possibly less populated zones regarding dataset elements, aiding in identifying patterns, clusters, and areas of greater relevance within the analyzed dataset.

3. Use of probiotics in metabolic syndrome

The use of probiotics in managing metabolic syndrome and its associated conditions, such as prediabetes and diabetes, has gained significant attention in recent research. Probiotics have been shown to have beneficial effects on various aspects of metabolic syndrome, including low-grade inflammation, immunity, oxidative stress, and lipid concentrations, as well as glycemic control [29–31]. Many studies have demonstrated the positive impact of specific bacterial strains on glycemic control in animal models, indicating the potential of probiotics in addressing metabolic disorders [29, 30].

Furthermore, probiotics have been associated with improvements in oxidative stress and inflammation markers, supporting their potential cardio-protective effects [31]. The regulation of probiotics on the immune system has also been highlighted as a method to prevent common diseases, indicating a broader impact beyond metabolic syndrome [32, 33]. Additionally, the modulation of lipid metabolism and lipid profiles, including improving HDL-C concentration, has been documented in individuals with type 2 diabetes [30, 34].

The potential of probiotics extends to other metabolic disorders, as evidenced by their ability to reduce homocysteine concentration in obese women, indicating a broader application in addressing metabolic abnormalities [35]. Additionally, the impact of glycemic control on various aspects of metabolic disorders, including lipid metabolism, immune response, and susceptibility to infections, underscores the interconnected nature of these conditions [36, 37].

While the evidence supporting the beneficial effects of probiotics on metabolic syndrome is substantial, it is essential to consider factors such as bacterial strains, dosage, and study heterogeneity when evaluating the effectiveness of probiotics in preventing or treating metabolic disorders [30, 38]. In a systematic review of randomized controlled trials that employed probiotics, prebiotics, or synbiotics for pre-diabetes treatment, the partial demonstration of benefits in modulating gut microbiota abundance has been observed. The authors emphasized that there is insufficient evidence to support the significant benefits of biotics in glucose metabolism, lipid metabolism, and body composition. Additionally, they highlighted the impact of small sample sizes and various study designs for comparing studies [39].

Recently, an umbrella meta-analysis was carried out to evaluate the effect on glycemia of the information available in databases such as Scopus, Embase, Pubmed, Web of Science, and Google Scholar on clinical studies on probiotic supplementation. The PRISMA methodology was followed, and a record was generated on the PROSPERO platform (Registration code: CRD42021286290). This work excluded observational papers, case reports, in vitro, ex vivo, in vivo, and quasi-experimental, controlled clinical trials, and articles in a language other than English. The AMSTAR methodology was used to evaluate the quality of work. The credibility of the meta-analyses was assessed using GRADE (Grading of Recommendations, Assessment, and Evaluation). Of 693 articles, only 48 met the inclusion criteria for the analysis and were published from 2013 to 2021. They concluded that probiotics benefit fasting plasma glucose, HbA1c, HOMA-IR, and insulin levels. A probiotic supplementation period of less than 8 weeks at moderate dosages (10^8 or 10^9 CFUs) was a more effective approach in improving these parameters [40].

In a PRISMA methodology umbrella meta-analysis (PROSPERO registration number = CRD42022304378), the effects of synbiotic supplementation on insulin, fasting blood sugar, and HOMA-IR were evaluated. For the selection and quality assessment of the included studies, AMSTAR2 checklist and GRADE were used. Of the total 156 articles, only 13 were selected. The study concluded that synbiotic supplementation can improve the glycemic indices studied and can be recommended as an adjunctive anti-hyperglycemic agent, particularly in diabetic and PCOS patients [41].

The therapeutic potential of probiotics in managing metabolic syndrome is supported by evidence of their positive impact on inflammation, immunity, oxidative stress, lipid concentrations, and glycemic control [42]. Probiotics have been shown to reduce systemic inflammation, decrease intestinal endotoxin, and lower insulin resistance and hyperglycemic incidences [43]. Furthermore, probiotics have demonstrated a glucose-lowering effect in participants with type 2 diabetes mellitus [44]. Studies have also indicated that probiotics, particularly *Lactobacillus* sub-strains, have beneficial effects on diabetes-related blood parameters, although more evidence from human trials is needed to confirm these effects [42]. Additionally, synbiotics have shown efficacy in improving glycemic indices, suggesting their use as a supplementary treatment for conditions like diabetes and polycystic ovary syndrome [39].

However, the efficacy of probiotics is influenced by the specific strains used, the dosage administered, and the variability among studies [43]. Future research should aim to standardize probiotic treatments and further elucidate the mechanisms by which they exert their beneficial effects on metabolic health [42]. It is important to note that the effects of probiotics on glycemic control and metabolic parameters in gestational diabetes mellitus are still being investigated, and further studies are warranted to address the limitations of existing evidence and better inform the management of this ailment [45, 46].

4. Dietary patterns in metabolic syndrome and their impact on the intestinal microbiota

Diet plays an essential role in the management of metabolic syndrome, directly influencing the composition and function of the intestinal microbiota [47]. Numerous dietary interventions have been proposed for patients with metabolic syndrome, emphasizing the importance of increased fiber consumption and analyzing the impact of lipids on the microbiome.

Numerous studies have demonstrated that dietary patterns emphasizing recommendations based on healthy high-fiber foods, such as the Mediterranean regional diet, plant-based diets, DASH diet, among others, are the gold standard for extending life expectancy and reducing the risks of cardiovascular diseases [48–53]. However, there are other dietary patterns that also have cardiovascular health benefits, such as intermittent fasting patterns. Many of these, as we will discuss later, contribute to or do not contribute to the improvement, balance, and diversity of the intestinal microbiome.

The Mediterranean diet is characterized by high consumption of virgin olive oil, whole grains, nuts, fruits, vegetables, and legumes, moderate consumption of fish, seafood, dairy products, and red wine, as well as a reduction in the consumption of red meats, processed meats, and sugar [52]. Numerous studies consistently demonstrate that the Mediterranean diet, especially when enriched with polyphenols and plant proteins, has a positive impact on reducing the risk of cardiovascular diseases (CVDs) and diabetes. These benefits result in a significant decrease in the incidence of cardiovascular events, improvement in lipoprotein function, and increased antioxidant capacity. However, it is crucial to emphasize that patient adherence to this diet and food choices play a crucial role in obtaining these benefits [54–56]. Beneficial modulation of the gastrointestinal microbiome and associated metabolomic profile has been found, including an increase in total bacteria, *Bifidobacterium*/*E. coli* ratio, lower amounts of *E. coli*, and the relative ratio of *Bacteroidetes*/short-chain fatty acids (SCFA) in feces [57]. Another study found that a Mediterranean diet partially restores the population of *P. distasonis*, *B. thetaiotaomicron*, *F. prausnitzii*, *B. adolescentis*, and *B. longum* in patients with metabolic syndrome [58] and *Eubacteria*, *Prevotella*, *Bifidobacteria*, and *Lactobacilli* in healthy subjects [59].

On the other hand, plant-based diets have gained popularity due to their potential health benefits and perceived environmental impact. While the term "plant-based" is sometimes used to refer to omnivorous diets with a relatively small component of animal foods, here it is understood to signify either vegetarian (plant-based plus dairy and/or eggs) or vegan (100% plant-based) diets, both characterized by maximal intake of plant products and the reduction or elimination of animal-derived food consumption. Additionally, vegetarian diets have been demonstrated to reduce body weight, fat mass, as well as blood lipids and glucose in patients with cardiovascular disease [56]. However, plant-based diets of low quality (e.g., refined cereals) have been associated with an increased risk of these pathologies [53]. Therefore, it is understood that achieving health benefits with such diets involves limiting animal-derived foods and making informed choices regarding the selection and quality of plant-based foods in the diet. Regarding the microbiome, conclusive findings are lacking; however, it is known that vegans exhibit higher proportions of *Bacteroides thetaiotaomicron*, *Bacteroides*/*Prevotella*, *Klebsiella pneumoniae*, *Faecalibacterium prausnitzii*, *Clostridium clostridioforme*; and lower proportions of *Bilophila wadsworthia*, *Clostridium* cluster XIVa [60]. However, another study found a lower count of *Bacteroides* and *Bifidobacterium* species, with no differences between vegans and non-vegans [61]. In another study involving a plant-based dietary intervention, the microbial community structure overcame interindividual differences in microbial gene expression but reverted to baseline values within 3 days [62].

DASH (Dietary Approaches to Stop Hypertension) diets represent a dietary pattern established for hypertension management, with a dietary structure similar to the Mediterranean diet. Given that an estimated 80% of individuals with metabolic syndrome also suffer from hypertension, DASH diets are highly relevant for metabolic syndrome treatment [63]. Rich in fruits and vegetables, skimmed milk, whole grains, and with moderate consumption of nuts and legumes, along with reduced amounts of red meats, fats, refined sugars, and sugary beverages, it results in significant blood pressure reduction compared to an American diet [50]. Subsequent clinical studies further confirmed the antihypertensive effects of this diet, expanding the list of positive effects to include improvements in other cardiovascular risk factors and comorbidities [64]. Likewise, systematic reviews and meta-analyses have demonstrated that the DASH diet significantly reduces body weight, improves lipid profile, blood glucose levels, insulin resistance, inflammatory response, and oxidative stress markers, as well as reduces the incidence of cardiovascular diseases, strokes, and type 2 diabetes [64, 65]. This diet has been observed to promote the expansion of protective microbes releasing intestinal metabolites such as SCFA [66] and showed a decrease in *Firmicutes* and *Bacteroidetes* and a significant reduction in lipopolysaccharide concentration [67].

The ketogenic diet is known as a very low-carbohydrate and high-fat diet, inducing ketosis [68]. Due to the negative reputation of fats regarding the risk of developing cardiovascular diseases, there is much controversy surrounding the impact of this diet on such conditions; however, ketogenic diets have been shown to improve cardiovascular risk factors, including blood glucose, body weight, triglycerides, and HDL levels, in studies lasting 6 months. However, most of these improvements were no longer significant after 12 months [69]. The impact of this diet on the microbiota is unclear, with some human and animal studies yielding different results, demonstrating positive effects on the remodeling of bacterial architecture and intestinal biological functions. In contrast, others report negative effects such as lower diversity and an increased amount of proinflammatory bacteria [70]. Additionally, with this diet, the intestinal microbiome structure in epileptic infants differs drastically from that of healthy infants. *Proteobacteria*, significantly higher in epileptic infants, decreased sharply after Crohn's disease. *Cronobacter* predominated in the epileptic infant group and remained at a low level in both healthy and epileptic infants after Crohn's disease. Bacteroides significantly increased in epileptic infants after Crohn's disease, whereas *Prevotella* and *Bifidobacterium* also grew in number and continued to increase [71]. The ketogenic diet strictly influences taxa, richness, and diversity of bacteria.

Fasting is the intentional cessation of solid food and stimulant intake over a limited period. Intermittent fasting has demonstrated beneficial effects on cardiovascular diseases, consistently showing a reduction in body weight, body fat mass, and BMI in individuals with obesity, type 2 diabetes, and high cardiovascular risk [72]. Time-restricted fasting enhances metabolic rhythms and prevents metabolic diseases such as obesity and inflammation, independently of caloric restriction [73]. The 5:2 diet (periodic fasting) has also proven effective in intermittent fasting programs for preventing and treating cardiometabolic diseases [72]. Some studies have shown that the 5:2 diet is more effective in glycemic control for patients with obesity, type 2 diabetes, and metabolic syndrome, achieving significant improvements in weight, blood pressure, and adiposity factors [74, 75]. Fasting may impact the composition and abundance of the human intestinal microbiota, with significant changes observed at the phylum, class, and species levels. One study identified changes in nine major phyla representing approximately 90% of operational taxonomic units in the intestinal microbiota, with Firmicutes and Bacteroidetes as predominant phyla. Additionally, a significant increase in the relative abundance of spirochetes was observed in the intermittent fasting group, while the majority of other phyla decreased. Furthermore, 23 species were identified as significantly affected after intermittent fasting intervention, with some species increasing in abundance (e.g., *Ruminococcus gnavus* and *Roseburia faecis*) and others decreasing [74].

Certain dietary patterns are less favorable for the microbiome and metabolic syndrome, as they are associated with obesity and subsequent diabetes and cardiovascular diseases. An example is the consumption of diets with artificial sweeteners, which may contribute to metabolic syndrome and obesity while negatively altering the host's microbiome [76]. Excessive consumption of simple carbohydrates can also pose problems, leading to reduced microbial diversity, particularly a decrease in *Bacteroidetes* and an increase in *Proteobacteria* [77]. There is also an increase in the *Firmicutes/Bacteroidetes* ratio, causing intestinal permeability disturbance and an increase in inflammatory cytokines (causing colitis) [78]. The American or Western diet (high in fat, animal protein, and sugar) induces dysbiosis, negative effects on gastrointestinal mucosa, inflammation, and an increase in bile-resistant microorganisms such as *Alistipes, Bilophila*, and *Bacteroides*, while reducing the levels of Firmicutes necessary for vegetable metabolism *(Roseburia, Eubacterium rectale, and Ruminococcus bromii*) [62]. Finally, alcohol consumption is associated with changes in the intestinal microbiota. Although evidence in humans is limited, various studies suggest that alcohol-induced alterations in the composition and metabolic function of the gastrointestinal microbiota may contribute to the well-established link between alcohol-induced oxidative stress, increased intestinal permeability to bacterial products, and the subsequent development of liver diseases and other conditions. Alcohol is associated with quantitative and qualitative changes in the intestinal microbiota. These changes may be linked to increased inflammation in the gastrointestinal tract, increased intestinal permeability resulting in the presence of bacterial toxins in the blood, systemic inflammation, and damage to tissues or organs [79].

5. Conclusions

Substantial evidence was provided by this chapter supporting the hypothesis that the gut microbiota could be beneficially modulated by probiotics, thereby positively influencing the management of metabolic syndrome. Aligned with the study's general objective, the significant scholarly focus on the interplay between diet, probiotics, and metabolic health was highlighted through bibliometric analysis and thematic exploration of research data from 2014 to 2023. The key findings emphasized the therapeutic potential of probiotics in inflammation reduction, immunity improvement, oxidative stress mitigation, and lipid concentration normalization, critical factors in the pathophysiology of metabolic syndrome. Additionally, dietary patterns, particularly Mediterranean and plant-based diets, were shown to positively impact cardiovascular health and diabetes management through their modulatory effects on the intestinal microbiota. These results validated the initial hypothesis and provided a comprehensive understanding of the current research landscape, offering valuable insights for future research directions and interventions to improve metabolic health through dietary and probiotic strategies.

The perspectives on this line of research are promising and suggest a dynamic and evolving field with a strong focus on the interplay between diet, probiotics, and metabolic health. The robust annual growth rate of 31.8% in scholarly output and the global dimension of international co-authorships at 23.91% indicate a burgeoning interest and collaborative efforts in this area. The significant attention given to the use of probiotics in managing metabolic syndrome and its associated conditions and the variability in study results points to the need for further research to solidify the evidence base and understand the mechanisms at play. The scientometric mapping and word cloud analysis reveal that cardiovascular and metabolic health, women's health, and gut microbiota are key thematic areas, suggesting these will continue to be significant topics of investigation. Systematic reviews and meta-analyses indicate an ongoing effort to synthesize and evaluate existing research, which is critical for advancing the field and informing clinical practice. Overall, the perspectives highlight the importance of continued research into the nuanced effects of probiotics on metabolic health, with an emphasis on experimental design, participant characteristics, probiotic strains, and dosages to address the current lack of consensus and to harness the full potential of probiotics in metabolic syndrome management.

Acknowledgements

This research received no specific grant from funding agencies in the public, commercial, or not-for-profit sectors.

Conflict of interest

The authors declare no conflict of interest.

Thanks

The authors thank the Sistema Nacional de Investigadoras e Investigadores (SNII-CONAHCyT), the Universidad Autónoma del Estado de Hidalgo (UAEH), the Instituto Tecnológico y de Estudios Superiores de Monterrey (ITESM) for the support provided to carry out this book chapter.

Author details

Laura García-Curiel[1,2*], Jesús Guadalupe Pérez Flores[1,3], Luis Guillermo González-Olivares[3], José Antonio Guerrero-Solano[4], Elizabeth Contreras-López[3], Emmanuel Pérez-Escalante[3], Lizbeth Anahí Portillo-Torres[3] and Jessica Lizbeth Sebastián-Nicolás[5]

1 Academic Area of Nursing, Institute of Health Sciences, Autonomous University of the State of Hidalgo, San Agustín Tlaxiaca, Mexico

2 Department of Biotechnology, Division of Biological and Health Sciences, Metropolitan Autonomous University, Iztapalapa, Mexico

3 Academic Area of Chemistry, Institute of Basic Sciences and Engineering, Autonomous University of the State of Hidalgo, Mineral de la Reforma, Mexico

4 Superior School of Tlahuelilpan, Autonomous University of the State of Hidalgo, Tlahuelilpan, Mexico

5 Science and Environment Division, Intercultural University of the State of Hidalgo, Tenango de Doria, Mexico

*Address all correspondence to: laura.garcia@uaeh.edu.mx

References

[1] Gourbeyre P, Denery S, Bodinier M. Probiotics, prebiotics, and synbiotics: Impact on the gut immune system and allergic reactions. Journal of Leukocyte Biology. 2011;**89**(5):685-695

[2] Markowiak P, Śliżewska K. Effects of probiotics, prebiotics, and Synbiotics on human health. Nutrients. 2017;**9**(9):1021

[3] Bilal M, Ashraf S, Zhao X. Dietary component-induced inflammation and its amelioration by prebiotics, probiotics, and synbiotics. Frontiers in Nutrition. 2022;**9**:931458

[4] Hedin C, Whelan K, Lindsay JO. Evidence for the use of probiotics and prebiotics in inflammatory bowel disease: A review of clinical trials. The Proceedings of the Nutrition Society. 2007;**66**(3):307-315. Available from: http://www.ncbi.nlm.nih.gov/pubmed/17637082

[5] Pérez-López E, Cela D, Costabile A, Mateos-Aparicio I, Rupérez P. In vitro fermentability and prebiotic potential of soyabean okara by human faecal microbiota. The British Journal of Nutrition. 2016;**116**(6):1116-1124

[6] Fallucca F, Porrata C, Fallucca S, Pianesi M. Influence of diet on gut microbiota, inflammation and type 2 diabetes mellitus. First experience with macrobiotic Ma-pi 2 diet. Diabetes/Metabolism Research and Reviews. 2014;**30**(S1):48-54

[7] Liao M, Zhang Y, Qiu Y, Wu Z, Zhong Z, Zeng X, et al. Fructooligosaccharide supplementation alleviated the pathological immune response and prevented the impairment of intestinal barrier in DSS-induced acute colitis mice. Food & Function. 2021;**12**(20):9844-9854

[8] Kim YA, Keogh JB, Clifton PM. Probiotics, prebiotics, synbiotics and insulin sensitivity. Nutrition Research Reviews. 2018;**31**(1):35-51

[9] Hill C, Guarner F, Reid G, Gibson GR, Merenstein DJ, Pot B, et al. The international scientific Association for Probiotics and Prebiotics consensus statement on the scope and appropriate use of the term probiotic. Nature Reviews. Gastroenterology & Hepatology. 2014;**11**(8):506-514

[10] Röder PV, Wu B, Liu Y, Han W. Pancreatic regulation of glucose homeostasis. Experimental & Molecular Medicine. 2016;**48**(3):e219

[11] Wastyk HC, Perelman D, Topf M, Fragiadakis GK, Robinson JL, Sonnenburg JL, et al. Randomized controlled trial demonstrates response to a probiotic intervention for metabolic syndrome that may correspond to diet. Gut Microbes. 2023;**15**(1):2178794

[12] Chen AC, Fang TJ, Ho HH, Chen JF, Kuo YW, Huang YY, et al. A multi-strain probiotic blend reshaped obesity-related gut dysbiosis and improved lipid metabolism in obese children. Frontiers in Nutrition. 2022;**9**:922993

[13] Zarezadeh M, Musazadeh V, Faghfouri AH, Sarmadi B, Jamilian P, Jamilian P, et al. Probiotic therapy, a novel and efficient adjuvant approach to improve glycemic status: An umbrella meta-analysis. Pharmacological Research. 2022;**183**:106397

[14] Santibañez-Gutierrez A, Fernández-Landa J, Calleja-González J, Delextrat A, Mielgo-Ayuso J. Effects of probiotic supplementation on exercise with predominance of aerobic

metabolism in trained population: A systematic review, Meta-analysis and Meta-regression. Nutrients. 2022;**14**(3):622

[15] Li Z, Li Y, Pan B, Wang X, Wu Y, Guo K, et al. The effects of Oral probiotic supplementation in postmenopausal women with overweight and obesity: A systematic review and Meta-analysis of randomized controlled trials. Probiotics and Antimicrobial Proteins. 2023;**15**(6):1567-1582

[16] Sivamaruthi BS, Bharathi M, Kesika P, Suganthy N, Chaiyasut C. The Administration of Probiotics against hypercholesterolemia: A systematic review. Applied Sciences. 2021;**11**(15):6913

[17] Çelik MN, Ünlü SM. Probiotics improve chemerin and metabolic syndrome parameters in obese rats. Balkan Medical Journal. 2019;**36**(5):270-275

[18] Dong Y, Xu M, Chen L, Bhochhibhoya A. Probiotic foods and supplements interventions for metabolic syndromes: A systematic review and Meta-analysis of recent clinical trials. Annals of Nutrition & Metabolism. 2019;**74**(3):224-241

[19] Gagnon E, Mitchell PL, Manikpurage HD, Abner E, Taba N, Esko T, et al. Impact of the gut microbiota and associated metabolites on cardiometabolic traits, chronic diseases and human longevity: A mendelian randomization study. Journal of Translational Medicine. 2023;**21**(1):60

[20] Green M, Arora K, Prakash S. Microbial medicine: Prebiotic and probiotic functional foods to target obesity and metabolic syndrome. International Journal of Molecular Sciences. 2020;**21**(8):2890. Available from: http://www.ncbi.nlm.nih.gov/pubmed/32326175

[21] Aron RAC, Abid A, Vesa CM, Nechifor AC, Behl T, Ghitea TC, et al. Recognizing the benefits of pre−/probiotics in metabolic syndrome and type 2 diabetes mellitus considering the influence of *Akkermansia muciniphila* as a key gut bacterium. Microorganisms. 2021;**9**(3):1-32

[22] Bock PM, Telo GH, Ramalho R, Sbaraini M, Leivas G, Martins AF, et al. The effect of probiotics, prebiotics or synbiotics on metabolic outcomes in individuals with diabetes: A systematic review and meta-analysis. Diabetologia. 2021;**64**(1):26-41

[23] Tenorio-Jiménez C, Martínez-Ramírez MJ, Gil Á, Gómez-Llorente C. Effects of probiotics on metabolic syndrome: A systematic review of randomized clinical trials. Nutrients. 2020;**12**(1):124. Available from: http://www.ncbi.nlm.nih.gov/pubmed/31906372

[24] Aria M, Cuccurullo C. bibliometrix: An R-tool for comprehensive science mapping analysis. Journal of Informetrics. 2017;**11**(4):959-975

[25] R Core Team. A Language and Environment for Statistical Computing. Vol. 3. Vienna, Austria; 2020. Available from: https://www.r-project.org

[26] R Studio Team. RStudio: Integrated Development Environment for R. Vol. 75. Boston, MA; 2022. Available from: http://www.rstudio.com/

[27] Sinkovics N. Enhancing the foundations for theorising through bibliometric mapping. International Marketing Review. 2016;**33**(3):327-350

[28] Pérez-Flores JG, García-Curiel L, Pérez-Escalante E, Contreras-López E, Olloqui EJ. Arabinoxylans matrixes as a potential material for drug delivery

systems development—A bibliometric analysis and literature review. Heliyon. 2024;**10**(3):e25445

[29] Alamdary SZ, Afifirad R, Asgharzadeh S, Asadollahi P, Mahdizade Ari M, Dashtibin S, et al. The influence of probiotics consumption on Management of Prediabetic State: A systematic review of clinical trials. International Journal of Clinical Practice. 2022;**2022**:1-14

[30] Cho YA, Kim J. Effect of probiotics on blood lipid concentrations. Medicine. 2015;**94**(43):e1714

[31] Khalesi S, Bellissimo N, Vandelanotte C, Williams S, Stanley D, Irwin C. A review of probiotic supplementation in healthy adults: Helpful or hype? European Journal of Clinical Nutrition. 2019;**73**(1):24-37

[32] Wang X, Zhang P, Zhang X. Probiotics regulate gut microbiota: An effective method to improve immunity. Molecules. 2021;**26**(19):6076

[33] Yan F, Polk DB. Probiotics and immune health. Current Opinion in Gastroenterology. 2011;**27**(6):496-501

[34] Ejtahed HS, Mohtadi-Nia J, Homayouni-Rad A, Niafar M, Asghari-Jafarabadi M, Mofid V, et al. Effect of probiotic yogurt containing *Lactobacillus acidophilus* and *Bifidobacterium lactis* on lipid profile in individuals with type 2 diabetes mellitus. Journal of Dairy Science. 2011;**94**(7):3288-3294

[35] Majewska K, Kręgielska-Narożna M, Jakubowski H, Szulińska M, Bogdański P. The multispecies probiotic effectively reduces homocysteine concentration in obese women: A randomized double-blind placebo-controlled study. Journal of Clinical Medicine. 2020;**9**(4):998

[36] Zhu J, Li W, Chen F, Xie Z, Zhuo K, Huang R. Impact of glycemic control on biventricular function in patients with type 2 diabetes mellitus: A cardiac magnetic resonance tissue tracking study. Insights Into Imaging. 2023;**14**(1):7

[37] Lee CH, Chen IL, Chuah SK, Tai WC, Chang CC, Chen FJ, et al. Impact of glycemic control on capsular polysaccharide biosynthesis and opsonophagocytosis of *Klebsiella pneumoniae*: Implications for invasive syndrome in patients with diabetes mellitus. Virulence. 2016;**7**(7):770-778

[38] Kandasamy S, Vlasova AN, Fischer DD, Chattha KS, Shao L, Kumar A, et al. Unraveling the differences between gram-positive and gram-negative probiotics in modulating protective immunity to enteric infections. Frontiers in Immunology. 2017;**8**:334

[39] Wang X, Yang J, Qiu X, Wen Q, Liu M, Zhou D, et al. Probiotics, pre-biotics and synbiotics in the treatment of pre-diabetes: A systematic review of randomized controlled trials. Frontiers in Public Health. 2021;**9**:645035

[40] Zarezadeh M, Musazadeh V, Faghfouri AH, Roshanravan N, Dehghan P. Probiotics act as a potent intervention in improving lipid profile: An umbrella systematic review and meta-analysis. Critical Reviews in Food Science and Nutrition. 2022;**63**(2):145-158

[41] Musazadeh V, Faghfouri AH, Kavyani Z, Dehghan P. Synbiotic as an adjunctive agent can be useful in the management of hyperglycemia in adults: An umbrella review and meta-research of meta-analysis studies. Journal of Functional Foods. 2022;**99**:105355

[42] Razmpoosh E, Javadi M, Ejtahed H, Mirmiran P. Probiotics as beneficial

agents in the management of diabetes mellitus: A systematic review. Diabetes/Metabolism Research and Reviews. 2016;**32**(2):143-168

[43] Ruan Y, Sun J, He J, Chen F, Chen R, Chen H. Effect of probiotics on Glycemic control: A systematic review and Meta-analysis of randomized, controlled trials. PLoS One. 2015;**10**(7):e0132121

[44] Rittiphairoj T, Pongpirul K, Janchot K, Mueller NT, Li T. Probiotics contribute to Glycemic control in patients with type 2 diabetes mellitus: A systematic review and Meta-analysis. Advances in Nutrition. 2021;**12**(3):722-734

[45] Zhang J, Ma S, Wu S, Guo C, Long S, Tan H. Effects of probiotic supplement in pregnant women with gestational diabetes mellitus: A systematic review and Meta-analysis of randomized controlled trials. Journal Diabetes Research. 2019;**2019**:1-12

[46] Yefet E, Bar L, Izhaki I, Iskander R, Massalha M, Younis JS, et al. Effects of probiotics on Glycemic control and metabolic parameters in gestational diabetes mellitus: Systematic review and Meta-analysis. Nutrients. 2023;**15**(7):1633

[47] Santos-Marcos JA, Perez-Jimenez F, Camargo A. The role of diet and intestinal microbiota in the development of metabolic syndrome. The Journal of Nutritional Biochemistry. 2019;**70**:1-27. Available from: https://linkinghub.elsevier.com/retrieve/pii/S0955286318309318

[48] Billingsley HE, Hummel SL, Carbone S. The role of diet and nutrition in heart failure: A state-of-the-art narrative review. Progress in Cardiovascular Diseases. 2020;**63**(5):538-551

[49] Butler T, Kerley CP, Altieri N, Alvarez J, Green J, Hinchliffe J, et al. Optimum nutritional strategies for cardiovascular disease prevention and rehabilitation (BACPR). Heart. 2020;**106**(10):724-731

[50] Campbell AP. DASH eating plan: An eating pattern for diabetes management. Diabetes Spectrum. 2017;**30**(2):76-81

[51] Casas R, Castro-Barquero S, Estruch R, Sacanella E. Nutrition and cardiovascular health. International Journal of Molecular Sciences. 2018;**19**(12):3988. Available from: https://www.mdpi.com/1422-0067/19/12/3988/htm

[52] Dernini S, Berry EM, Serra-Majem L, La Vecchia C, Capone R, Medina FX, et al. Med diet 4.0: The Mediterranean diet with four sustainable benefits. Public Health Nutrition. 2017;**20**(7):1322-1330

[53] Jafari S, Hezaveh E, Jalilpiran Y, Jayedi A, Wong A, Safaiyan A, et al. Plant-based diets and risk of disease mortality: A systematic review and meta-analysis of cohort studies. Critical Reviews in Food Science and Nutrition. 2022;**62**(28):7760-7772. Available from: https://www.tandfonline.com/doi/abs/10.1080/10408398.2021.1918628

[54] Delgado-Lista J, Alcala-Diaz JF, Torres-Peña JD, Quintana-Navarro GM, Fuentes F, Garcia-Rios A, et al. Long-term secondary prevention of cardiovascular disease with a Mediterranean diet and a low-fat diet (CORDIOPREV): A randomised controlled trial. The Lancet. 2022;**399**(10338):1876-1885

[55] RAH S. Primary prevention of cardiovascular disease with a Mediterranean diet supplemented with extra-virgin olive oil or nuts. The New England Journal of Medicine.

2018;**379**(14):1388. Available from: http://www.ncbi.nlm.nih.gov/pubmed/30285333

[56] Wang W, Liu Y, Li Y, Luo B, Lin Z, Chen K, et al. Dietary patterns and cardiometabolic health: Clinical evidence and mechanism. MedComm (Beijing). 2023;**4**(1):e212

[57] Mitsou EK, Kakali A, Antonopoulou S, Mountzouris KC, Yannakoulia M, Panagiotakos DB, et al. Adherence to the Mediterranean diet is associated with the gut microbiota pattern and gastrointestinal characteristics in an adult population. British Journal of Nutrition. 2017;**117**(12):1645-1655

[58] Haro C, Garcia-Carpintero S, Alcala-Diaz JF, Gomez-Delgado F, Delgado-Lista J, Perez-Martinez P, et al. The gut microbial community in metabolic syndrome patients is modified by diet. Journal of Nutritional Biochemistry. 2016;**27**:27-31

[59] Del Chierico F, Vernocchi P, Dallapiccola B, Putignani L. Mediterranean diet and health: Food effects on gut microbiota and disease control. International Journal of Molecular Sciences. 2014;**15**(7):11678-11699

[60] Matijašić BB, Obermajer T, Lipoglavšek L, Grabnar I, Avguštin G, Rogelj I. Association of dietary type with fecal microbiota in vegetarians and omnivores in Slovenia. European Journal of Nutrition. 2014;**53**(4):1051-1064

[61] Zimmer J, Lange B, Frick JS, Sauer H, Zimmermann K, Schwiertz A, et al. A vegan or vegetarian diet substantially alters the human colonic faecal microbiota. European Journal of Clinical Nutrition. 2012;**66**(1):53-60

[62] David LA, Corinne FM, Rachel NC, David BG, Julie EB, Benjamin EW, et al. Diet rapidly and reproducibly alters the human gut microbiome. Nature. 2014;**505**:559-563

[63] Katsimardou A, Imprialos K, Stavropoulos K, Sachinidis A, Doumas M, Athyros V. Hypertension in metabolic syndrome: Novel insights. Current Hypertension Reviews. 2019;**16**(1):12-18

[64] Chiavaroli L, Viguiliouk E, Nishi SK, Mejia SB, Rahelić D, Kahleová H, et al. DASH dietary pattern and cardiometabolic outcomes: An umbrella review of systematic reviews and meta-analyses. Nutrients. 2019;**11**(2):338

[65] Lari A, Sohouli MH, Fatahi S, Cerqueira HS, Santos HO, Pourrajab B, et al. The effects of the dietary approaches to stop hypertension (DASH) diet on metabolic risk factors in patients with chronic disease: A systematic review and meta-analysis of randomized controlled trials. Nutrition, Metabolism and Cardiovascular Diseases. 2021;**31**(10):2766-2778. Available from: https://linkinghub.elsevier.com/retrieve/pii/S0939475321002532

[66] Jama HA, Beale A, Shihata WA, Marques FZ. The effect of diet on hypertensive pathology: Is there a link via gut microbiota-driven immunometabolism? Cardiovascular Research. 2019;**115**(9):1435-1447

[67] Diao Z, Molludi J, Latef Fateh H, Moradi S. Comparison of the low-calorie DASH diet and a low-calorie diet on serum TMAO concentrations and gut microbiota composition of adults with overweight/obesity: A randomized control trial. International Journal of Food Sciences and Nutrition. 2023:1-14 [Online ahead of print]

[68] Batch JT, Lamsal SP, Adkins M, Sultan S, Ramirez MN. Advantages and disadvantages of the ketogenic diet: A review article. Cureus. 2020;**12**(8):e9639

[69] Mohammadifard N, Haghighatdoost F, Rahimlou M, Rodrigues APS, Gaskarei MK, Okhovat P, et al. The effect of ketogenic diet on shared risk factors of cardiovascular disease and cancer. Nutrients. 2022;**14**(17):3499

[70] Paoli A, Mancin L, Bianco A, Thomas E, Mota JF, Piccini F. Ketogenic diet and microbiota: Friends or enemies? Genes (Basel). 2019;**10**(7):534

[71] Xie G, Zhou Q, Qiu CZ, Dai WK, Wang HP, Li YH, et al. Ketogenic diet poses a significant effect on imbalanced gut microbiota in infants with refractory epilepsy. World Journal of Gastroenterology. 2017;**23**(33):6164-6171

[72] Varady KA, Cienfuegos S, Ezpeleta M, Gabel K. Clinical application of intermittent fasting for weight loss: Progress and future directions. Nature Reviews. Endocrinology. 2022;**18**(5):309-321

[73] Dorighello GG, Rovani JC, Luhman CJF, Paim BA, Raposo HF, Vercesi AE, et al. Food restriction by intermittent fasting induces diabetes and obesity and aggravates spontaneous atherosclerosis development in hypercholesterolaemic mice. British Journal of Nutrition. 2014;**111**(6):979-986

[74] Guo Y, Luo S, Ye Y, Yin S, Fan J, Xia M. Intermittent fasting improves cardiometabolic risk factors and alters gut microbiota in metabolic syndrome patients. Journal of Clinical Endocrinology and Metabolism. 2021;**106**(1):64-79

[75] Hajek P, Przulj D, Pesola F, McRobbie H, Peerbux S, Phillips-Waller A, et al. A randomised controlled trial of the 5:2 diet. PLoS One. 2021;**16**(11 November):e0258853

[76] Pearlman M, Obert J, Casey L. The association between artificial sweeteners and obesity. Current Gastroenterology Reports. 2017;**19**(12):64

[77] Khan S, Waliullah S, Godfrey V, Khan MAW, Ramachandran RA, Cantarel BL, et al. Dietary simple sugars alter microbial ecology in the gut and promote colitis in mice. Science Translational Medicine. 2020;**12**(567):eaay6218

[78] Do MH, Lee E, Oh MJ, Kim Y, Park HY. High-glucose or-fructose diet cause changes of the gut microbiota and metabolic disorders in mice without body weight change. Nutrients. 2018;**10**(6):761

[79] Engen PA, Green SJ, Voigt RM, Forsyth CB, Keshavarzian A. The gastrointestinal microbiome: Alcohol effects on the composition of intestinal microbiota. Alcohol Research: Current Reviews. 2015;**37**(2):223-236

Section 2

Obesity and Metabolic Disorders

Chapter 4

Obesity in Low-Income Communities

Amardeep Shrestha and Prakriti Singh Shrestha

Abstract

The relationship between income levels and obesity is complex. Obesity has historically been a disease in affluent countries. Hence it is thought that greater wealth brings greater obesity. However, data suggested overall obesity prevalence decreased with increased levels of income. This observation proved that obesity as a disease is complex and not a simple calorie-in and calorie-out equation. Low socioeconomic communities suffer from inequalities and health disparities that we need to amend by reforming our healthcare delivery system. We will discuss why obesity is a problem in low-income communities and what preventive and treatment strategies we would need to implement to combat this.

Keywords: food insecurity, obesity, low income, food stamp program, health disparity

1. Introduction

The prevalence of obesity has increased over time [1]. It is now a major public health risk factor that has been linked to several non-communicable diseases such as diabetes, hypertension, cardiovascular disease, obstructive sleep apnea, etc. [1]. It has also been related to increased all-cause mortality and reduced quality of life [1]. To better understand obesity, several studies and research have been ongoing looking at correlations. Epidemiological research depicting the relationship with the socio-economic status of the community has been ongoing and several hypotheses have been laid out [1]. Socioeconomic status includes the household income level as well as their level of education [2]. The relationship between income levels and obesity is complex [2]. We reviewed current and previous literature depicting this relationship with a thorough web search of journal articles, books, and statistical data from national surveys. These included any articles that appeared on the search criteria including low income and obesity.

The pattern of relation was noted to vary between high-income and low-income countries [1, 2]. In low-income countries, it has been noted to be a disease of the rich [2]. Hence, a thought that greater wealth brings greater obesity [3]. The relationship, however, did not stay the same in medium- to high-income countries. It was the opposite [1, 2]. Obesity prevalence decreased with increased levels of income in affluent countries [1–3]. This observation also proved that obesity as a disease is complex and not a simple calorie-in and calorie-out equation [2, 4].

Review of NHANES (National Health and Nutrition Examination Survey) 2011–2014 data [4] categorized income levels into three categories: Highest (federal poverty level FPL >350%), middle-income levels (FPL > 130% to <350%), and lowest-income group (FPL ≤ 130%). The data revealed the overall prevalence of obesity was comparatively lower in the highest-income group (31.2%) as compared to middle-income group (40.8%) and lowest-income group (39%) [4].

Various other concomitant determinants such as gender, ethnicity, etc., affected the prevalence in a community [5]. On a gender level, obesity decreased with increased levels of income among women, consistent with overall prevalence [5]. It was 29.7% in FPL > 350% whereas it increased to 42.9% in FPL >130% to <350% group and 45.2% in FPL < 130% group [4]. However, this relationship was complex among men. Men had lower prevalence in both the lowest-income group (31.5%) and the highest-income group (32.6%) but affected middle-income group the most (38.5%) (**Figure 1**). One of the explanations for this is that men in low-income groups are involved in more labor-intensive jobs [4, 5].

The relationship between obesity and income levels also varied by race and ethnicity. As shown in **Table 1**, obesity prevalence decreased as income increased in non-Hispanic whites (30.6% in FPL >350% vs. 35.8% in FPL < 130% and 40.2% in FPL > 130 to <350%). A similar relation was noted in the Asian population with an obesity prevalence of 10.7% in FPL > 350% vs. 15% in FPL < 130% and 11.2% in FPL > 130 to <350%; in the Hispanic population with 39.1% in FPL > 50% vs. 42.6% in FPL < 130 and 45% in FPL > 130 to <350%. Among, non-Hispanic Black men, there was no significant difference in obesity prevalence per poverty level (**Table 1**).

2. Understand the health disparity

There are lots of disparities and inequalities in our community. People living in low-income communities are one of the groups that suffer from these disparities. They suffer from a higher prevalence of obesity as discussed earlier. They also lack access to effective treatment and preventive measures. They suffer from overall lower levels of education

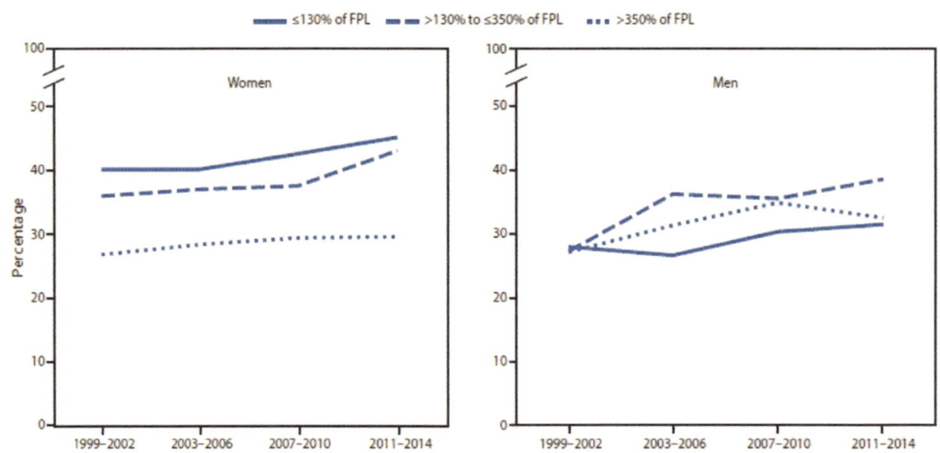

Figure 1.
Obesity prevalence among adults, by household income (percentage of FPL) and sex—National Health and Nutrition Examination Survey, 1999–2002 to 2011–2014.

		Race/Hispanic origin				
		Overall	White, non–Hispanic	Black, non–Hispanic	Asian, non–Hispanic	Hispanic
Characteristic	**No.**	**% (95% CI)**	**% (95% CI)**	**% (95% CI)**	**% (95% CI)**	**% (95% CI)**
Overall	10,636	36.3 (34.7–38.0)	34.5 (32.4–36.7)	48.1 (45.5–50.7)	11.7 (9.8–13.7)	42.5 (39.8–45.3)
Women	5413	38.3 (36.1–40.5)	35.5 (32.4–38.6)	56.9 (54.2–59.7)	11.9 (8.8–15.1)	45.7 (42.2–49.2)
Men	5223	34.3 (32.6–36.1)	33.6 (31.4–35.7)	37.5 (34.3–40.8)	11.2 (8.8–13.6)	39.0 (35.4–42.5)
Household income, both sexes						
≤130% FPL	3462	39.0 (36.9–41.0)	35.8 (32.8–38.7)	46.6 (43.2–50.0)	15.0 (9.7–20.3)	42.6 (38.1–47.1)
>130 to ≤350% FPL	3331	40.8 (38.2–43.4)	40.2 (36.5–43.9)	48.8 (44.6–52.9)	11.2 (6.6–15.8)	45.0 (40.7–49.2)
>350% FPL	2992	31.2 (28.3–34.2)[†,§]	30.6 (27.3–34.0)[†,§]	49.3 (43.4–55.1)	10.7 (8.3–13.1)	39.1 (33.9–44.3)
Household income, women						
≤130% FPL	1835	45.2 (42.5–48.0)	42.0 (37.4–46.5)	55.8 (52.2–59.4)	17.2 (10.3–24.1)	48.7 (43.1–54.4)
>130 to ≤350% FPL	1702	42.9 (40.1–45.8)	42.5 (38.8–46.1)	59.4 (53.7–65.2)	11.7 (5.6–17.7)	44.6 (37.4–51.8)
>350% FPL	1453	29.7 (26.1–33.3)[†,§]	27.9 (24.0–31.9)[†,§]	56.7 (50.0–63.5)	9.7 (5.8–13.7)	42.9 (35.2–50.5)
Household income, men						
≤130% FPL	1627	31.5 (28.5–34.4)	28.5 (24.4–32.6)	33.8 (28.9–38.6)	11.8 (4.7–18.9)	35.9 (30.9–40.8)
>130 to ≤350% FPL	1629	38.5 (35.1–41.9)[†]	37.8 (32.7–43.0)[†]	35.6 (30.7–40.5)	10.3 (5.6–15.0)	44.6 (40.1–49.2)[†]
>350% FPL	1539	32.6 (29.4–35.8)[§]	32.9 (29.2–36.6)	42.7 (35.8–49.6)[†]	11.8 (7.9–15.7)	35.6 (27.8–43.4)[§]
Education, both sexes						
High school graduate or less	4714	40.0 (37.9–42.2)	38.1 (34.5–41.6)	46.6 (42.8–50.4)	11.5 (7.6–15.5)	43.8 (40.6–47.0)
Some college	3231	40.6 (38.1–43.1)	39.2 (35.9–42.5)	50.5 (46.3–54.7)	12.4 (8.9–15.8)	42.9 (38.2–47.5)
College graduate	2683	27.8 (25.0–30.7)[¶,**]	27.5 (24.1–30.9)[¶,**]	47.3 (43.3–52.1)	11.1 (8.7–13.6)	36.9 (30.6–43.2)[¶]
Education, women						
High school graduate or less	2227	45.3 (42.3–48.3)	43.3 (38.7–47.8)	57.9 (53.2–62.6)	11.4 (6.1–16.7)	49.6 (45.6–53.7)

		Race/Hispanic origin				
		Overall	White, non-Hispanic	Black, non-Hispanic	Asian, non-Hispanic	Hispanic
Characteristic	**No.**	**% (95% CI)**	**% (95% CI)**	**% (95% CI)**	**% (95% CI)**	**% (95% CI)**
Some college	1777	41.2 (38.5–43.9)	38.9 (35.1–42.7)	58.8 (53.8–63.9)	13.3 (7.6–19.0)	43.0 (36.3–49.8)
College graduate	1355	27.8 (24.1–31.5)¶,**	27.0 (22.3–31.6)¶,**	52.1 (47.4–56.8)**	11.3 (7.6–15.0)	36.1 (26.5–45.6)¶
Education, men						
High school graduate or less	2437	35.5 (33.0–37.9)	34.1 (29.7–38.5)	36.0 (30.7–41.2)	11.0 (5.7–16.2)	37.7 (34.0–41.4)
Some college	1454	40.0 (35.9–44.1)	39.9 (34.7–45.1)	38.2 (32.7–43.7)	10.3 (5.6–15.1)	42.9 (36.0–49.9)
College graduate	1328	27.9 (24.3–31.5)¶,**	28.1 (24.1–32.1)**	40.4 (32.4–48.3)	11.0 (7.9–14.1)	38.5 (28.1–48.8)

Abbreviations: CI = confidence interval; FPL = federal poverty level. *Age adjusted by the direct method to the 2000 projected U.S census population using the age groups 20–30, 40–59, and ≤ 60 years.*

†*Significantly different from ≤130% FPL, $p < 0.05$.*

§*Significantly different from >130 to ≤350% FPL, $p < 0.05$.*

¶*Significantly different from high school graduates or less, $p < 0.05$.*

***Significantly different from some colleges, $p < 0.05$.*

Table 1.

*Prevalence of obesity among adults, *by race/Hispanic origin, sex, household income (percentage of FPL), and education—National Health and Nutrition Examination Survey, 2011–2014.*

and get lower occupational and other opportunities. This same group also includes certain racial and ethnic minorities, which are already a disadvantaged group [6].

Since obesity prevalence has been on the rise, there is undoubtedly a major need to effectively combat the obesity epidemic. The focus of implementing effective strategies in low-income populations can be challenging. The first step to being able to reform and create equity for this community is understanding this inequity and disparity exist. This understanding will help to allocate resources appropriately among these disadvantaged groups and close the healthcare gap.

3. Understand potential etiologies

For the implementation of health reform, we need to know why such problems exist. So, let us dig in deeper. Several factors lead to an increased prevalence of obesity in low-income communities. In most cases, there is a combination of factors that contribute. A lot of these factors are also interconnected with each other.

3.1 Financial crunch

Obesity in a low-income population comes down to a lack of money for healthy food options. Low income leads to low-quality food. To eat a decent quality meal every day, it can cost significantly more for a person who is living on a minimum wage. Many people in this society barely make their ends meet taking in the cheapest food and drink which include inferior-quality nutrients. Unfortunately, good and healthy food are more expensive options [2], which leads these folks to steer away from these options.

3.2 Lack of education

There are also a lot of nutritional misconceptions in low-income populations. This unfortunately flows through their successive generations. There is a lack of education on how food creates good health versus makes you sick. Children learn from adults as they also lack getting a good education. When adults in families do not eat vegetables daily and have sugary beverages [6], the following generation feels it is acceptable to eat junk food and then the tradition continues.

3.3 Food insecurity

Low-income communities suffer from food insecurity. Food insecurity is the uncertainty of having or inability to acquire sufficient food [2, 3, 6]. It leads to several unhealthy behaviors. They grab and consume what they get. Families mostly choose energy-dense food such as sugars, cereals, potatoes, and processed meat products as these foods are more affordable, readily available, and last longer than fresh vegetables, fruits, lean meats, and fish. The food stamp program, now known as the Supplemental Nutritional Assistance Program (SNAP), was developed to combat food insecurity in low-income communities [6]. SNAP program provides mostly energy-dense food and lacks fresh and healthful food options [6].

Furthermore, food-insecure families also have limited knowledge, time, and resources to engage in healthful eating and exercise. They are all busy running around and working hard to provide for themselves and their families.

3.4 Poor access/resources to fresh food

This is the most saddening part. Not only do they not know what healthy food is, but people who live in poor communities also have poor access to fresh food. These areas are hence termed "food deserts" [3]. The food stamp program developed to combat food insecurity in low-income populations has poorer access to fresh food, and increased access to energy-dense food. Food insecurity has improved since then with a surplus of food, though mostly processed [6]. However, there has been very little change in how the SNAP program rolls out since its inception [6]. This leads to continued poor access to the resources to fresh food in low-income populations.

3.5 Stressful life

Economic insecurity due to low income leads to increased stress. The society they live in is also crime-ridden [3]. Many people are worried about their own or their family's survival, about gunshots, police abuse, and about society holding them down and not educating them and therefore the jobs they deserve. They sleep with one eye open, in fear, night terrors, and fear due to an insecure society and environment. We all know how stress and anxiety play a role in our hormonal control and hormonal aberrations leading to obesity. People cope with stress by eating unhealthy high-fat sugary and processed food. They also lack adequate sleep. This disrupts their circadian rhythm leading to hormonal aberrations and eventually obesity.

3.6 Sedentary lifestyle

Several factors play a role in this. Low-income communities are crime-ridden, preventing people from being active outdoors. There are also fewer available parks and sports facilities in those communities [3]. Due to a lack of income, affording a gym membership, sports clothing, and exercise equipment are also out of the question [2, 3]. There might be people who are working double shifts to provide for their families, leaving very much less time to indulge in their well-being.

3.7 Racial/ethnic effect

Low-income communities also have a higher number of ethnic minority populations and hence incorporate all the racial or ethnic health disparities. As we all know, obesity is more common in certain racial and ethnic minatory groups [6].

4. Understand potential solutions

As complex as the disease of obesity is, equally complex is its management. Prevention is undoubtedly the best strategy. Not one strategy leads to success in combating obesity in low-income communities but requires a combination of strategies. Failure of certain focused studies like COPTR studies, and the GEMS trial [7] emphasizes how important it is that a combined broader focus on the social, economic, and physical environment is needed to prevent obesity in low-income communities.

This was described by Kumanyika et al. with their equity-oriented obesity prevention framework (**Figure 2**) [7, 8]. The framework involves four different quadrants with each quadrant specifically addressing different intervention approaches. The

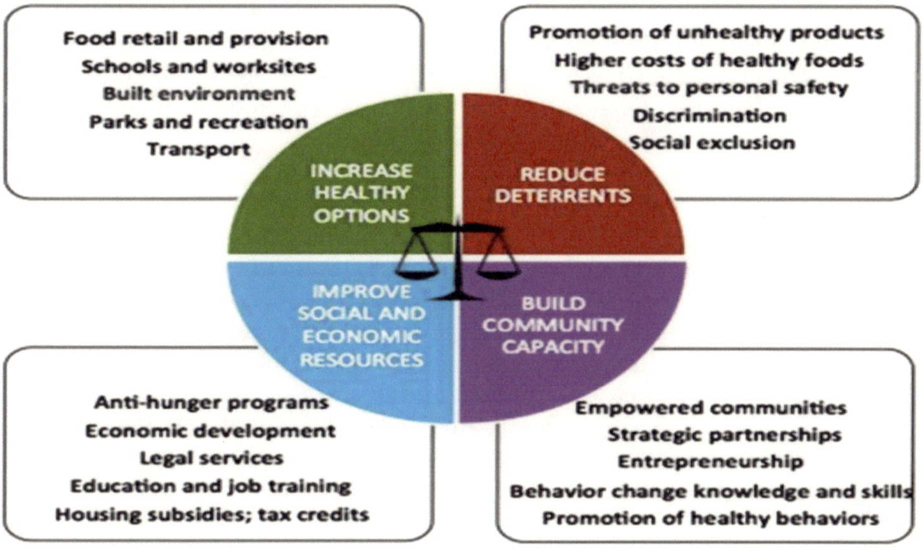

Figure 2.
The equity-oriented obesity prevention framework. Adapted from Kumanyika et al. [8].

upper quadrants include how to increase healthy eating options and improve physical activity along with how to reduce deterrents leading to unhealthy eating and reduced physical activity. The bottom quadrants include improving individual and community resources and the capacity to support them. These focus on addressing health disparities and food insecurities with the development of different public health policies to improve social determinants of health.

4.1 Preventive strategies

The preventive strategies include not only dietary and physical activities but also include various regulatory and educational strategies [7].

4.1.1 Dietary strategies

Different educational and environmental dietary interventions can be implemented at multiple levels [9]. At a consumer level, different strategies that can be used or tried are price manipulation to promote healthier food, posters/flyers/shelf labels, interactive sessions like taste testing healthier food, and promotional give-aways /incentivizing healthier food purchases with point of purchase promotions [9].

Improvising policy-level reforms such as increasing the availability of targeted food items, implementing a food labeling system to increase awareness of food ingredients with the number of calories, sugar, saturated fat, and sodium in a product, and increasing access to healthy food by incorporating healthy food supply chain rather than processed food [9]. Improved access to healthy food could reduce food insecurity. The New York Green Carts program used mobile food carts to offer fresh produce in certain poor neighborhoods. Understandably, this will involve extensive collaborations and planning with city council members, city health authorities, department leaders, local and regional retailers, and local community organization representatives [9].

Regulatory strategies at certain places such as schools could also be taken up to combat this problem. Eliminating soft drink vending machines in school, regulating food advertising to children in school, and mandating nutrition labeling can be some reforms that can be made. These are to educate people from low-income communities regarding their healthful vs. unhealthful food choices.

4.1.2 Physical activity strategies

Texts, letters, or telephone calls to promote playground use (as used in COPTR trial) [7]; school hip hop and African and step dance classes (as used in GEMS trials) [7] are different strategies used in different low-income community-based studies. Family-based intervention is used to reduce screen media time.

Furthermore, children may not be physically active unless efforts to improve neighborhood safety are made or provide them with places to play. Individuals do not improve until the community is strong and improved. We need to provide the community with adequate resources, safety, and opportunities [2].

4.1.3 Redesigning food stamp program

Redesigning the food stamp program could have a widespread impact on the health of food stamp recipients, who are the low-income communities. The food stamp program was first established as a pilot project to stabilize agricultural prices by stimulating the consumption of surplus farm commodities and alleviating hunger by providing additional calories to the recipients. Nutritional needs have now changed, nevertheless, the food stamp program operates for the same traditional norm. There needs to be a shift in emphasis on the program from calories to diet quality, from low-nutrient high energy-dense food to high-nutrient low energy-dense food. E.g., whole wheat bread instead of doughnuts. This change will lead the food industry to create low-cost palatable food products that are healthier and provide more fresh fruits and vegetables as options for consumers.

4.1.4 Improving school and head start programs

Schools and Head Start programs which include comprehensive health, nutrition, and education services to children are key influencers to combat childhood and youth obesity. Our youngsters spend a lot of time in them, and these are valued community institutions. Incorporating physical activities and good nutrition into school and preschool programs can create an enormous difference.

4.2 Treatment strategies

The leading strategy to help obesity in a poor environment is counseling. Dietary counseling and educating them about different diets and their nutritional values is especially important [10]. We need to provide all the education as this is their only resource. A randomized trial testing a high-intensity, lifestyle-based treatment program delivered in an underserved community showed a significant weight loss at 24 months [10]. Behavioral treatment strategies to steer them from fast food and get them to cook meals at home and hunt for vegetables in the grocery store remain the mainstay strategy for obesity management in low-income populations.

Most of the low-income individuals will be covered under the medical health plan from the state. Unfortunately, obesity care is still not an approved condition for which they can seek care under these plans. Hence the struggle for management is still present. Some medications are approved to be used for obesity. However, insurance coverage and costs associated with these medications are still outrageous and out of reach for these folks. Phentermine and topiramate are generic medications and certainly can be an option for treatment. Another combination of medication which includes bupropion and naltrexone can also be a cost-effective option for treatment. GLP1 receptor agonists and now GIP agonists are novel agents for obesity management, however, these are expensive and not always covered under the medical card. Semaglutide, one of the newest GLP1 receptor agonists, is approved for diabetes management in a lower dose. These have recently been placed under the formulary and can be used but most of the time these require prior authorization. The process of prior authorization is cumbersome and since care and coverage for obesity is still not an approved condition, these will still be unreachable goals at this time. This can delay the promptness in instituting these medications for the management of their weight, unfortunately. Some of the other GLP1 receptor agonists, like dulaglutide, though not approved for weight loss, can be used for treatment as these have more recently been under formulary in Medicaid plans. Metformin can be used off-label for weight loss, which can offset some of their weight, but it has not been shown to have a significant decrease in weight.

The low-income folks also suffer from grief, depression, anxiety, insomnia, weight stigma, and discrimination. They might be on multiple different medications that can cause weight gain. Working with them and tapering or adjusting some medications to counteract their weight gain side effects can be a helpful strategy to help with their obesity. Metformin can be used to counteract the weight-gaining properties of some psychotropic medications.

Surgery for obesity is not covered under a lot of health plans and particularly for the low income, it is still out of the question.

Furthermore, follow-up care in low-income populations is scarce. The no-show rate is plentiful. Their priority for self-care is low. These may not be entirely because of their choice. Their jobs may not offer time off; patients may be working two full-time jobs just to make enough to pay the bills. These all come into play.

Moreover, there might also be this weight stigma and discrimination that discourages them from seeking care. We also need to understand this. Our goal is to be nonjudgmental about their weight in our day-to-day practice, respect them, and understand these social determinants of health. No one wants to be unhealthy. We need to provide adequate guidance and create a supporting community that they can rely on to achieve their goals. Instead of pointing it out, let us help them to fight this battle.

The Healthcare Reform (The Patient Protection and Affordable Care Act P.L. 111-148) was devised in 2010 to help bridge these gaps to help care for obesity in the United States [11].

5. The cause or the effect?

There has also been a concept of reverse causality [1]. People suffering from obesity tend to also suffer from labor discrimination [1]. They are likely to be perceived as lazy, unsuccessful, weak-willed, and undisciplined [1]. This leads them to conquer low-income jobs in a labor market leading to poverty [1]. These negative energies in the community among people who suffer from obesity further increase higher levels of psychosocial stressors, higher insecurity, social isolation, and mental disorders [1]. This further leads to increased poverty and a higher risk of obesity. One systematic literature search which included 21 studies, from January 2017 suggested strong reverse causality than the causality [1]. However, more studies are needed to further elaborate this relationship [1].

6. Conclusion

Whether it is the cause or effect that came first, one thing is for fact from our observations that these create a cycle of events. The low-income communities experience disparity in health leading to obesity and experience inequity in their obesity care. Inequity in obesity care further leads to obesity. Health reforms involving a combination of strategies at social, economic, and community levels are required to break this cycle and create equity.

Conflict of interest

The authors declare no conflict of interest.

Author details

Amardeep Shrestha[1]* and Prakriti Singh Shrestha[2]

1 Family Medical Clinic, O'Fallon, IL, USA

2 Department of Family Medicine, Larkin Community Hospital Family Medicine Residency Program, South Miami, FL, USA

*Address all correspondence to: amardeepshrestha@hotmail.com

References

[1] Kim TJ, von dem Knesebeck O. Income and obesity: What is the direction of the relationship? A systematic review and meta-analysis. BMJ Open. 2018;**8**:e019862. DOI: 10.1136/bmjopen-2017-019862

[2] Adams J. Addressing socioeconomic inequalities in obesity: Democratizing access to resources for achieving and maintaining a healthy weight. PLoS Medicine. 2020;**17**(7):e1003243. DOI: 10.1371/journal. pmed.1003243

[3] Levine JA. Poverty and obesity in the U.S. Diabetes. 2011;**60**(11):2667-2668. DOI: 10.2337/db11-1118

[4] Ogden CL, Fakhouri TH, Carroll MD, et al. Prevalence of obesity among adults, by household income and education—United States, 2011-2014. MMWR Morbidity and Mortality Weekly Report. 2017;**66**:1369-1373. DOI: 10.15585/mmwr.mm6650a1

[5] Fan JX, Wen M, Li K. Associations between obesity and neighborhood socioeconomic status: Variations by gender and family income status. SSM Population Health. 2019;**10**(10):100529. DOI: 10.1016/j.ssmph.2019.100529

[6] Townsend MS. Obesity in low-income communities: Prevalence, effects, a place to begin. Journal of the American Dietetic Association. 2006;**106**(1):34-37. DOI: 10.1016/j.jada.2005.11.008

[7] William H. Dietz; we need a new approach to prevent obesity in low-income minority populations. Pediatrics. 2019;**143**(6):e20190839. DOI: 10.1542/peds.2019-0839

[8] Kumanyika SK. A framework for increasing equity impact in obesity prevention. American Journal of Public Health. 2019;**109**(10):1350-1357. DOI: 10.2105/AJPH.2019.305221. Epub 2019 Aug 15

[9] Gittelsohn J, Trude A. Diabetes and obesity prevention: Changing the food environment in low-income settings. Nutrition Reviews. 2017;**75**(suppl 1):62-69. DOI: 10.1093/nutrit/nuw038

[10] Katzmarzyk PT, Martin CK, Newton RL Jr, Apolzan JW, Arnold CL, Davis TC, et al. Weight loss in underserved patients—A cluster-randomized trial. The New England Journal of Medicine. 2020;**383**(10):909-918. DOI: 10.1056/NEJMoa2007448

[11] Levine JA, Koepp GA. Federal health-care reform: Opportunities for obesity prevention. Obesity (Silver Spring). 2011;**19**(5):897-899. DOI: 10.1038/oby.2010.281

Chapter 5

Understanding and Managing Obesity: A Multidisciplinary Approach

Maryam Alkhatry

Abstract

Obesity emerges as a critical public health threat, with numerous nations witnessing a staggering surge in prevalence over recent decades. This escalating health crisis increases the risk of diseases, including type 2 diabetes mellitus, fatty liver disease, hypertension, cardiovascular diseases, dementia, osteoarthritis, and various cancers, contributing to morbidity and mortality. The consequences of obesity extend beyond health, including unemployment, social disparities, and impaired quality of life. The ineffectiveness of conventional methods to control obesity highlights the need for a new approach to public policy that shifts away from an emphasis on individual behavior change toward strategies that address environmental factors. The role of a multidisciplinary team, including nurses, dietitians, and psychologists, to support patients through their weight loss journey should not be neglected. Multidisciplinary management of obesity has been recognized as an effective means to improve weight loss and associated health outcomes.

Keywords: obesity, weight loss, multidisciplinary, comorbidities, prevention

1. Introduction

Obesity, defined as an excess accumulation of body fat, is a serious health condition and a public health threat that continues to be on the rise worldwide [1]. In 2016, more than 1.9 billion adults worldwide were overweight, and 650 million of them, accounting for 15% of the world's adult population, were classified as obese by the WHO Global Health Observatory [2, 3]. Owing to the significant and rapid increase in obesity prevalence globally, the condition has been classified as a pandemic, similar to the COVID-19 pandemic [2].

The alarming increase in the prevalence of obesity could be attributed to multiple factors such as urbanization, sedentary lifestyle, and the consumption of high-calorie processed foods. Unfortunately, childhood obesity rates are also increasing, which could lead to a greater burden on healthcare systems in the future [1]. Around 38.2 million children under the age of five were considered obese in 2019, and more than 340 million children and adolescents between the ages of 5–19 were overweight or obese in 2016 [3]. Obesity is no longer considered a disease specific to high-income countries. Overweight and obesity are increasing in low- and middle-income countries all the same [2–4].

Obesity contributes to global morbidity and mortality, with around 2.8 million people dying yearly due to overweight or obesity [2]. Preventing obesity is crucial in reducing the risk of developing related health issues such as diabetes, cardiovascular disease, stroke, hypertension, cancer, and psychological problems [1].

The ineffectiveness of conventional methods to control obesity highlights the need for a new approach to public policy that is non-stigmatizing. This requires shifting away from an emphasis on individual behavior change toward strategies that address environmental factors. Another significant challenge related to overweight, and obesity is weight bias and discrimination. Obese individuals often experience discrimination in various public settings such as work environments, healthcare facilities, and educational institutions [1].

This chapter explores the burden imposed by obesity, its consequences, current management strategies, and the pivotal role of a multidisciplinary approach in addressing this pressing global health challenge.

2. Obesity: the global pandemic

2.1 Definition and classification

A little over a decade ago, the American Medical Association (AMA) officially declared obesity as a chronic disease that requires treatment and prevention [5]. Obesity has been identified as a chronic relapsing progressive disease similar to other chronic disorders, such as hypertension [5, 6].

In order to evaluate the impact of obesity, it is important to first understand what obesity is. According to the World Health Organization (WHO), obesity is "abnormal or excessive fat accumulation that may impair health, caused by energy imbalance between calories consumed and calories expended" [3, 7].

Obesity can be diagnosed using the "body mass index" (BMI), which is measured by calculating [(weight in kg)/(height in m^2)]. Although there are some debates regarding the use of BMI, it remains the most common and the simplest tool used to classify adults into one of three categories: "underweight," "overweight," or "obese" (**Table 1**) [7, 8].

This WHO classification can detect individuals at increased risk of developing associated comorbidities and, consequently, death due to obesity [7, 8].

BMI (kg/m^2)	**Class**
25–29.9	Overweight
30–34.9	Class I obesity
35–39.9	Class II obesity
≥40	Class III obesity

Table 1.
Classes of obesity in adults.

2.2 Underlying factors and causes

Obesity is a complex problem that cannot be solved with a single or simple solution. It is a multifactorial issue that requires a multifactorial approach. The causes of obesity are extremely intricate, but they ultimately result in an energy imbalance between the calories consumed and the calories expended. Societal and environmental changes cannot be ignored as they lead to changes in dietary habits and physical activity. Other factors that contribute to obesity include gender, ethnicity, socioeconomic status, and genetics [7].

Despite recent research on obesity's genetic and epigenetic influences, obesity is still regarded as an acquired disease that develops due to lifestyle patterns and personal choices, including sedentary lifestyles and a tendency to overeat [7].

It is also worth mentioning that binge eating disorder (BED) is often linked to obesity [9, 10]. BED is the most prevalent eating disorder among the general population, and those who have it are more likely to experience both physical and psychiatric comorbidities. BED is known to be associated with an earlier onset of being overweight and a history of obesity. Furthermore, it is independently linked to an increased risk of physical comorbidities such as diabetes, hypertension, back/neck pain, chronic headaches, and various other types of chronic pain [10].

It is crucial to comprehend the root causes and contributing factors that lead to obesity. This understanding is vital for the creation of effective policies and programs aimed at preventing obesity and its associated complications. Without a detailed, science-based understanding of the risk factors and their interconnections, efforts to combat obesity are unlikely to succeed [7].

3. Obesity burden

3.1 Health consequences of obesity

Obesity has been linked to various health consequences and comorbidities. Overweight and obesity are the most common risk factors for the development of numerous associated health conditions that not only adversely affect individuals but also create significant challenges for healthcare systems (**Figure 1**) [1, 7, 8].

3.1.1 Cardiovascular diseases

Obesity significantly raises the risk of cardiovascular diseases (CVDs), including hypertension, coronary artery disease, and stroke [3, 8]. The surplus adipose tissue contributes to increased blood pressure, dyslipidemia, and systemic inflammation, collectively fostering the development of atherosclerosis [11].

3.1.2 Type 2 diabetes

The correlation between obesity and type 2 diabetes is firmly established. Excessive adipose tissue, particularly visceral fat, plays a role in insulin resistance and the onset of diabetes [12]. The escalating prevalence of obesity has substantially fueled the global diabetes epidemic [13].

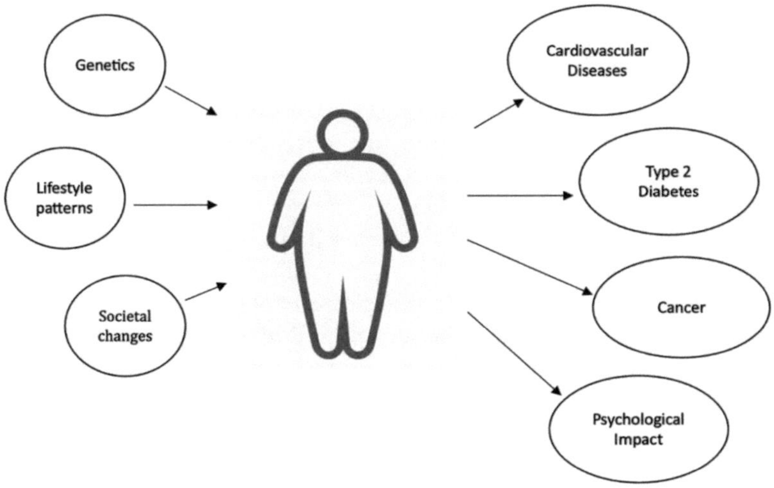

Figure 1.
Underlying causes and consequences of obesity.

3.1.3 Cancer

Recent data suggests that approximately 4–8% of all cancer cases are connected to obesity. Although the exact mechanism remains unclear, obesity has been correlated with various prevalent cancers such as those affecting the liver, breast, colorectal, and endometrium [14].

3.1.4 Psychological impact

Obesity is linked to an elevated risk of mental health disorders, including depression and anxiety [15]. Stigma and discrimination related to body weight can intensify psychological distress, creating a challenging cycle for individuals dealing with obesity [15].

3.1.4.1 Depression and anxiety

Obesity is strongly associated with an increased risk of depression and anxiety disorders. The stigma and societal prejudice faced by individuals with obesity can lead to negative self-perception and contribute to the development or exacerbation of mental health conditions [15]. Coping with body image issues, societal pressures, and discrimination can result in heightened levels of stress, leading to a vicious cycle of emotional distress.

3.1.4.2 Eating disorders

Obesity is linked to various eating disorders, including binge eating disorder (BED) and emotional eating. The interplay between psychological factors and disordered eating behaviors can contribute to the maintenance of obesity and hinder successful weight management efforts [16].

3.1.4.3 Low self-esteem and body image disturbances

Individuals with obesity often face challenges related to body image and self-esteem. Social comparisons and unrealistic societal standards can contribute to negative body image, impacting self-worth and self-perception [17].

3.1.5 Obesity in women

Obesity has a significant impact on reproductive health in women, and one of the most common reproductive disorders is PCOS, which can be impaired or even caused by visceral obesity [18]. Obesity negatively affects fertility and contraception in women due to hormonal and metabolic alterations.

During pregnancy, obesity is associated with various complications. It increases the risk of early loss of pregnancy, higher rates of cesarean section, and high-risk obstetrical conditions. Maternal and neonatal mortality rates are also higher in obese women, and there is an increased risk of congenital malformations. Abnormal weight gain during pregnancy further worsens maternal health.

In addition to these reproductive health issues, obesity in women is closely linked to other health problems. It is associated with an increased risk of certain types of cancer, including breast, endometrial, gallbladder, esophageal, and renal cancer. Obesity is also closely linked to mental health disorders such as depression, anxiety disorders, neurodegenerative diseases, and sleep disorders.

Overall, obesity in women has significant consequences for both physical and mental health, and it is important to address and manage obesity to prevent these complications and improve overall well-being [18].

3.2 Economic and societal implications

1. *Healthcare costs*: the economic repercussions of obesity extend to healthcare costs, with obesity-related illnesses significantly contributing to global medical expenses [19]. Direct medical costs for treating obesity and indirect costs related to productivity losses constitute a considerable economic burden.

2. *Workplace productivity*: obesity is associated with reduced workplace productivity due to absenteeism, presenteeism, and disability [20]. Health-related limitations imposed by obesity can impede individuals' full participation in work-related activities, affecting overall productivity.

3. *Social stigma and discrimination*: individuals with obesity often experience societal prejudice and discrimination, leading to social exclusion and negative impacts on mental health [17]. Stigmatization can impede efforts to seek healthcare and perpetuate a cycle of weight gain.

4. Consequences of inaction

4.1 Escalating public health challenges

Despite the well-documented health risks associated with obesity, a failure to address this global issue leads to escalating public health challenges. The rising prevalence of obesity contributes to a higher incidence of chronic conditions, putting an additional strain on healthcare systems worldwide [21]. This inaction exacerbates the burden of preventable diseases, contributing to increased mortality rates and reduced overall life expectancy [22].

4.2 Long-term effects on individuals and communities

Inaction regarding obesity has profound long-term effects on both individuals and communities. Individuals with untreated obesity face a heightened risk of developing severe health complications, including cardiovascular diseases, diabetes, and certain cancers [23]. Moreover, the intergenerational transmission of unhealthy lifestyles perpetuates the cycle of obesity, leading to a compounding effect on future generations [24].

5. Current treatment approaches

Management is a challenging task as weight loss is often followed by weight regain. Due to the associated metabolic changes that co-occur, obesity has been labeled a "chronic relapsing progressive disease" [6]. Eating less and exercising are not enough to achieve sustainable results. The management of obesity has included an array of interventions in recent years, including pharmacological treatment, endoscopic and surgical interventions, alongside dietary changes, other lifestyle changes such as exercise, and counseling [8].

While procedural interventions, such as bariatric surgery and endoscopic therapy, offer numerous advantages in terms of weight loss and reducing comorbidities, they are accompanied by side effects and may not be a viable option for every patient [8]. Therefore, these interventions should be employed not as substitutes but as complementary measures to other nonoperative approaches in the management of obesity. This includes incorporating dietary and lifestyle modifications, providing psychosocial counseling, and considering pharmacotherapy [8].

While it might seem like individuals are mainly responsible for their habits, such as eating and exercising, these behaviors are often shaped by the society we belong to. Changes in our surroundings, such as health policies, transportation, and education, can significantly affect our habits. In the absence of supportive policies in different sectors such as health, agriculture, and education, simply advising people to eat better or exercise more may not be very effective. The World Health Organization (WHO) emphasizes the need to encourage healthy eating and more physical activity for everyone through policies and actions in society [8].

5.1 Lifestyle interventions

There is evidence to support the role of lifestyle and behavioral intervention in weight loss. Obesity management should include monitoring caloric intake, physical exercise, and exercising control over food through behavioral therapy [25]. A comprehensive lifestyle intervention through diet, exercise, and behavioral modifications is recommended for individuals with a BMI ≥ 25 kg/m^2 [25]. It is built on three pillars:

5.1.1 Diet

The rapid urbanization has led to a predominant diet of fast foods, sweets, and processed snacks [26]. Patients aiming to lose weight should seek the help of a nutrition specialist or an expert dietitian who would be able to prescribe an individualized and tailored meal plan specific to their needs, health conditions, and food preferences. The diet should aim to elicit an energy deficit of 500–750 kcal/day compared to the patient's current calorie intake. Overall guidance would be to prescribe 1200–1500 kcal/day for women and 1500–1800 kcal/day for men. Regular follow-up and assessment of patient adherence to the meal plan is recommended, and changes should be implemented depending on their ability to follow the diet.

5.1.2 Physical activity

Physical activity and movement are part of comprehensive lifestyle interventions for effective weight loss. Increased aerobic physical activity (such as brisk walking) is recommended for ≥150 min/week. Higher levels of physical activity, approximately 200–300 min/week, are recommended to maintain lost weight or minimize weight regain in the long term (>1 year). A combination of a moderately reduced caloric diet and exercise is more effective at reducing weight and maintaining weight loss compared to either intervention alone.

5.1.3 Behavioral therapy

A comprehensive lifestyle intervention usually includes a structured behavior change program that includes regular self-monitoring of food intake, physical activity, and weight. These same behaviors are recommended to maintain lost weight with the addition of frequent monitoring of body weight.

An in-depth psychological assessment is necessary to identify factors that may hinder goals for weight loss. While some patients can achieve their weight loss goals with little to no psychological intervention, others need psychological support to resolve factors that can pose a risk to the weight loss plan. Common psychiatric disorders that may coexist with obesity are depression, anxiety, and binge eating disorder. These disorders can affect patients' eating habits and lower their tendency to follow a weight loss program.

A multifactorial, comprehensive lifestyle program that revolves around the three above pillars, which include a reduction in calorie intake, an increase in physical activity, and measures to support behavioral change, is recommended as a baseline therapy in all overweight and obese patients according to the guidelines reviewed.

5.2 Pharmacological weight reduction

All recent guidelines mention pharmacologic therapy as an effective treatment modality for obesity [8, 27–29]. The guidelines recommend pharmacotherapy for the treatment of obesity to be considered in patients with a BMI > 30 kg/m^2 with no comorbidities or BMI ≥ 27 kg/m^2 with comorbidities and used in addition to lifestyle intervention. When lifestyle interventions alone fail at reducing a patient's weight, pharmacotherapy is also recommended. Pharmacological weight reduction should only be maintained when a person has lost at least 5% of their initial body weight during the first 3 months or at least 2 kg during the first 4 weeks of treatment. In some patients with obesity, anti-obesity medications should be considered for chronic weight maintenance.

The choice of weight loss medication should take into account multiple factors, including contraindications and safety profile, associated comorbidities, efficacy, cost, and availability [25].

5.3 Bariatric surgery

The American Society for Metabolic and Bariatric Surgery (ASMBS) and the International Federation for the Surgery of Obesity and Metabolic Disorders (IFSO) have released new guidelines for metabolic and bariatric surgery in 2022. The recommendations state that individuals with a BMI of ≥35 kg/m^2 should consider metabolic and bariatric surgery, regardless of any comorbidities. Metabolic and bariatric surgery should also be considered for individuals with metabolic disease and a BMI of 30–34.9 kg/m^2 [30].

Long-term data consistently demonstrate the safety, efficacy, and durability of metabolic bariatric surgeries in the treatment of severe obesity and its comorbidities, resulting in reduced mortality compared to conventional treatment approaches. It has been proved that bariatric surgeries provide superior weight loss outcomes compared to nonsurgical approaches. Benefits beyond weight loss, including improvement of metabolic disease and decrease in overall mortality, were also observed [30, 31]. On the other side, it is worth mentioning that patients need to go through a strict assessment to be eligible for surgery. Patients must be physically and psychologically capable of undergoing surgery and comply with post-surgery instructions. Common complications of surgery include weight regain and surgical complications such as hemorrhage, anastomotic leak, bowel perforation, and bowel obstruction [32]. While the cost of bariatric surgery is higher compared to conventional treatment, studies have investigated the cost-effectiveness of this therapeutic modality. Bariatric surgery might be a cost-effective intervention for moderately to severely obese people as opposed to nonsurgical interventions. However, more data is needed to establish conclusions [32, 33].

5.4 Endoscopic management of obesity

One of the recent interventions recommended for the management of obesity is endoscopic bariatric therapies (EBTs). EBTs are considered a treatment option that provides superior efficacy to pharmacotherapy and a safer and less invasive alternative to traditional surgical treatment. The cost of some endoscopic treatments may also be lower than those of bariatric surgery [34].

EBTs increase the total body weight loss and improve metabolic profile as observed with bariatric surgeries.

Even though there are no formal guidelines for EBTs, the American Society for Gastrointestinal Endoscopy (ASGE) has issued a guidance on the use of EBTs in patients with obesity [35]. According to their recommendations, EBTs are recommended for patients who have failed nonsurgical weight loss or weight maintenance with lifestyle intervention alone and have medical conditions requiring weight loss for additional benefits [35].

Recently published guidelines of the American Association of Clinical Endocrinologists (AACE), the Obesity Society (TOS), and the American Society for Metabolic and Bariatric Surgery (ASMBS) have also included endoscopic bariatric and metabolic therapies as part of their recommendations [30]. The 2022 American Society for Metabolic and Bariatric Surgery (ASMBS) and International Federation for the Surgery of Obesity and Metabolic Disorders (IFSO) guidelines recommended metabolic and bariatric surgery (MBS) for individuals with a body mass index (BMI) 35 kg/m^2, regardless of presence, absence, or severity of comorbidities.

MBS should be considered for individuals with metabolic disease and a BMI of 30–34.9 kg/m^2 [30].

Endoscopic bariatric therapies (EBTs) mainly involve the stomach, but they also include remodeling procedures for the duodenum or small bowel [28]. Gastric interventions work on the receptors in the gastric fundus to delay gastric emptying and alter orexigenic hormones, whereas small bowel interventions act by bypassing the stomach to affect satiety and gastric motility [34].

The currently available EBTs include endoluminal procedures such as an intragastric balloon (IGB) placement, endoscopic sleeve gastroplasty (ESG), gastric bypass revision, and aspiration therapy, among others. These procedures are divided into two categories based on the mechanism of action into restrictive or malabsorptive. Both methods enhance weight loss by altering gastric motility, hormones, and function [34].

6. Multidisciplinary management of obesity

Addressing obesity requires a comprehensive and integrated approach that involves collaboration among various healthcare professionals. A multidisciplinary management strategy acknowledges the multifaceted nature of obesity and tailors interventions to individual needs, considering both physical and psychological aspects. Healthcare providers, medical authorities, governments, and insurers should recognize and treat obesity as a chronic disease, using a multidisciplinary team approach similar to that used for other chronic diseases, such as diabetes and cancer.

Since obesity is a leading cause of chronic disease, disability, and increased healthcare costs, all medical and public authorities should cooperate to address this problem systematically.

7. The role of healthcare professionals

7.1 Physicians and nurses

Physicians play a pivotal role in diagnosing and treating obesity-related comorbidities. Nurses, as frontline healthcare providers, contribute significantly to patient education and follow-up care [36]. Together, they form the primary healthcare team responsible for coordinating patient care and monitoring progress.

7.2 Dietitians and nutritionists

Dietitians and nutritionists focus on developing personalized dietary plans, considering nutritional needs, preferences, and cultural factors. Nutritional guidance is essential for sustainable weight management and overall well-being [37].

7.3 Psychologists and mental health experts

Psychological factors contribute significantly to obesity, and psychologists play a crucial role in addressing emotional eating, body image issues, and underlying mental health concerns. Integrating mental health expertise into obesity management enhances treatment outcomes [38].

7.4 Physical therapists and exercise specialists

Physical activity is a cornerstone of obesity management, and the expertise of physical therapists and exercise specialists is invaluable. Tailored exercise programs not only contribute to weight loss but also improve overall fitness and reduce obesity-related health risks [39].

Effective obesity management requires seamless communication and collaboration among healthcare professionals. Regular interdisciplinary team meetings facilitate a holistic understanding of the patient's needs and enhance treatment strategies [8]. A patient-centered approach is fundamental to successful multidisciplinary management. Involving patients in decision-making, setting realistic goals, and considering their preferences enhances treatment adherence and long-term success [40].

Several initiatives have been taken by globally recognizable bodies to halt the progress of the obesity epidemic [41–43]. Interventions, such as dietary modifications, physical activity, lifestyle changes, pharmacologic treatment, bariatric surgery, and minimally invasive endoscopic surgery, are recommended for people who are overweight or obese [27]. Family physicians and primary healthcare physicians play an essential role in helping patients achieve their weight loss goals. The role of a multidisciplinary team, including nurses, dietitians, and psychologists to support patients through their weight loss journey, should not be neglected [44].

Multidisciplinary management of obesity has been recognized as an effective means to improve weight loss and associated health outcomes [45, 46]. The need for multiple stakeholders in this process is rooted in the multifactorial nature of the disease, which has genetic, social, dietary, cultural, and psychological factors [47]. There is a need to create policies that lead to social and behavioral changes that sustainably impact obesity. In addition, there is an emphasis on the importance of tackling obesity through collaboration across multiple domains between healthcare professionals (HCPs). At the same time, a broader strategy incorporating multiple disciplines acting on implementing lifestyle changes produces more tangible and long-lasting outcomes [44]. Effective approaches to tackling obesity in the early stages include one-to-one sessions for over six months led by various healthcare team members because weight loss requires commitment from the client and the specialist [44–48]. Group-based interventions have also proved beneficial for patients in terms of weight loss, providing group support, and other therapeutic benefits, including HbA1c and systolic pressure improvement. From a socioeconomic perspective, group-based interventions facilitate access to care for a large number of patients at the same time while efficiently utilizing staff efforts [49].

In some patients, medication and lifestyle changes have been shown to have a minor impact on weight loss. Although bariatric surgery has been demonstrated to be effective in the treatment of obesity, many patients are afraid of surgeries and dread their long-term side effects [34]. Using state-of-the-art technology, bariatric endoscopy can replicate weight reduction surgery without the comorbidities [34].

According to the latest guidelines from the Obesity Medicine Association, obesity management follows a pathway that starts with data collection and ends with interventions provided by HCPs at various levels, including dietitians, behavioral therapists, physicians, surgeons, and other professionals [50].

8. Conclusion

In this book chapter, we embarked on a comprehensive exploration of the multifaceted landscape of obesity, delving into its burden, consequences, current management approaches, and the pivotal role of multidisciplinary care. Our exploration of the complex relationship between biology, behavior, and societal factors uncovered the impact of obesity on physical and mental health.

From the epidemiological rise of obesity to its profound consequences on cardiovascular health, mental well-being, and societal structures, it became evident that obesity extends far beyond a mere issue of body weight. The economic burdens, workplace implications, and the perpetuation of a cycle of chronic diseases underscored the urgency of addressing this global health challenge.

Navigating through different management approaches, we analyzed lifestyle interventions, medications, and surgeries. Each option has its own considerations and effectiveness, emphasizing the need for personalized treatment plans.

In our exploration of multidisciplinary management, we emphasized the indispensable roles of healthcare professionals from diverse fields—physicians, nurses, dietitians, psychologists, physical therapists, and more. The collaborative efforts of these professionals create a holistic framework, addressing not only the physical aspects of obesity but also the psychological and behavioral components crucial for sustained success.

As we conclude this chapter, we stand at the intersection of challenges and opportunities in the realm of obesity. The path forward demands a united front—researchers, healthcare professionals, policymakers, and communities—to unravel the complexities of obesity and forge innovative solutions. With a commitment to multidisciplinary care, a deep understanding of the social determinants at play, and a focus on prevention and early intervention, we can envision a future where the burden of obesity is mitigated, and individuals thrive in both physical and mental well-being.

As we continue working toward a healthier world, our combined efforts can bring about significant change, freeing ourselves from the weight of obesity and building a society where everyone can enjoy a lively and fulfilling life.

Author details

Maryam Alkhatry
Division of Gastroenterology and Endoscopy, Ibrahim Bin Hamad Obaidullah Hospital (IBHO), Emirates Health Services, Ras Al Khaimah, United Arab Emirates

*Address all correspondence to: dr.maryam.alkhatry@gmail.com

References

[1] Tiwari A, Balasundaram P. Public health considerations regarding obesity. StatPearls. 2023. Available from: https://www.ncbi.nlm.nih.gov/books/NBK572122/

[2] The Lancet Gastroenterology & Hepatology. Obesity: Another ongoing pandemic. The Lancet Gastroenterology & Hepatology. 2021;**6**:411

[3] Obesity and overweight. Available from: https://www.who.int/news-room/fact-sheets/detail/obesity-and-overweight

[4] Blüher M. Obesity: Global epidemiology and pathogenesis. Nature Reviews Endocrinology. 2019;**15**:288-298. Available from: https://www.nature.com/articles/s41574-019-0176-8

[5] Rosen H. Is obesity a disease or a behavior abnormality? Did the AMA get it right? Missouri Medicine. 2014;**111**:104. Available from: /pmc/articles/PMC6179496/

[6] Bray GA, Kim KK, Wilding JPH. Obesity: A chronic relapsing progressive disease process. A position statement of the world obesity federation. Obesity Reviews. 2017;**18**:715-723. Available from: https://onlinelibrary.wiley.com/doi/full/10.1111/obr.12551

[7] Safaei M, Sundararajan EA, Driss M, Boulila W, Shapi'i A. A systematic literature review on obesity: Understanding the causes & consequences of obesity and reviewing various machine learning approaches used to predict obesity. Computers in Biology and Medicine. 2021;**136**:104754

[8] International Federation for the Surgery of Obesity and Metabolic Diseases (IFSO) and World Gastroenterology Organisation. Guidelines on Obesity. 2023. Available from: https://www.worldgastroenterology.org/UserFiles/file/guidelines/obesity-english-2022.pdf

[9] Abdulla ZARA, Almahmood HO, Alghasra RR, Alherz ZAS, Alsharifa HAG, Qamber SJ, et al. Prevalence and associated factors of binge eating disorder among Bahraini youth and young adults: A cross-sectional study in a self-selected convenience sample. Journal of Eating Disorders. 2023;**11**:1-10. Available from: https://jeatdisord.biomedcentral.com/articles/10.1186/s40337-022-00726-3

[10] McCuen-Wurst C, Ruggieri M, Allison KC. Disordered eating and obesity: Associations between binge eating-disorder, night-eating syndrome, and weight-related co-morbidities. Annals of the New York Academy of Sciences. 2018;**1411**:96. Available from: /pmc/articles/PMC5788730/

[11] Powell-Wiley TM, Poirier P, Burke LE, Després JP, Gordon-Larsen P, Lavie CJ, et al. Obesity and cardiovascular disease: A scientific statement from the American Heart Association. Circulation. 2021;**143**:e984. Available from: /pmc/articles/PMC8493650/

[12] Hossain P, Kawar B, El Nahas M. Obesity and diabetes in the developing world--a growing challenge. The New England Journal of Medicine. 2007;**356**:213-215. Available from: https://pubmed.ncbi.nlm.nih.gov/17229948/

[13] International Diabetes Federation. IDF Diabetes Atlas.... - Google Scholar. Available from: https://scholar.google.com/scholar?hl=en&q=International+Diabetes+Federation.+IDF+Diabetes+Atlas.+9th+ed.+Brussels%2C+Belgium%

3A+International+Diabetes+Federation%3B+2019.#d=gs_cit&t=1705953912877&u=%2Fscholar%3Fq%3Dinfo%3AGoa9NZBfdCIJ%3Ascholar.google.com%2F%26output%3Dcite%26scirp%3D0%26hl%3Den

[14] Pati S, Irfan W, Jameel A, Ahmed S, Shahid RK. Obesity and cancer: A current overview of epidemiology, pathogenesis, outcomes, and management. Cancers (Basel). 2023;**15**(2):485. Available from: /pmc/articles/PMC9857053/

[15] Luppino FS, De Wit LM, Bouvy PF, Stijnen T, Cuijpers P, Penninx BWJH, et al. Overweight, obesity, and depression: A systematic review and meta-analysis of longitudinal studies. Archives of General Psychiatry. 2010;**67**:220-229. Available from: https://pubmed.ncbi.nlm.nih.gov/20194822/

[16] Ricca V, Castellini G, Lo Sauro C, Ravaldi C, Lapi F, Mannucci E, et al. Correlations between binge eating and emotional eating in a sample of overweight subjects. Appetite. 2009;**53**:418-421. Available from: https://pubmed.ncbi.nlm.nih.gov/19619594/

[17] Puhl RM, Heuer CA. The stigma of obesity: A review and update. Obesity (Silver Spring). 2009;**17**:941-964. Available from: https://pubmed.ncbi.nlm.nih.gov/19165161/

[18] Weschenfelder J, Bentley J, Himmerich H, Weschenfelder J, Bentley J, Himmerich H. Physical and mental health consequences of obesity in women. Adipose Tissue. 2018. Available from: https://www.intechopen.com/chapters/59223

[19] Cawley J, Meyerhoefer C. The medical care costs of obesity: An instrumental variables approach. Journal of Health Economics. 2012;**31**:219-230. Available from: https://pubmed.ncbi.nlm.nih.gov/22094013/

[20] Gates DM, Succop P, Brehm BJ, Gillespie GL, Sommers BD. Obesity and presenteeism: The impact of body mass index on workplace productivity. Journal of Occupational and Environmental Medicine. 2008;**50**:39-45. Available from: https://pubmed.ncbi.nlm.nih.gov/18188080/

[21] Noncommunicable Diseases Progress Monitor. 2017. Available from: https://www.who.int/publications/i/item/9789241513029

[22] Afshin A, Forouzanfar MH, Reitsma MB, Sur P, Estep K, Lee A, et al. Health effects of overweight and obesity in 195 countries over 25 years. The New England Journal of Medicine. 2017;**377**:13-27. Available from: https://pubmed.ncbi.nlm.nih.gov/28604169/

[23] Bentham J, Di Cesare M, Bilano V, Bixby H, Zhou B, Stevens GA, et al. Worldwide trends in body-mass index, underweight, overweight, and obesity from 1975 to 2016: A pooled analysis of 2416 population-based measurement studies in 128·9 million children, adolescents, and adults. The Lancet. 2017;**390**:2627-2642. Available from: http://www.thelancet.com/article/S0140673617321293/fulltext

[24] Lobstein T, Jackson-Leach R, Moodie ML, Hall KD, Gortmaker SL, Swinburn BA, et al. Child and adolescent obesity: Part of a bigger picture. Lancet. 2015;**385**:2510. Available from: /pmc/articles/PMC4594797/

[25] Abusnana S, Fargaly M, Alfardan SH, Al Hammadi FH, Bashier A, Kaddaha G, et al. Clinical practice recommendations for the Management of Obesity in the United Arab Emirates. Obesity Facts. 2018;**11**:413-428

[26] Fox A, Feng W, Asal V. What is driving global obesity trends? Globalization or "modernization"?

Globalization and Health. 2019;**15**:1-16. Available from: https://globalizationandhealth.biomedcentral.com/articles/10.1186/s12992-019-0457-y

[27] Semlitsch T, Stigler FL, Jeitler K, Horvath K, Siebenhofer A. Management of overweight and obesity in primary care—A systematic overview of international evidence-based guidelines. Obesity Reviews. 2019;**20**:1218-1230

[28] Garvey WT, Mechanick JI, Brett EM, Garber AJ, Hurley DL, Jastreboff AM, et al. American Association of Clinical Endocrinologists and American College of endocrinology comprehensive clinical practice guidelines for medical care of patients with obesity. Endocrine Practice. 2016;**22**:1-203

[29] Wharton S, Lau DCW, Vallis M, Sharma AM, Biertho L, Campbell-Scherer D, et al. Obesity in adults: A clinical practice guideline. Canadian Medical Association Journal. 2020;**192**:E875-E891

[30] Eisenberg D, Shikora SA, Aarts E, Aminian A, Angrisani L, Cohen RV, et al. 2022 American Society of Metabolic and Bariatric Surgery (ASMBS) and International Federation for the Surgery of Obesity and Metabolic Disorders (IFSO) indications for metabolic and bariatric surgery. Obesity Surgery. 2023;**33**:3-14

[31] Abu Dayyeh BK, Bazerbachi F, Vargas EJ, Sharaiha RZ, Thompson CC, Thaemert BC, et al. Endoscopic sleeve gastroplasty for treatment of class 1 and 2 obesity (MERIT): A prospective, multicentre, randomised trial. The Lancet. 2022;**400**:441-451

[32] Neff KJ, Olbers T, le Roux CW. Bariatric surgery: The challenges with candidate selection, individualizing treatment and clinical outcomes. BMC Medicine. 2013;**11**:8. Available from: https://pubmed.ncbi.nlm.nih.gov/23302153/

[33] Picot J, Jones J, Colquitt J, Gospodarevskaya E, Loveman E, Baxter L, et al. The clinical effectiveness and cost-effectiveness of bariatric (weight loss) surgery for obesity: A systematic review and economic evaluation. Health Technology Assessment. 2009;**13**(41):1-iv

[34] Goyal H, Kopel J, Perisetti A, Mann R, Ali A, Tharian B, et al. Endobariatric procedures for obesity: Clinical indications and available options. Therapeutic Advances in Gastrointestinal Endoscopy. 2021;**14**:263177452098462

[35] Sullivan S, Kumar N, Edmundowicz SA, Abu Dayyeh BK, Jonnalagadda SS, Larsen M, et al. ASGE position statement on endoscopic bariatric therapies in clinical practice. Gastrointestinal Endoscopy. 2015;**82**:767-772

[36] Butryn ML, Webb V, Wadden TA. Behavioral treatment of obesity. The Psychiatric Clinics of North America. 2011;**34**:841-859. Available from: https://pubmed.ncbi.nlm.nih.gov/22098808/

[37] Jensen MD, Ryan DH, Apovian CM, Ard JD, Comuzzie AG, Donato KA, et al. 2013 AHA/ACC/TOS guideline for the management of overweight and obesity in adults: A report of the American College of Cardiology/American Heart Association Task Force on Practice Guidelines and The Obesity Society. Circulation. 2014;**129**. Available from: https://pubmed.ncbi.nlm.nih.gov/24222017/

[38] Pagoto S, Schneider KL, Whited MC, Oleski JL, Merriam P, Appelhans B, et al. Randomized controlled trial of behavioral treatment for comorbid obesity and depression in women: The

be active trial. International Journal of Obesity. 2013;**37**:1427-1434. Available from: https://pubmed.ncbi.nlm.nih.gov/23459323/

[39] Swift DL, Johannsen NM, Lavie CJ, Earnest CP, Church TS. The role of exercise and physical activity in weight loss and maintenance. Progress in Cardiovascular Diseases. 2014;**56**:441-447. Available from: https://pubmed.ncbi.nlm.nih.gov/24438736/

[40] Wadden TA, Butryn ML, Hong PS, Tsai AG. Behavioral treatment of obesity in patients encountered in primary care settings: A systematic review. Journal of the American Medical Association. 2014;**312**:1779-1791. Available from: https://pubmed.ncbi.nlm.nih.gov/25369490/

[41] Hazlehurst JM, Logue J, Parretti HM, Abbott S, Brown A, Pournaras DJ, et al. Developing integrated clinical pathways for the management of clinically severe adult obesity: A critique of NHS England policy. Current Obesity Reports. 2020;**9**:530-543

[42] Curry SJ, Krist AH, Owens DK, Barry MJ, Caughey AB, Davidson KW, et al. Behavioral weight loss interventions to prevent obesity-related morbidity and mortality in adults. Journal of the American Medical Association. 2018;**320**:1163

[43] Alkharaiji M, Anyanwagu U, Donnelly R, Idris I. Tier 3 specialist weight management service and pre-bariatric multicomponent weight management programmes for adults with obesity living in the UK: A systematic review. Endocrinology, Diabetes & Metabolism. 2019;**2**:e00042

[44] Blackburn GL, Greenberg I, McNamara A, Rooks D, Fischer S, Day K. The multidisciplinary approach to weight loss: Defining the roles of the necessary providers : Bariatric Times [Internet]. [Cited 2024 Feb 21]. Available from: https://bariatrictimes.com/the-multidisciplinary-approach-to-weight-loss-defining-the-roles-of-the-necessary-providers/

[45] Yu B, Chen Y, Qin H, Chen Q, Wang J, Chen P. Using multi-disciplinary teams to treat obese patients helps improve clinical efficacy: The general practitioner's perspective. American Journal of Translational Research. 2021;**13**:2571-2580

[46] Zolotarjova J, ten Velde G, Vreugdenhil ACE. Effects of multidisciplinary interventions on weight loss and health outcomes in children and adolescents with morbid obesity. Obesity Reviews. 2018;**19**:931-946

[47] Orlando G, Gervasi R, Luppino IM, Vitale M, Amato B, Silecchia G, et al. The role of a multidisciplinary approach in the choice of the best surgery approach in a super-super-obesity case. International Journal of Surgery. 2014;**12**:S103-S106

[48] Kelley CP, Sbrocco G, Sbrocco T. Behavioral modification for the management of obesity. Primary Care: Clinics in Office Practice. 2016;**43**:159-175

[49] Swancutt D, Tarrant M, Pinkney J. How group-based interventions can improve services for people with severe obesity. Current Obesity Reports. 2019;**8**:333-339

[50] Fitch AK, Bays HE. Obesity definition, diagnosis, bias, standard operating procedures (SOPs), and telehealth: An Obesity Medicine Association (OMA) Clinical Practice Statement (CPS) 2022. Obesity Pillars. 2022;**1**:100004

Chapter 6

The Badly Behaving Brain: How Ultra-Processed Food Addiction Thwarts Sustained Weight Loss

Susan Peirce Thompson and Andrew Kurt Thaw

Abstract

Global obesity rates continue to rise, despite billions spent annually on weight loss. Sustained success is rare; recidivism is the most common feature of weight loss attempts. According to the DSM-5 criteria for substance use disorders, the pattern of ultra-processed food (UPF) overconsumption is best characterized as an addiction. There is significant overlap in how UPF and drugs of abuse impact many brain systems. Over time, neurological changes result in overpowering cravings, insatiable hunger, and a willpower gap. The Yale Food Addiction Scale 2.0 is a validated and widely used tool for the diagnosis of UPF addiction. Research on treatment is nascent, but two weight loss approaches that directly target addiction, GLP-1 agonists and Bright Line Eating, both decrease hunger and cravings and result in significantly greater sustained weight loss than other methods. Addressing addiction is an avenue to weight loss that warrants further study.

Keywords: ultra-processed food addiction, UPF addiction, food addiction, DSM-5 substance use disorder criteria, dopamine downregulation, leptin resistance, impulse control, cue reactivity, GLP-1 agonists, semaglutide, wegovy, ozempic, bright line eating, abstinence-based treatment, yale food addiction scale, weight loss

1. Introduction

The World Health Organization declared obesity to be a global epidemic in 1997 [1]. In 2013, the Member States of the World Health Assembly unanimously agreed to adopt the target that rises in childhood, adolescent, and adult obesity should be halted at 2010 levels by 2025 [2]. But the rise has not abated; instead, we are on pace to see a doubling of obesity by 2025 [3]. It is now projected that by 2035, one half of all people worldwide will be living with overweight or obesity [4]. Co-occurring with this rise in obesity has been a steady increase in UPF consumption [5]. Mounting evidence indicates that these trends are related [6–8].

Meanwhile, sustained weight loss is rare [9]. Dieters repeatedly "fall off" and "get back on" the wagon just like smokers and others with a substance use disorder who are trying to quit [10]. The extremely poor results of nearly every type of weight loss approach do not make sense, given how motivated people are to not be overweight [11] and how much time and money they spend to lose weight [12].

Even people attempting to lose weight for a needed surgery or to avoid a second limb amputation due to type 2 diabetes are not likely to be successful [13, 14]. Many researchers are concluding that addiction is the framework that best explains this pattern of behavior [15].

Since there is little consensus, currently, regarding whether the proper term should be "food addiction," "processed food addiction," "ultra-processed food addiction," or something else (like "eating addiction"), in this article we will use these terms interchangeably, while defaulting to "ultra-processed food addiction" or UPFA. Irrespective of the term used, the reality is, as one group of researchers put it, that "the neurological evidence for overeating as an addiction is extensive" [15]. In this chapter we will review this evidence, and the implications it has, both for a person trying to lose weight and a global society trying to support people in being healthy.

First, we will discuss new research on the relationship between UPF and weight gain. Then we will outline the many brain changes that co-occur with repeated intake of all drugs of abuse, including UPF. We will discuss fMRI research that sheds light on the specific elements of UPF that are driving the addictive response, versus those contributing to overeating more broadly. Then we will outline the three main phenomena that impact people trying to lose weight, which together hijack sound reasoning and create the "badly behaving brain" that thwarts long-term adherence to a healthy eating regimen: overpowering cravings, insatiable hunger, and the willpower gap.

The second half of the chapter will explore the diagnosis and treatment of UPFA, beginning with a review of the diagnostic criteria for substance use disorders in the DSM-5 and the evidence that excess food consumption meets these criteria. We will discuss research on the Yale Food Addiction Scale 2.0 and data showing the extent to which UPFA correlates with BMI, various eating disorders, and type 2 diabetes. Then we will discuss treatment options for those afflicted. Interestingly, the two current weight loss approaches that most directly target addiction, GLP-1 weight loss drugs and Bright Line Eating, are the two non-surgical approaches with the highest rates of sustained weight loss. Finally, we will explore eight distinct reasons why UPFA is uniquely challenging and difficult to overcome.

2. Ultra-processed food addiction (UPFA)

The question of whether UPF consumption is a causal contributor to the obesity pandemic is logically distinct from the question of whether UPF is addictive. Research shows that both are true [6, 16], and, of course, because many of the features of addiction—like an inability to control consumption, including difficulty quitting or moderating—drive UPF overconsumption, these phenomena are deeply related. We will first address the relationship between the processing of food and its impact on human weight.

2.1 UPF and weight gain

Until recently, it was unclear that the processing of food was a driver of human weight gain, separate and apart from its energy density, sugar content, lack of fiber, or the like. But in 2019, Hall and colleagues published a randomized controlled trial of ad libitum food intake in 20 weight-stable adults (average BMI 27) who spent 4 weeks in a metabolic ward [17]. They were randomly assigned to eat either an ultra-processed diet or a diet of entirely unprocessed foods for 2 weeks; the groups switched diets for the remaining 2 weeks. Importantly, the diets were matched for presented calories, energy density, protein, carbohydrate, fat, sugar, sodium, and fiber. Subjects could eat as much as they wanted from the diet they were on, in a structured setting of meals and snacks. Over the 2 weeks, subjects on the ultra-processed diet ate an average of 508 extra calories daily and gained significant weight, while subjects on the unprocessed diet lost significant weight. Subjects did not report preferring the ultra-processed diet nor enjoying it over the unprocessed diet [17, 18]. Despite the small sample size, the tightly controlled conditions of this experiment shed light on the power of food processing, in and of itself, to drive overconsumption and weight gain. Further evidence of the impact of UPF consumption on weight gain can be found in the increase of overweight and obesity as fast food outlets and snack foods become more available within a population [18, 19].

The impact of UPF consumption on weight is sobering, considering that two-thirds of the calories that children and adolescents consume in the USA today are UPF [20, 21] and that the prevalence of UPF is rapidly increasing worldwide [19]. For example, in China alone, over 2000 new McDonalds, Pizza Hut, and KFC outlets opened over the most recent calendar year (2023)—an average of one new fast food restaurant every 5 hours [22]. Given that the constraints of food delivery and storage result in ultra-processing being required to optimize profits, these trends are not likely to decline anytime soon [18].

2.2 UPF and addiction

The earliest studies on the dopamine response curve and addiction in rats did not use alcohol, opioids, stimulants, caffeine, or tobacco as the addictive agent, they used glucose [23]. Results showed that dopamine receptor downregulation occurred after repeated exposure, resulting in cravings. Thereafter, cues that predicted the addictive reward caused a spike in dopamine, while actual delivery of the addictive agent produced less and less of an effect [23, 24]. Sweet taste alone drives an addictive response: consumption of a sweet beverage activates dopaminergic neurons in the midbrain and then the ventral striatum, wiring the brain to remember the cues associated with that reward [25]. Rats, when not hungry nor thirsty, who are offered a forced-choice between a bolus of cocaine or some sips of sweetened water (whether sweetened with saccharin or sucrose) so strongly prefer the sweet taste that they nearly ignore the cocaine [26].

In humans, an fMRI study with a crossover design explored whether it was sugar, fat, or both, that drives the addictive response in the brain. Subjects were given a sample of a chocolate milkshake matched for flavor but containing high vs. low sugar and high vs. low fat in a 2x2 design. The presence of high sugar, but not fat, activated the insula and the associated reward centers of the brain [27]. Salt drives passive overconsumption of calories but not an addictive response [28]. But foods containing flour, and other forms of glucose unmitigated by significant fiber (like potato chips or popcorn), repeatedly score among the most addictive foods [29]. Combinations of ultra-processed carbohydrates and fats appear to be the most rewarding [30].

As with all addictions, key features of the neurological changes associated with UPFA include dopamine receptor downregulation [31–33] as well as opiate [34–36], endocannabinoid [37, 38], and serotonin [39, 40] receptor downregulation. People with a substance use disorder tend to experience reduced inhibition around their drug of choice, and this holds true for UPFA and UPF [41]. People with a drug addiction experience an increased stress response, specifically heightened release of corticotropin releasing factor; this same response has been found in those addicted to UPF [42]. Many entire textbooks and review articles catalog the broad and consistent body of literature, now totaling thousands of articles, accepting that UPF is addictive and is associated with the same pattern of neurological and behavioral changes as drugs of abuse [16, 43–46].

Heightened cue reactivity, especially in early abstinence, is another common feature of both drug addiction and UPFA [47]. Much like addictive drug use, the consumption of UPF sensitizes dopaminergic systems [48]. Thus, environmental cues associated with UPF can both evoke cravings and initiate episodes of binge consumption [49]. In studies examining the neural response to food cues, the brain areas known to be involved in cue reactivity in response to drugs showed higher activation with UPF compared to minimally processed foods [50]. In addition, studies using MRI revealed that both food and smoking cues were associated with increased activation in almost identical areas—namely the left amygdala, bilateral insula, bilateral orbitofrontal cortex, and striatum [51, 52]. A wide and heavily replicated literature shows that the cue reactivity and cue-induced cravings produced by drug and food cues are nearly identical [53].

Finally, specific impairments in cognitive function are found with extensive use of both addictive drugs and UPF. For example, exposure to UPF early in life predicts long-term deficits in both learning and memory [54]. In addition, childhood obesity is associated with cognitive deficits that may last into adulthood [55–57]. In adults, UPF consumption impairs cognition [58, 59], and binge eating is associated with deficits in attention, memory, and inhibition [60].

3. The badly behaving brain

Millions of people are spending time, money, and significant effort trying to lose weight, only to fail repeatedly. The average dieter makes four or five new attempts each year [61]. Many experience the strange phenomenon where they launch a new attempt with confidence and excitement, watch it work awhile, and then find themselves heavier than they were before, without a clear idea of what made it all unravel [62]. Three phenomena—all related to UPF consumption and how it impacts the brain—are driving this pattern of behavior and experience. We call them overpowering cravings, insatiable hunger, and the willpower gap.

3.1 Overpowering cravings

Dopamine downregulation is the neural substrate of cravings [63]. Initial exposure to an addictive substance causes a spike in dopamine [64]. The dopamine response to UPF is not as large as the dopamine response to heroin or cocaine; it's more like the response to alcohol or tobacco [65]. Yet, it is larger than the dopamine response to broccoli or blueberries [66–68], and, over time, it causes downregulation of the dopamine receptors [69]. This, combined with the downregulation of serotonin, endocannabinoid, and opiate receptors that also occurs with UPFA [34–40], leaves a person in a state of discomfort and malaise unless and until they consume more UPF to get relief [70]. In other words, cravings are both an effort, driven by positive reinforcement, to experience the release of dopamine, and an effort, driven by negative reinforcement, to seek relief from a now-unpleasant baseline state [71, 72]. Behavioral examples of such cravings are: driving across town for a specific food to scratch a specific itch or wandering through grocery store aisles (or scrolling through food delivery apps or staring into the refrigerator) wondering what will "hit the spot."

What makes the cravings "overpowering" is that, with the development of UPFA, decision making is impaired [58, 59] and inhibition is reduced [41], leaving the prefrontal cortex unable to effectively counteract the urges generated by the reward centers of the midbrain [73]. In addition, as addiction develops, the wanting of UPF increases while the liking of it decreases [74], leaving a person in a chronic state of yearning that is never satisfied. Over time, as UPF consumption leads to depression and increased days of poor mental health [75, 76], this pattern becomes increasingly difficult to break.

3.2 Insatiable hunger

Hunger is thought of as a helpful physiological drive, a signal that more fuel is needed. Someone starts a meal hungry, and over the course of the meal, the hunger diminishes or perhaps goes away entirely [77, 78]. The modern hunger that accompanies UPFA, however, is "insatiable" precisely because it does not go away over the course of a meal [79–81]. People eat an entire dinner and then, still wanting more, sit on the couch with a family-sized bag of chips. Chips gone, they go to the freezer for ice cream. This is insatiable hunger.

Under normal circumstances, leptin triggers the ventromedial nucleus of the hypothalamus to signal that adequate fuel has been consumed, effectively regulating energy homeostasis [82]. Both current consumption of fuel and overall increased adiposity trigger leptin release from fat cells [83]. Several factors result in leptin resistance, the inability of the hypothalamus to sense circulating leptin and register its signal: high baseline insulin levels [84], high triglycerides [85] and inflammation, especially of the ventromedial nucleus of the hypothalamus [86]. Since UPF consumption causes all three [87–89], regular UPF consumption, with or without addiction, can result in insatiable hunger. This is confirmed by clinical experience—many people in modern society report that they never, or rarely, feel full [90, 91].

UPF also often delivers a mismatch between what it promises in the mouth and what it delivers to the stomach, with non-nutritive sweeteners signaling a big bolus of calories that never arrives and flavor profiles cueing the stomach to expect, for example, large amounts of fat from a fat-free product. Over time, this disparity also contributes to insatiable hunger [92, 93].

When leptin was discovered in 1994, pharmaceutical companies spent small fortunes attempting to patent the perfect leptin pill or injection that would take away the desire to eat [94]. But because the problem is leptin resistance, not leptin deficiency, no amount of exogenous leptin produces satiety [95]. Very low levels of leptin signal starvation, an urgent situation causing a cascade of hormonal changes that compels the consumption of large amounts of fuel [96]. Given that leptin resistance mimics this state in the brain [97], the resulting insatiable hunger makes perfect sense. Furthermore, leptin does not just act on the hypothalamus, it also acts on the brain stem [98], making prolonged calorie restriction in the face of insatiable hunger about as doable as holding your breath while slowly climbing a long flight of stairs.

3.3 The willpower gap

In an experience sampling study published in 2012, Hofmann and colleagues concluded that people are resisting temptations an average of 4 hours per day, that they give in to their temptations about half the time, and that the urge to eat is the number one temptation people are trying to resist [99]. Further, resisting temptations, making decisions, and regulating emotions all require effective functioning of the anterior cingulate cortex [100], which after 15 minutes of effort is depleted to the point of significantly diminished functioning [101, 102], resulting in a marked inability to restrain impulses—a willpower gap. This willpower gap impacts people without an addiction to UPF (and may help to explain the significant rates of overweight and obesity, and dieting recidivism, in those populations), but for people with UPFA, several additional factors are operative. First, as previously discussed, both inhibition [41] and decision making are significantly impaired [58, 59], widening the willpower gap. And second, cue reactivity is stronger, especially during early abstinence [47], making the person with UPFA extra sensitive to the myriad temporal, spatial, visual, auditory, and olfactory cues to eat in the modern obesogenic environment [103], greatly increasing the frequency of encountering the willpower gap throughout the day. Astute bariatric surgeons, dieticians, and general practitioners have sensed for decades that increased information or education alone is not the solution to the obesity pandemic, as they have little lasting effect [104]. When it comes to weight loss, the willpower gap helps explain the chasm between knowledge and volition on the one hand, and sustained execution on the other.

4. The diagnosis of ultra-processed food addiction

For both individuals wanting support and clinicians trying to help them, effective and accurate diagnosis is the first step in the treatment journey. There are dozens, if not hundreds, of online quizzes and self-assessments to help someone get a sense of whether they have an addictive relationship with sugar, UPF, or food more generally, but there is currently only one validated diagnostic tool: the Yale Food Addiction Scale (YFAS) [105], now in its second iteration (YFAS 2.0) [106], discussed in greater detail below. The YFAS 2.0 is based on the diagnostic criteria for substance use disorders in the DSM-5 section on Substance-Related Addictive Disorders [107, 108], which we will review next.

4.1 The DSM-5 criteria for substance use disorders

In the DSM-5, there are 11 criteria for a substance use disorder. Diagnosis is given along a continuum, with the presence of 2–3 symptoms indicating a mild disorder, 4–5 symptoms a moderate disorder, and 6 or more symptoms a severe disorder. In each case, however, the pattern of use must also lead to "clinically significant impairment or distress" [108]. Research shows that the use and abuse of UPF meets each of these 11 criteria, with examples and prevalence as follows.

4.1.1 Criterion 1: consuming more than intended

UPF is eaten in larger amounts or over a longer period than was intended.

Consuming more UPF than intended is a common, perhaps even universal, experience [109]; in fact, irresistibility and overconsumption are features that UPF manufacturers tout, as with the Lay's potato chip slogan, "Betcha can't eat just one!" With UPFA, this overconsumption can reach levels that cause significant impairment and distress [76, 110]. Increases in diagnosis of UPFA correlate with increases in the frequency of binge episodes [106]. Because UPFA is associated with gradually impaired impulse control [41, 60], this symptom is progressive [16]. Prevalence: in the general population, 19.3% of people have this symptom [106].

4.1.2 Criterion 2: desiring yet unable to cut down, stop, or stay stopped

There is a persistent desire or unsuccessful efforts to cut down or control UPF consumption.

On the surface, this criterion seems easily met by the vast majority of people, as it is plausible to imagine that most everyone, at one time or another, has attempted to diet or control their food intake. However, very few diets require abstinence from all UPF; indeed, the sale and distribution of branded UPF is a core component of many diets. Further, attempting to stop consuming an addictive, injurious substance is not the same as attempting to lose weight [111, 112]. Yet, market research shows that the average dieter makes four or five new attempts each year, highlighting the difficulty people have in staying "on the wagon" once they stop eating certain foods [61]. The evidence is clear that UPF is not only difficult to resist, it is also specifically engineered to enhance palatability and desire [113]. Prevalence: in the general population, 25% of people have this symptom [106].

4.1.3 Criterion 3: significant time spent

A great deal of time is spent in activities necessary to obtain UPF, consume UPF, and recover from its effects.

Clearly, if the average dieter is making four or five attempts to lose weight each year, they are spending significant time (and likely significant money) preparing for, launching, failing at, and recovering from their attempts to control their food consumption [61]. People also report spending a lot of time driving to get specific foods, significant time eating certain foods throughout the day, and a lot of time feeling tired and sluggish from overeating [114]. In the later stages of UPFA, the impact can expand to nearly 24 hours each day if disrupted sleep and night eating infiltrate the overnight hours and mental obsession with procuring and consuming UPF and managing weight and health symptoms dominate during the day [115]. Even among those with UPFA who do not have a weight problem, the time spent obsessing about what they have eaten or not eaten, what they plan to eat or not eat, and whether they are on their food plan or off their food plan can nearly consume the day [116]. Prevalence: in the general population, 18.7% of people have this symptom [106].

4.1.4 Criterion 4: craving

Craving, or a strong desire or urge to consume UPF.

Of all food, UPF has the highest likelihood of being consumed in an addictive manner and the highest likelihood of being craved [117]. Not only does the experience of craving UPF parallel the experience of craving drugs of abuse, but the activation pattern in neural structures associated with craving shows significant overlap across various addictive substances, including UPF [52, 118]. In self-reported data, overeating is linked to more intense and frequent instances of food craving among individuals with binge eating disorder, bulimia nervosa, and obesity [119]. Similarly, food addiction, as gauged by the Yale Food Addiction Scale, correlates with elevated self-reported food craving [120]. Thus, the criterion of frequently experiencing craving or a strong urge to consume a substance can be extended to UPF and represents an observable symptom in the context of UPFA. Prevalence: in the general population, 20.3% of people have this symptom [106].

4.1.5 Criterion 5: failure to fulfill roles

Recurrent UPF consumption resulting in a failure to fulfill major role obligations at work, school, or home.

There is a significant literature confirming that obesity hampers people's ability to fulfill their role obligations at work, school, and home [121], and given the correlation between UPFA and obesity [106, 122], some of that impact is likely stemming from addiction. But even people who are not carrying excess weight can struggle to perform their major role obligations due to the impact of food obsession and the negative consequences of overconsuming UPF such as remorse, shame, sluggishness, and a desire to isolate [123]. In the general population, the prevalence of this symptom is 21.5% [106], which means that more than one in five people is agreeing that, over the prior 12 months, "My overeating got in the way of me taking care of my family or doing household chores" and "I didn't do well at work or school because I was eating too much" [124].

4.1.6 Criterion 6: use despite social or interpersonal problems

Continued UPF consumption despite having persistent or recurrent social or interpersonal problems caused or exacerbated by the effects of UPF.

Social and interpersonal challenges manifest distinctly within the realm of eating behavior. Notably, obese individuals report heightened levels of social isolation compared to those with normal weight [125]. While this can be attributed to weight gain accompanying excess consumption of UPF, research indicates a significant connection between interpersonal problems—such as distrust, social insecurity, or hostility—and binge eating behavior, independent of body mass [125, 126]. Experimental research focusing on UPFA and social or interpersonal problems is just emerging and future studies are needed to establish a causal link between the two. Preliminary data indicate that others' disapproval of food choices and eating behaviors contributes to interpersonal conflict [117]. Prevalence: in the general population, 19.4% of people have this symptom [106], which means they agree that they have problems with family and friends because of how much they overeat and their friends and family worry about how much they overeat [127].

4.1.7 Criterion 7: important activities given up

Important social, occupational, or recreational activities are given up or reduced because of UPF consumption.

As noted above, individuals with obesity often report heightened levels of social isolation that may be attributed to body weight, but also to eating behaviors [125]. Disordered eating can also lead to decreases in exercise and other physical activities [128]. Recent findings demonstrate that the obesity epidemic is a direct result of the prevalence of UPF in our diets [129]. Regardless of BMI, people with UPFA endorse statements like: "I eat certain foods so often or in such large amounts that I stop doing other important things like working or spending time with family or friends" and "I avoid work, school, or other activities because I'm afraid I will overeat there" and "I felt so bad about overeating that I didn't do other important things like working or spending time with family or friends" [130]. Prevalence: in the general population, 11.9% of people have this symptom [106].

4.1.8 Criterion 8: hazardous use

Recurrent UPF consumption in situations in which it is physically hazardous.

The symptom of hazardous use typically pertains to the risks associated with intoxication, such as driving or using heavy machinery, or even simpler situations such as crossing a busy street on foot. Clearly, eating does not involve the same level of intoxication as alcohol or opiates. However, a parallel can be drawn with tobacco, where the DSM-5 suggests that this criterion may encompass smoking in bed, posing a fire risk. Extending this analogy, the hazards of UPF consumption include eating while driving, which is known to impair performance and increase crash risks [131–133]. Indeed, approximately one in four people agree that, over the past 12 months, they have been so distracted, either by thinking about food or by eating food, that they could have been hurt (e.g., when driving a car, crossing the street, or operating machinery) [106, 134]. Prevalence: in the general population, 24.8% of people have this symptom [106].

4.1.9 Criterion 9: Use despite physical or emotional consequences

UPF consumption is continued despite knowledge of having a persistent or recurrent physical or psychological problem that is likely to have been caused or exacerbated by UPF.

This particular criterion involves continued excess consumption of UPF despite an acute health condition exacerbated by UPF. This is a relatively widespread phenomenon, as individuals with diabetes often continue to consume excessive sugar despite knowing that it is injurious [135, 136] and individuals who have recently had a medical procedure (such as bariatric surgery) often continue to overeat despite the contraindications [137]. In fact, of people who have just had a limb amputated due to unmanaged type 2 diabetes, 55% will have a second limb amputated within 2 years [14]. Additionally, persons with both UPFA and certain eating disorders with psychologically harmful comorbidities are seen to persist in detrimental eating, resisting dietary recommendations that could potentially reduce their symptoms and accompanying psychological distress [138]. In short, physical and psychological problems are often not sufficient to reduce the consumption of UPF. Prevalence: in the general population, 23.5% of people have this symptom [106].

4.1.10 Criterion 10: tolerance

Tolerance, as defined by either of the following:

a. A need for markedly increased amounts of UPF to achieve intoxication or desired effect.

b. A markedly diminished effect with continued use of the same amount of UPF.

Individuals with UPFA report diminished enjoyment of UPF over time [113]. Considering that psychological changes, as well as physiological and behavioral changes, accompany tolerance [139], a decrease in the subjective reward value of UPF over time is a marker of the development of tolerance. In the general population, 17.4% of people have this symptom [106], which means they agree with statements like, "eating the same amount of food did not give me as much enjoyment as it used to" and, "I needed to eat more and more to get the feelings I wanted from eating" [140].

4.1.11 Criterion 11: withdrawal

Withdrawal, as manifested by either of the following:

a. The characteristic withdrawal syndrome for UPF.

b. UPF (or closely related substances) are taken to relieve or avoid withdrawal symptoms.

Mounting evidence indicates that withdrawal effects are indeed observed with UPF [10, 141]. Specific foods, particularly those highly processed with added sweeteners and fats, exhibit heightened addictive potential [44, 70]. While both behavioral and substance-related factors play significant roles in the addictive process for food, UPFA symptoms more closely align with the criteria for substance use disorder [141], and withdrawal symptoms are a defining feature. Classic withdrawal symptoms such as anxiety, headaches, irritability, and unstable mood appear for many individuals upon decreasing or stopping consumption of UPF [142]. In addition, the time-scale of withdrawal symptoms is the same as for tobacco, opiates, stimulants, and alcohol [142]. Prevalence: in the general population, 29.7% of people have this symptom [106].

4.1.12 The requirement of significant impairment or distress

In the general population, the average person has 2.38 of these 11 symptoms, which would qualify them for a diagnosis of mild UPFA, except that only 12.5% of people in the mild symptom range meet the criteria for a pattern of use that causes "clinically significant impairment or distress," which is also required for diagnosis. In the moderate range of 4–5 symptoms, only 19.6% of people meet this threshold, while in the severe range of 6 or more symptoms, 61.5% of people have significant impairment or distress [106].

There is a significant implication of the "impairment or distress" requirement on weight gain and weight loss trends. The data show that most people in Western society can be said to have *an addictive relationship with food*, as evidenced by manifesting multiple symptoms of UPFA [106], but they will not meet the criteria for an addiction diagnosis because it is not bothering them badly enough or inhibiting their functioning to a significant extent [106]. However, the addictive symptoms may very well be contributing to their weight gain and hindering their efforts to lose weight—and to maintain that weight loss once it is achieved. This would help to explain abysmal weight loss results [9] and widespread diet recidivism [10]. It would also predict that weight loss approaches taking an abstinence-based approach to UPFA, rather than building consumption of UPF into their plans, would be significantly more successful than average. This turns out to be the case, and is the subject of Section 5.

4.2 The Yale food addiction scale

The original Yale Food Addiction Scale (YFAS) to diagnose food addiction was released in 2009 by Yale University's Rudd Center for Food Policy and Obesity [105]. It was a 25-item self-report Likert-scale questionnaire examining eating behaviors over the prior 12 months, based on the DSM-4 criteria for substance dependence. A shorter, modified YFAS (mYFAS) with only 9 items was released in 2014 and was shown to yield similar results to the original [143]. In 2013, a version for children, the YFAS-C, was released [144].

In May of 2013, the DSM-5 was published with significant updates to the DSM-4. The section on Substance Use Disorders was renamed Substance-Related and Addictive Disorders. Substance abuse and substance dependence were combined, and the new substance use disorders diagnosis could now be made along a continuum: mild (2–3 symptoms), moderate (4–5 symptoms), or severe (6–11 symptoms). The symptom of legal consequences was removed and the symptom of craving was added. In 2016, the YFAS 2.0 was released to conform to the new DSM-5 structure and thereby update the instrument to reflect the latest thinking in substance use diagnosis [106]. Shortly thereafter, the mYFAS 2.0 and mYFAS-C 2.0 were released to offer an updated shorter screening tool and an updated version suitable for children, respectively [145, 146].

The YFAS 2.0 was shown to have convergent validity by measuring associations with scores on other instruments assessing problematic eating behaviors such as the Three Factor Eating Questionnaire (TFEQ) disinhibition, TFEQ hunger, current BMI, highest BMI, and frequency of binge eating episodes [106]. Food addiction scores increase with BMI [106]. Discriminant validity was shown by demonstrating that YFAS 2.0 scores are not significantly correlated with TFEQ dietary restraint, as food addiction and dietary restraint are unrelated [106, 147]. Incremental validity was shown using hierarchical multiple regression, looking at YFAS 2.0 scores and binge eating frequency as predictors of BMI. YFAS 2.0 scores predicted BMI above and beyond the contributions of binge eating frequency [106].

A meta-analysis reviewing 6425 abstracts of studies assessing food addiction using the YFAS and its derivatives and including 272 studies in its analysis showed a weighted mean prevalence of food addiction diagnosis of 20% [122], meaning that, in the general population, about 20% of people likely qualify for a diagnosis of UPFA.

4.3 Correlations with eating disorders and weight

Numerous studies show that UPFA is related to, but distinct from, eating disorders [106, 122, 148]. Although the standard deviation is large as findings vary widely, a meta-analysis that calculated weighted pooled averages showed that the prevalence of UPFA, according to the YFAS and its derivatives, is roughly 44% among people with a clinical diagnosis of anorexia nervosa, 48% among people with a clinical diagnosis of bulimia nervosa, and 55% among people with a clinical diagnosis of binge eating disorder [122].

Importantly, UPFA is distinct from obesity and the propensity to gain weight [106, 122]. While UPFA is positively correlated with weight [106], according to a meta-analysis [122], the pooled prevalence of UPFA among people with no weight disorder is 17%, among people with overweight is 24%, among people with obesity is 28%, and among those who have had bariatric surgery is 28%. UPFA is a contributor to weight gain but not the sole driver. In addition, UPFA is strongly associated with type 2 diabetes in a dose-response like manner [149].

5. The treatment of ultra-processed food addiction

The scientific literature on the neurobiological similarity between addictive drugs and UPF as substances of abuse is large [150]. The literature on diagnosis is robust as well [122]. Between the two, several hundred new studies are being published every year, and that number has been increasing dramatically and linearly since 2010 [122]. In comparison, there are still relatively few published studies evaluating the treatment of UPFA [16]. One factor is that it is difficult to treat a condition that is still not formally recognized by the DSM or the ICD, especially since proper treatment, like treatment for drug or alcohol addiction, can be expensive, and governments and insurance companies typically will not cover it. Studies on treatment are also expensive and time consuming. But avenues of treatment do exist, and there is a nascent literature attempting to evaluate the results, which we review below. In addition, there are weight loss approaches that, intentionally or unintentionally, target addiction, and it turns out that they are significantly more effective than other weight loss approaches. We will cover those findings in the following sections as well.

5.1 Treatment centers and food addiction professionals

Perhaps the longest running treatment center for UPFA is Shift Recovery by Acorn, which was founded in the United States in 1993 and offers online and in-person intensive treatment programs for UPFA [151]. Bitten Jonsson Center opened in Sweden in 1999 and offered an inpatient UPFA treatment program until 2005 [152]. MFM in Iceland was founded in 2006 and offers outpatient UPFA treatment [153]. And in the United States, Milestones in Recovery [154] and Turning Point of Tampa [155] both offer inpatient treatment for individuals with co-occurring eating disorders and UPFA.

In 2016, the International School for Food Addiction Counseling and Treatment (INFACT) was established to train professionals in the core functions, clinical guidelines, and best practices of food addiction treatment. Graduates are certified in Europe by the European Certification Board and in the USA by the Addiction Professionals Certification Board as Certified Food Addiction Professionals [156]. The Food Addiction Institute (FAI) aims to advance awareness [157] and the Food Addiction Professionals Network (FAPN) provides clinicians ongoing education and peer support. In addition, many 12-step programs, such as Food Addicts in Recovery Anonymous (FA) offer comprehensive recovery programs for people with UPFA [158]. An individual looking for treatment could reach out to any of these organizations to get help.

Until recently, there was either no data or very little published data on the efficacy of these programs and approaches. But a multi-center study is underway, and their preliminary findings are promising. Across 103 participants receiving treatment from Certified Food Addiction Professionals offering online treatment group programs based in North America, Sweden, and the United Kingdom, results showed that, over 10–14 weeks of treatment, food addiction symptoms went significantly down (as measured by the YFAS 2.0 and the CRAVED instrument which measures symptoms according to the ICD-10 criteria), weight went down slightly (weight loss was not a focus of treatment), and well-being went significantly up [159]. Monthly follow-up sessions are a part of these treatment protocols, and future publications will analyze longer-term data.

5.2 Bariatric surgery

Bariatric surgery is not intended as a treatment for UPFA, but studies have shown that most post-surgical patients do experience initial remission of UPFA symptoms

[160, 161]. Unfortunately, practitioners in the field do not typically observe sustained remission, though no long-term data have yet been published [162]. Studies show that significant weight regain 5–6 years post-operatively affects as many as three-quarters of surgical patients [163] and revision surgery is becoming increasingly common [164]. Two of the most common causes of weight regain post-surgery are thought to be out-of-control eating and a return to previous eating habits [163], indicating that lasting remission of UPFA symptoms after bariatric surgery is not the norm.

5.3 GLP-1 weight loss drugs

Science declared GLP-1 therapies for obesity to be the 2023 Breakthrough of the Year, for both their weight loss results and additional health benefits like reduction in heart attacks, strokes, and liver disease [165]. GLP-1 agonists such as semaglutide (marketed as Ozempic for diabetes and Wegovy for weight loss in the USA) not only help regulate blood sugar in people with diabetes and curb appetite in people with obesity, but they decrease cravings for UPF, cigarettes, alcohol, and other drugs of abuse as well. Over 100 studies in both humans and rodents have demonstrated the effects of GLP-1s on the reward pathways of the brain [166]. These drugs both decrease activity to the left insula, reducing the anticipated reward from eating UPF, and improve activity deficits in the insula, hypothalamus, and orbitofrontal cortex [166].

Clinical trials show that patients taking semaglutide lose approximately 15% of their bodyweight within 1 year [167] and maintain that weight loss at 2 years [168]. Drug use must be continued, or an average of two-thirds of lost weight will be regained within 1 year [169]. The combination of suppressed appetite and reduced addictive cravings on GLP-1 drugs produces weight loss results that are far larger than what standard weight loss approaches produce.

5.4 Bright line eating

Bright Line Eating (BLE) is an online weight-loss program within a food addiction recovery framework that teaches clients to abstain from UPF, eat three meals a day, and engage in ongoing education and peer support [170]. Research shows that, from weeks two through eight on the program, participants' hunger and cravings decrease linearly, reaching an average rating of just 1.4 (on a Likert scale of 1 through 5, with 5 being high) at 8 weeks [171]. The average eight-week weight loss result on BLE is 7.8% of initial body weight [170], the average one-year weight loss result is 16.8% [172], and the average two-year weight loss result is 14.3% [172].

Interestingly, studies show that the process of mastication releases GLP-1 and thus contributes to satiety [173]. UPF is manufactured to require minimal chewing [18, 174] while raw vegetables and many of the other whole foods on the BLE food plan require significant chewing. Research also shows that fiber releases GLP-1 and peptide YY, another satiety hormone [175]. These factors together may play a role in the semaglutide-like appetite-suppression effects of a whole-foods, zero UPF approach to eating.

5.5 The impact of treating UPFA on weight loss

There are relatively few peer-reviewed studies on commercial weight loss programs, and even fewer randomized clinical trials. Results are notoriously poor, so

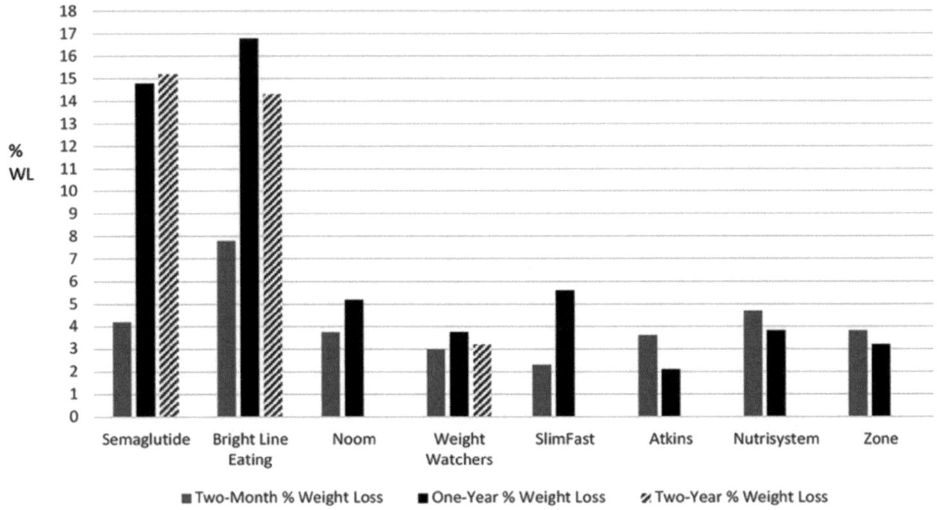

Figure 1.
A comparison of data from twelve peer-reviewed studies reporting weight loss results from semaglutide and various commercial weight loss programs [167, 168, 170, 172, 177–184]. (No studies reporting two-year % weight loss data were found for Noom, SlimFast, Atkins, Nutrisystem, or Zone diets).

there is little commercial benefit to documenting the results [176]. A direct comparison of the studies that do exist is both difficult and problematic due to differences in design, methods, variables measured, and lack of randomized assignment of participants to conditions across studies. However, despite these significant issues, a visual comparison of the weight loss data that do exist yields an interesting pattern. With these caveats in mind, **Figure 1** aggregates data from 12 published papers on commercial weight loss programs and demonstrates a clear demarcation between approaches that allow (or even encourage) the consumption of UPF versus the two approaches that target addiction, whether behaviorally or pharmacologically [167, 168, 170, 172, 177–184].

6. The hardest addiction?

UPF does not deliver a dopamine reward comparable with opiates or stimulants [185], nor are the withdrawal symptoms from UPF as severe as the withdrawal symptoms from most drugs [10, 70], yet, for eight distinct reasons, it could be argued that UPFA is uniquely difficult to overcome.

First, for no other substance addiction is the average age of first exposure so young, nor the rate of early exposure so frequent. Infant formula is UPF, so babies who are formula-fed are exposed to UPF multiple times a day, from birth or shortly thereafter. Even breastfed babies are typically exposed to UPF at around 6 months of age, as UPF cereal is the most commonly recommended first baby food [186]. Regular exposure continues from there, with research showing that 60.6% of infants and 98.3% of toddlers in the USA are consuming added sugars every day [187].

Second, UPFA is the result of a hijacking of neural circuits whose original function was to make the procurement and consumption of calories an organism's top priority. Every other substance addiction hijacks these same circuits, but no organism's brain prioritizes the procurement of alcohol, cocaine, or tobacco the way it prioritizes the consumption of energy dense, highly rewarding food.

Third, UPFA is a substance addiction [188] that has so many features of a behavioral addiction (such as shopping or gambling) that it is often categorized as such [189], meaning that the process of eating is rewarding and cue-laden enough to carry the addiction on its own. One could effectively argue that UPFA is actually both a substance addiction and a behavioral addiction, as people addicted to UPF often eat excessive quantities of regular foods and demonstrate an addiction to the process of eating itself [190].

Fourth, and perhaps most perniciously, UPFA is unique among all addictions in causing a health-deteriorating side effect (excess weight) that, when addressed, re-triggers the original addiction. Alcohol causes liver damage, but when the liver heals, it does not release a cascade of hormones that cause intense cravings for alcohol. Smoking causes lung damage, but when the lungs heal, nicotine cravings are not a direct result. But weight loss causes a barrage of hormonal changes that lead to overeating and weight regain [191], meaning the person with UPFA who is carrying excess weight is caught in a pernicious cycle unlike anything else in the addiction-recovery landscape.

Fifth, unique among all substance addictions, we cannot simply stop eating. People addicted to alcohol, nicotine, caffeine, or drugs can abstain completely, and feel highly confident that they are successfully abstaining, as the category definitions are quite clear. But the person addicted to UPF must continue eating on a daily basis, which raises the question, at every eating opportunity, of whether a specific food is likely to trigger an addictive response. The NOVA definition for UPF is many pages long [192] and has poor inter-rater reliability [193], highlighting that even experts find it difficult to articulate or agree on the category definition. Furthermore, some foods like peanut butter, made from just peanuts and salt, routinely trigger overconsumption [194], illustrating that, once the addiction is established, abstinence from all UPF may not be sufficient for full recovery. Lack of certainty about where to draw the line of abstinence creates a slippery slope that heightens the likelihood of relapse.

Sixth, the multi-trillion-dollar UPF industry is highly invested in our ongoing addiction, and there are currently very few limits on their reach. They use fMRI to ensure their snack formulations and commercials optimally stimulate the mesolimbic reward pathways [195]. Brains healing from addiction are extra-sensitive to these cues, especially in early recovery [47, 49–52], and the bombardment of commercials, billboards, jingles, and logos for UPF can make living in modern society torturous. Certainly, decades ago, before limits on alcohol and cigarette advertising, or in a hypothetical world where drug cartels had free reign to advertise their products, we might imagine a quasi-comparable situation, but in actual modern-day society, UPF is unique in the magnitude of the advertising dollars promoting it.

Seventh, UPF consumption occurs in more locations, and more frequently throughout the day, than the use of any other addictive substance. This is significant, because relapse is often based on a specific temporal or location-based cue, as any former smoker walking out of a movie theater can attest. Most people start eating within minutes of first waking up and consume their final calories mere minutes before falling asleep [196]. From the temptation to put a scoop of sugar or packet of non-nutritive sweetener into the first morning cup of coffee, to the drive-through on the way to work, to the doughnuts in the break room, to the vending machine outside the office, to the pizza and chips in the lunch line, living an average day means encountering literally hundreds of temporal and location-based cues to consume UPF [103].

And quitting means facing all of those same cues and being well-resourced enough to not succumb, each and every time.

Eighth and finally, the social pressures to eat [197, 198], and to not consider food of any sort to be an addiction [199], are immense. The person addicted to stimulants or opiates can get out of rehab and form myriad associations where no one uses drugs and there is zero pressure to return to their addiction; even the person addicted to alcohol who misses pub culture can form plentiful associations with groups who do not blend alcohol consumption with their fellowship. But the person addicted to UPF will find that nearly every gathering of every sort involves the consumption of food and that the pressure to eat all things in moderation is immense [200]. Furthermore, bonding over food is, and always has been, woven into our very ways of experiencing togetherness and community [201].

For all these reasons, recovery from UPFA, especially if it coincides with a desire to lose weight, is especially difficult and will require an intensive and multifaceted approach.

7. Conclusion

Years ago, the construct of UPFA was hotly debated [202] and the words "food addiction" nearly always had quotes around them or were qualified with adjectives like "controversial" and "purported." Indeed, such qualifiers will likely persist until UPFA receives official standing as a diagnosis in the DSM and the ICD. It is difficult to predict when that will be, but applications to these committees for official diagnoses are in progress.

However, during the late 2010s and early 2020s, the rate of published papers on the topic of food addiction escalated dramatically [122] and in the thousands of papers published on this topic over the past several years, two trends are marked. First, the neurobiological evidence substantiating the impact of UPF as an addictive drug in the brain, across multiple structures and impacting many cognitive functions, has become very convincing [16]. Second, there is great utility and empirical productivity in applying the DSM-5 criteria for a substance use disorder to UPF consumption [106, 122]. In a word, it fits.

More research is needed, especially controlled trials on each of the 11 criteria for a substance use disorder as applied to UPF, and also, perhaps most urgently, more research in the domain of treatment. Research shows that 30% of people receiving treatment for an eating disorder are not improving with the current standard of care [203]. Studies examining whether those individuals are more likely to have undiagnosed UPFA, and randomized, controlled trials exploring whether an abstinence-based treatment approach (rather than an all-foods-fit-for-all-people treatment approach) would help them, are badly needed. These studies are likely to be conducted over the next few years, as the field is maturing now quite rapidly.

While many will wait for an official diagnosis in the DSM or the ICD to drop the quotes and stop using the word "controversial," the reality is that the existence of UPFA will long precede any official seal of validation. No longer is the question, "Is UPF addictive like alcohol, tobacco, stimulants, and opiates?" but rather, "How can we best treat UPFA?" and, "What are the implications?"

Clearly, as is true for alcohol, caffeine, nicotine, and all drugs, not everyone is equally susceptible to the addictive pull of UPF. But the average person has at least some degree of addictive susceptibility [106]. Two weight loss approaches—GLP-1

DOI: http://dx.doi.org/10.5772/intechopen.1004428

drugs for weight loss and Bright Line Eating—that each target UPFA directly and both decrease hunger and cravings, offer promise for people wanting to lose weight and health care practitioners looking to help them. But the average person with obesity is likely aiming for far better results than merely losing 15% of their current body weight. Perhaps if a pharmacological solution was paired with an abstinence-based approach to eating, much higher average weight loss percentages could be achieved.

We must remember that the "badly behaving brain" is performing exquisitely well, for the conditions in which it evolved. But the food environment has changed dramatically. There are good reasons why fewer than 1% of those living with obesity have reached a normal BMI within any given year [204]. Until just recently, there were no weight loss approaches that targeted UPFA. But today there are, and we now know that addressing UPFA results in far greater weight loss than ignoring it. That is important, because as our collective body mass continues to rise, we need a framework to reinvent how we approach weight loss in the twenty-first century.

Acknowledgements

Dr. Mark Goetting, Dr. Cynthia Prehar, and Joseph Fleischman provided detailed feedback and excellent copy edits of this chapter. It was a better manuscript because of their contributions.

Conflict of interest

Susan Peirce Thompson is the founder and CEO of Bright Line Eating. Andrew Kurt Thaw declares no conflict of interest.

Author details

Susan Peirce Thompson[1*] and Andrew Kurt Thaw[2]

1 University of Rochester, Rochester, NY, USA

2 Millsaps College, Jackson, MS, USA

*Address all correspondence to: sthomps4@ur.rochester.edu

References

[1] World Health Organization. Obesity: Preventing and Managing the Global Epidemic. Report of a WHO consultation on Obesity. World Health Organization Technical Report Series. 2000;**894**(i-xii):1-253

[2] McGuire S. World Health Organization. Comprehensive implementation plan on maternal, infant, and Young child nutrition. Geneva, Switzerland. Advances in Nutrition. 2015;**6**(1):134-135. DOI: 10.3945/an.114.007781

[3] NCD Risk Factor Collaboration (NCD-RisC). Worldwide trends in body-mass index, underweight, overweight, and obesity from 1975 to 2016: A pooled analysis of 2416 population-based measurement studies in 128·9 million children, adolescents, and adults. Lancet. 2017;**390**(10113):2627-2642. DOI: 10.1016/S0140-6736(17)32129-3

[4] Lobstein T, Jackson-Leach R, Powis J, Brinsden H, Gray M. World Obesity Atlas 2023, World Obesity Federation. United Kingdom. 2023. Available from: https://policycommons.net/artifacts/3454894/untitled/4255209/. [Accessed: 05 Mar, 2024]. CID: 20.500.12592/hrmxx8

[5] Juul F, Parekh N, Martinez-Steele E, Monteiro CA, Chang VW. Ultra-processed food consumption among US adults from 2001 to 2018. The American Journal of Clinical Nutrition. 2022;**115**(1):211-221. DOI: 10.1093/ajcn/nqab305

[6] Harb AA, Shechter A, Koch PA, St-Onge MP. Ultra-processed foods and the development of obesity in adults. European Journal of Clinical Nutrition. 2023;**77**(6):619-627. DOI: 10.1038/s41430-022-01225-z

[7] Rauber F, Steele EM, Louzada ML, Millett C, Monteiro CA, Levy RB. Ultra-processed food consumption and indicators of obesity in the United Kingdom population (2008-2016). Public Librbary of Science. 2020;**15**(5):e0232676. DOI: 10.1371/journal.pone.0232676

[8] Poti JM, Braga B, Qin B. Ultra-processed food intake and obesity: What really matters for health-processing or nutrient content? Current Obesity Reports. 2017;**6**(4):420-431. DOI: 10.1007/s13679-017-0285-4

[9] Ng M, Fleming T, Robinson M, Thomson B, Graetz N, Margono C, et al. Global, regional, and national prevalence of overweight and obesity in children and adults during 1980-2013: A systematic analysis for the global burden of disease study 2013. The Lancet. 2014;**384**(9945):766-781. DOI: 10.1016/S0140-6736(14)60460-8

[10] Schulte EM, Smeal JK, Lewis J, Gearhardt AN. Development of the highly processed food withdrawal scale. Appetite. 2018;**131**:148-154. DOI: 10.1016/j.appet.2018.09.013

[11] Teixeira PJ, Going SB, Sardinha LB, Lohman TG. A review of psychosocial pre-treatment predictors of weight control. Obesity Reviews. 2005;**6**(1):43-65. DOI: 10.1111/j.1467-789X.2005.00166.x

[12] Ward ZJ, Bleich SN, Long MW, Gortmaker SL. Association of body mass index with health care expenditures in the United States by age and sex. Public Librbary of Science. 2021;**16**(3):e0247307. DOI: 10.1371/journal.pone.0247307

[13] Peyrot M, Rubin RR, Lauritzen T, Snoek FJ, Matthews DR, Skovlund S. Psychosocial problems and barriers to improved diabetes management: Results of the cross-National Diabetes Attitudes, wishes and needs (DAWN) study. Diabetic Medicine. 2005;**22**(10):1379-1385. DOI: 10.1111/j.1464-5491.2005.01644.x

[14] Ziegler-Graham K, MacKenzie EJ, EphraimPL TTG, Brookmeyer R. Estimating the prevalence of limb loss in the United States: 2005 to 2050. Archives of Physical Medicine and Rehabilitation. 2008;**89**(3):422-429. DOI: 10.1016/j.apmr.2007.11.005

[15] Peeke P, Ifland J. Overlap between drug and processed food addiction. In: Ifland J, Marcus M, Preuss H, editors. Processed Food Addiction: Foundations, Assessment, and Recovery. 1st ed. Boca Raton, Florida: CRC Press; 2018. p. 6. 978-0367503420

[16] Ifland J, Marcus M, Preuss H. Processed Food Addiction: Foundations, Assessment, and Recovery. 1st ed. Boca Raton, Florida: CRC Press; 2018. 462 p. ISBN: 978-0367503420

[17] Hall KD, Ayuketah A, Brychta R, Cai H, Cassimatis T, Chen KY, et al. Ultra-processed diets cause excess calorie intake and weight gain: An inpatient randomized controlled trial of ad libitum food intake. Cell Metabolism. 2019;**30**(1):67-77. DOI: 10.1016/j.cmet.2019.05.008

[18] Van Tulleken C. Ultra-Processed People: The Science behind Food That Isn't Food. New York City, New York: W. W. Norton & Company; 2023. 384 p. ISBN: 9781529900057

[19] Zobel EH, Hansen TW, Rossing P, von Scholten BJ. Global changes in food supply and the obesity epidemic. Current Obesity Reports. 2016;**5**:449-455. DOI: 10.1007/s13679-016-0233-8

[20] Crino M, Sacks G, Vandevijvere S, et al. The influence on population weight gain and obesity of the macronutrient composition and energy density of the food supply. Current Obesity Reports. 2015;**4**:1-10. DOI: 10.1007/s13679-014-0134-7

[21] Wang L, Martínez Steele E, Du M, Pomeranz JL, O'Connor LE, Herrick KA, et al. Trends in consumption of Ultraprocessed foods among US youths aged 2-19 years, 1999-2018. Journal of the American Medical Association. 2021;**326**(6):519-530. DOI: 10.1001/jama.2021.10238

[22] Website: China Daily. Fast Food Players Eye Formidable 2023 Sales. [Internet] 2023. Available from: https://www.chinadaily.com.cn/a/202302/10/WS63e584eaa31057c47ebadf66.html [Accessed: 2024-03-04]

[23] Westerink BH, Spaan SJ. Effect of glucose on dopamine metabolism in the rat striatum. Journal of Pharmacy and Pharmacology. 1981;**33**(1):601-602. DOI: 10.1111/j.2042-7158.1981.tb13876.x

[24] Koshimura K, Tanaka J, Murakami Y, Kato Y. Effect of high concentration of glucose on dopamine release from pheochromocytoma-12 cells. Metabolism. 2003;**52**(7):922-926. DOI: 10.1016/s0026-0495(03)00059-3

[25] Mirenowicz J, Schultz W. Preferential activation of midbrain dopamine neurons by appetitive rather than aversive stimuli. Nature. 1996;**379**(6564):449-451. DOI: 10.1038/379449a0

[26] Ahmed S. Is sugar as addictive as cocaine? In: Brownell K, Gold M, editors.

Food and Addiction: A Comprehensive Handbook. 1st ed. Oxford, England: Oxford University Press; 2012. pp. 231-238. 978-0199738168

[27] Stice E, Burger KS, Yokum S. Relative ability of fat and sugar tastes to activate reward, gustatory, and somatosensory regions. The American Journal of Clinical Nutrition. 2013;**98**(6):1377-1384. DOI: 10.3945/ajcn.113.069443

[28] Bolhuis DP, Costanzo A, Newman LP, Keast RS. Salt promotes passive overconsumption of dietary fat in humans. Journal of Nutrition. 2016;**146**(4):838-845. DOI: 10.3945/jn.115.226365

[29] Schulte EM, Avena NM, Gearhardt AN. Which foods may Be addictive? The roles of processing, fat content, and Glycemic load. Public Librbary of Science. 2015;**10**(2):e0117959. DOI: 10.1371/journal.pone.0117959

[30] DiFeliceantonio AG, Coppin G, Rigoux L, Edwin Thanarajah S, Dagher A, Tittgemeyer M, et al. Supra-additive effects of combining fat and carbohydrate on food reward. Cell Metabolism. 2018;**28**(1):33-44.e3. DOI: 10.1016/j.cmet.2018.05.018

[31] Lustig RH. Ultraprocessed food: Addictive, toxic, and ready for regulation. Nutrients. 2020;**12**(11):3401. DOI: 10.3390/nu12113401

[32] Jastreboff AM, Sinha R, Arora J, Giannini C, Kubat J, Malik S, et al. Altered brain response to drinking glucose and fructose in obese adolescents. Diabetes. 2016;**65**(7):1929-1939. DOI: 10.2337/db15-1216

[33] Kelley AE, Baldo BA, Pratt WE, Will MJ. Corticostriatal-hypothalamic circuitry and food motivation: Integration of energy, action and reward. Physiology & Behavior. 2005;**86**(5):773-795. DOI: 10.1016/j.physbeh.2005.08.066

[34] Winterdahl M, Noer O, Orlowski D, Schacht AC, Jakobsob S, Alstrup AKO, et al. Sucrose intake lowers μ-opioid and dopamine D2/3 receptor availability in porcine brain. Scientific Reports. 2019;**9**:16918. DOI: 10.1038/s41598-019-53430-9

[35] Maldonado R, Saiardi A, Valverde O, Somad TA, Roques BP, Barrelli E. Absence of opiate rewarding effects in mice lacking dopamine D2 receptors. Nature. 1997;**388**:586-589. DOI: 10.1038/41567

[36] Mikus N, Korb S, Massaccesi C, Gausterer C, Graf I, Willeit M, et al. Effects of dopamine D2/3 and opioid receptor antagonism on the trade-off between model-based and model-free behaviour in healthy volunteers. eLife. 2022;**11**:e79661. DOI: 10.7554/eLife.79661

[37] Pertwee RG. The diverse CB_1 and CB_2 receptor pharmacology of three plant cannabinoids: Δ^9-tetrahydrocannabinol, cannabidiol and Δ^9-tetrahydrocannabivarin. British Journal of Pharmacology. 2008;**153**:199-215. DOI: 10.1038/sj.bjp.0707442

[38] Bloomfield MA, Ashok AH, Volkow ND, Howes OD. The effects of Δ^9-tetrahydrocannabinol on the dopamine system. Nature. 2016;**539**(7629):369-377. DOI: 10.1038/nature20153

[39] Contreras-Rodriguez O, Solanas M, Escorihuela RM. Dissecting ultra-processed foods and drinks: Do they have a potential to impact the brain? Reviews in Endocrine and Metabolic Disorders. 2022;**23**:697-717. DOI: 10.1007/s11154-022-09711-2

[40] van Galen KA, ter Horst KW, Serlie MJ. Serotonin, food intake, and obesity. Obesity Reviews. 2021;**22**:e13210. DOI: 10.1111/obr.13210

[41] Mesas AE, Girotto E, Rodrigues R, Martinez-Vizcairio V, Jimenez-Lopez E, Lopez-Gil J. Ultra-processed food consumption is associated with alcoholic beverage drinking, tobacco smoking, and illicit drug use in adolescents: A Nationwide population-based study. International Journal of Mental Health Addiction. 2023;**21**(6):1-24. DOI: 10.1007/s11469-023-01059-1

[42] Hecht EM, Rabil A, Martinez Steele E, Abrams GA, Ware D, Landy DC, et al. Cross-sectional examination of ultra-processed food consumption and adverse mental health symptoms. Public Health Nutrition. 2022;**25**(11):3225-3234. DOI: 10.1017/S1368980022001586

[43] Brownell K, Gold M. Food and Addiction: A Comprehensive Handbook. 1st ed. Oxford, England: Oxford University Press; 2012. 496 p. ISBN: 978-0199374571

[44] Cottone P, Moore CF, Sabino V, Koob GF. Compulsive Eating Behavior and Food Addiction: Emerging Pathological Constructs. 1st ed. Cambridge, Massachusettes: Academic Press; 2019. 496 p. ISBN: 978-0128162071

[45] Gearhardt AN, Schulte EN. Is food addictive? A review of the science. Annual Review of Nutrition. 2021;**41**:387-410. DOI: 10.1146/annurev-nutr-110420-111710

[46] Schiestl ET, Rios JM, Parnarouskis L, Cummings JR, Gearhardt AN. A narrative review of highly processed food addiction across the lifespan. Progress in Neuro-Psychopharmacology & Biological Psychiatry. 2020;**106**:110152. DOI: 10.1016/j.pnpbp.2020.110152

[47] Uhl GR, Koob GF, Cable J. The neurobiology of addiction. Annals of the New York Academy of Sciences. 2019;**1451**(1):5-28. DOI: 10.1111/nyas.13989

[48] Berridge KC, Ho CY, Richard JM, DiFeliceantonio AG. The tempted brain eats: Pleasure and desire circuits in obesity and eating disorders. Brain Research. 2010;**1350**:43-64. DOI: 10.1016/j.brainres.2010.04.003

[49] Johnson AW. Eating beyond metabolic need: How environmental cues influence feeding behavior. Trends in Neurosciences. 2013;**36**(2):101-109. DOI: 10.1016/j.tins.2013.01.002

[50] Jansen A. A learning model of binge eating: Cue reactivity and cue exposure. Behaviour Research and Therapy. 1998;**36**(3):257-272. DOI: 10.1016/s0005-7967(98)00055-2

[51] Schulte EM, Yokum S, Jahn A, Gearhardt AN. Food cue reactivity in food addiction: A functional magnetic resonance imaging study. Physiology & Behavior. 2019;**208**:112574. DOI: 10.1016/j.physbeh.2019.112574

[52] Tang DW, Fellows LK, Small DM, Dagher A. Food and drug cues activate similar brain regions: A meta-analysis of functional MRI studies. Physiology & Behavior. 2012;**106**(3):317-324. DOI: 10.1016/j.physbeh.2012.03.009

[53] Boswell RG, Kober H. Food cue reactivity and craving predict eating and weight gain: A meta-analytic review. Obesity Reviews. 2016;**17**(2):159-177. DOI: 10.1111/obr.12354

[54] Noble EE, Kanoski SE. Early life exposure to obesogenic diets and learning and memory dysfunction. Current Opinion in Behavioral

Sciences. 2016;**9**:7-14. DOI: 10.1016/j.cobeha.2015.11.014

[55] Burns SF. Nutrition to raise childhood cognition. In: WLD H, Jamaludin A, Rahman AA, editors. Applying the Science of Learning to Education: An Insight into the Mechanisms That Shape Learning. 1st ed. Vol. 1. Singapore: Springer; 2024. pp. 187-223. DOI: 10.1007/978-981-99-5378-3_9

[56] Afzal AS, Gortmaker S. The relationship between obesity and cognitive performance in children: A longitudinal study. Childhood Obesity. 2015;**11**(4):466-474. DOI: 10.1089/chi.2014.0129

[57] Li Y, Dai Q, Jackson JC, Zhang J. Overweight is associated with decreased cognitive functioning among school-age children and adolescents. Obesity. 2008;**16**(8):1809-1815. DOI: 10.1038/oby.2008.296

[58] Weinstein G, Vered S, Ivancovsky-Wajcman D, Ravona-Springer R, Heymann A, Zelber-Sagi S, et al. Consumption of ultra-processed food and cognitive decline among older adults with type-2 diabetes. The Journals of Gerontology: Series A. 2023;**78**(1):134-142. DOI: 10.1093/gerona/glac070

[59] Gonçalves NG, Ferreira NV, Khandpur N, Steele EM, Levy RB, Lotufo PA, et al. Association between consumption of ultraprocessed foods and cognitive decline. Journal of the American Medical Association Neurology. 2023;**80**(2):142-150. DOI: 10.1001/jamaneurol.2022.4397

[60] Kittel R, Brauhardt A, Hilbert A. Cognitive and emotional functioning in binge-eating disorder: A systematic review. International Journal of Eating Disorders. 2015;**48**(6):535-554. DOI: 10.1002/eat.22419

[61] The U.S. Weight Loss & Diet Control Market Report. 2023. 427 p. Marketdata LLC. ID: 5313560. Available from: https://www.researchandmarkets.com/reports/5313560/the-u-s-weight-loss-and-diet-control-market

[62] Anderson JW, Konz EC, Frederich RC, Wood CL. Long-term weight-loss maintenance: A meta-analysis of US studies. The American Journal of Clinical Nutrition. 2001;**74**(5):579-584. DOI: 10.1093/ajcn/74.5.579

[63] Self DW. Neural substrates of drug craving and relapse in drug addiction. Annals of Medicine. 1998;**30**(4):379-389. DOI: 10.3109/07853899809029938

[64] NIDA. Understanding Drug Use and Addiction DrugFacts. National Institute on Drug Abuse website. 2018. Available from: https://nida.nih.gov/publications/drugfacts/understanding-drug-use-addiction [Accessed: January 30, 2024]

[65] Koob GF, Volkow ND. Neurobiology of addiction: A neurocircuitry analysis. Lancet Psychiatry. 2016;**3**(8):760-773. DOI: 10.1016/S2215-0366(16)00104-8

[66] Wise RA. Role of brain dopamine in food reward and reinforcement. Philosophical Transactions of the Royal Society of London. 2006;**B361**:1149-1158. DOI: 10.1098/rstb.2006.1854

[67] Volkow ND, Wang GJ, Baler RD. Reward, dopamine and the control of food intake: Implications for obesity. Trends in Cognitive Science. 2011;**15**(1):37-46. DOI: 10.1016/j.tics.2010.11.001

[68] Vucetic Z, Reyes TM. Central dopaminergic circuitry controlling

food intake and reward: Implications for the regulation of obesity. Wiley Interdisciplinary Reviews – Mechanism of Disease. 2010;**2**(5):577-593. DOI: 10.1002/wsbm.77

[69] Calcaterra V, Cena H, Rossi V, Santero S, Bianchi A, Zuccotti G. Ultra-processed food, reward system and childhood obesity. Children. 2023;**10**(5):804. DOI: 10.3390/children10050804

[70] Parnarouskis L, Leventhal AM, Ferguson SG, Gearhardt AN. Withdrawal: A key consideration in evaluating whether highly processed foods are addictive. Obesity Reviews. 2022;**23**(11):e13507. DOI: 10.1111/obr.13507

[71] Wise RA. The neurobiology of craving: Implications for the understanding and treatment of addiction. Journal of Abnormal Psychology. 1988;**97**(2):118-132. DOI: 10.1037/0021-843X.97.2.118

[72] Cho SB, Su J, Kuo SI-C, Bucholz KK, Chan G, Edenberg HJ, et al. Positive and negative reinforcement are differentially associated with alcohol consumption as a function of alcohol dependence. Psychology of Addictive Behaviors. 2019;**33**(1):58-68. DOI: 10.1037/adb0000436

[73] Arnsten AF. Stress signalling pathways that impair prefrontal cortex structure and function. Nature Reviews Neuroscience. 2009;**10**(6):410-422. DOI: 10.1038/nrn2648

[74] Rogers PJ, Vural Y, Berridge-Burley N, Butcher C, Cawley E, Gao Z, et al. Evidence that carbohydrate-to-fat ratio and taste, but not energy density or NOVA level of processing, are determinants of food liking and food reward. Appetite. 2024;**193**:107124. DOI: 10.1016/j.appet.2023.107124

[75] Samuthpongtorn CS, Nguyen LH, Okereke OI, Wang DD, Song M, Chan AT, et al. Consumption of ultraprocessed food and risk of depression. Journal of the American Medical Association Network Open. 2023;**6**(9):e2334770. DOI: 10.1001/jamanetworkopen.2023.34770

[76] Lane MM, Gamage E, Travica N, Dissanayaka T, Ashtree DN, Gauci S, et al. Ultra-processed food consumption and mental health: A systematic review and Meta-analysis of observational studies. Nutrients. 2022;**14**(13):2568. DOI: 10.3390/nu14132568

[77] Davis J. Hunger, ghrelin and the gut. Brain Research. 2018;**1693**(Pt B):154-158. DOI: 10.1016/j.brainres.2018.01.024

[78] Klok MD, Jakobsdottir S, Drent ML. The role of leptin and ghrelin in the regulation of food intake and body weight in humans: A review. Obesity Reviews. 2007;**8**(1):21-34. DOI: 10.1111/j.1467-789X.2006.00270.x

[79] Barr SB, Wright JC. Postprandial energy expenditure in whole-food and processed-food meals: Implications for daily energy expenditure. Food and Nutrition Research. 2010;**54**:1-9. DOI: 10.3402/fnr.v54i0.5144

[80] Crimarco A, Landry MJ, Gardner CD. Ultra-processed foods, weight gain, and Co-morbidity risk. Current Obesity Reports. 2022;**11**(3):80-92. DOI: 10.1007/s13679-021-00460-y

[81] Fazzino TL, Dorling JL, Apolzan JW, Martin CK. Meal composition during an ad libitum buffet meal and longitudinal predictions of weight and percent body fat change: The role of hyper-palatable, energy dense, and ultra-processed foods. Appetite. 2021;**167**:105592. DOI: 10.1016/j.appet.2021.105592

[82] Pandit R, Beerens S, Adan RAH. Role of leptin in energy expenditure: The hypothalamic perspective. American Journal of Physiology-Regulatory, Integrative and Comparative Physiology. 2017;**312**(6):R938-R947. DOI: 10.1152/ajpregu.00045.2016

[83] Martelli D, Brooks VL. Leptin increases: Physiological roles in the control of sympathetic nerve activity, energy balance, and the hypothalamic-pituitary-thyroid Axis. International Journal of Molecular Sciences. 2023;**24**(3):2684. DOI: 10.3390/ijms24032684

[84] Wang J, Obici S, Morgan K, Barzilai N, Feng Z. Luciano Rossetti; overfeeding rapidly induces leptin and insulin resistance. Diabetes. 2001;**50**(12):2786-2791. DOI: 10.2337/diabetes.50.12.2786

[85] Banks WA, Coon AB, Robinson SM, Moinuddin A, Shultz JM, Nakaoke R, et al. Triglycerides induce leptin resistance at the blood-brain barrier. Diabetes. 2004;**53**(5):1253-1260. DOI: 10.2337/diabetes.53.5.1253

[86] Barlampa D, Bompoula MS, Bargiota A, Kalantaridou S, Mastorakos G, Valsamakis G. Hypothalamic inflammation as a potential pathophysiologic basis for the heterogeneity of clinical, hormonal, and metabolic presentation in PCOS. Nutrients. 2021;**13**(2):520. DOI: 10.3390/nu13020520

[87] Almarshad MI, Algonaiman R, Alharbi HF, Almujaydil MS, Barakat H. Relationship between ultra-processed food consumption and risk of diabetes mellitus: A Mini-review. Nutrients. 2022;**14**(12):2366. DOI: 10.3390/nu14122366

[88] Rico-Campà A, Martínez-González MA, Alvarez-Alvarez I, Mendonça RD, de la Fuente-Arrillaga C, Gómez-Donoso C, et al. Association between consumption of ultra-processed foods and all cause mortality: SUN prospective cohort study. British Medical Journal. 2019;**365**:l1949. DOI: 10.1136/bmj.l1949

[89] Dionysopoulou S, Charmandari E, Bargiota A, Vlahos NF, Mastorakos G, Valsamakis G. The role of hypothalamic inflammation in diet-induced obesity and its association with cognitive and mood disorders. Nutrients. 2021;**13**(2):498. DOI: 10.3390/nu13020498

[90] Yanovski SZ, Leet M, Yanovski JA, Flood M, Gold PW, Kissileff HR, et al. Food selection and intake of obese women with binge-eating disorder. The American Journal of Clinical Nutrition. 1992;**56**(6):975-980. DOI: 10.1093/ajcn/56.6.975

[91] Wiss D. Clinical considerations of ultra-processed food addiction across weight classes: An eating disorder treatment and care perspective. Current Addiction Reports. 2022;**9**:255-267. DOI: 10.1007/s40429-022-00411-0

[92] Mattes RD, Popkin BM. Nonnutritive sweetener consumption in humans: Effects on appetite and food intake and their putative mechanisms. American Journal of Clinical Nutrition. 2009;**89**(1):1-14. DOI: 10.3945/ajcn.2008.26792

[93] Alfenas RCG, Mattes RD. Effect of fat sources on satiety. Obesity Research. 2012;**11**(2):183-187. DOI: 10.1038/oby.2003.29

[94] Karlsson C. Leptin – A slimmer's dream that crashed? The electronic Journal of the International Federation of Clinical Chemistry and Laboratory Medicine (EJIFCC). 2000;**12**(3):73-81. Available from: http://www.ifcc.org/ejifcc/vol12no3/leptin.htm

[95] Izquierdo AG, Crujeiras AB, Casanueva FF, Carreira MC. Leptin, obesity, and leptin resistance: Where are we 25 years later? Nutrients. 2019;**11**(11):2704. DOI: 10.3390/nu11112704

[96] Obradovic M, Sudar-Milovanovic E, Soskic S, Essack M, Arya S, Stewart AJ, et al. Leptin and obesity: Role and clinical implication. Frontiers in Endocrinology (Lausanne). 2021;**12**:585887. DOI: 10.3389/fendo.2021.585887

[97] Liu J, Lai F, Hou Y, Zheng R. Leptin signaling and leptin resistance. Medical Review. 2022;**2**(4):363-384. DOI: 10.1515/mr-2022-0017

[98] Hosoi T, Kawagishi T, Okuma Y, Tanaka J, Nomura Y. Brain stem is a direct target for leptin's action in the central nervous system. Endocrinology. 2002;**143**(9):3498-3504. DOI: 10.1210/en.2002-220077

[99] Hofmann W, Baumeister RF, Förster G, Vohs KD. Everyday temptations: An experience sampling study of desire, conflict, and self-control. Journal of Personality and Social Psychology. 2012;**102**(6):1318-1335. DOI: 10.1037/a0026545

[100] Rolls ET. The cingulate cortex and limbic systems for emotion, action, and memory. Brain Structure and Function. 2019;**224**(9):3001-3018. DOI: 10.1007/s00429-019-01945-2

[101] Baumeister RF, Bratslavsky E, Muraven M, Tice DM. Ego depletion: Is the active self a limited resource? Journal of Personality and Social Psychology. 1998;**74**(5):1252-1265. DOI: 10.1037//0022-3514.74.5.1252

[102] Clewett D, Schoeke A, Mather M. Amygdala functional connectivity is reduced after the cold pressor task. Cognitive, Affective, & Behavioral Neuroscience. 2013;**13**(3):501-518. DOI: 10.3758/s13415-013-0162-x

[103] Kanoski SE, Boutelle KN. Food cue reactivity: Neurobiological and behavioral underpinnings. Reviews in Endocrine and Metabolic Disorders. 2022;**23**(4):683-696. DOI: 10.1007/s11154-022-09724-x

[104] Walls HL, Peeters A, Loff B, Crammond BR. Why education and choice won't solve the obesity problem. American Journal of Public Health. 2009;**99**(4):590-592. DOI: 10.2105/AJPH.2008.156232

[105] Gearhardt AN, Corbin WR, Brownell KD. Preliminary validation of the Yale food addiction scale. Appetite. 2009;**52**(2):430-436. DOI: 10.1016/j.appet.2008.12.003

[106] Gearhardt AN, Corbin WR, Brownell KD. Development of the Yale food addiction scale version 2.0. Psychology of Addictive Behaviors. 2016;**30**(1):113-121. DOI: 10.1037/adb0000136

[107] Pape M, Herpertz S, Schroeder S, Seiferth C, Färber T, Wolstein J, et al. Food addiction and its relationship to weight- and addiction-related psychological parameters in individuals with overweight and obesity. Frontiers in Psychology. 2021;**12**:736454. DOI: 10.3389/fpsyg.2021.736454

[108] American Psychiatric Association. Diagnostic and Statistical Manual of Mental Disorders. 5th ed. text rev. (DSMV-TR)2022. DOI: 10.1176/appi.books. 9780890425787

[109] Ayton A, Ibrahim A, Dugan J, Galvin E, Wright OW. Ultra-processed foods and binge eating: A retrospective observational study. Nutrition. 2021;**84**:111023. DOI: 10.1016/j.nut.2020.111023

[110] Lane MM, Davis JA, Beattie S, Gómez-Donoso C, Loughman A, O'Neil A, et al. Ultraprocessed food and chronic noncommunicable diseases: A systematic review and meta-analysis of 43 observational studies. Obesity Reviews. 2021;**22**:e13146. DOI: 10.1111/obr.13146

[111] De Almeida R, Kamath G, Cabandugama P. Food addiction in application to obesity management. Missouri Medicine. 2022;**119**(4):372-378

[112] Barbarich-Marsteller NC, Foltin RW, Walsh BT. Does anorexia nervosa resemble an addiction? Current Drug Abuse Reviews. 2011;**4**(3):197-200. DOI: 10.2174/1874473711104030197

[113] Schulte EM, Smeal JK, Gearhardt AN. Foods are differentially associated with subjective effect report questions of abuse liability. Public Library of Science One. 2017;**12**(8):e0184220. DOI: 10.1371/journal.pone.0184220

[114] Schulte EM, Gearhardt AN. Yale Food Addiction Scale 2.0, questions 5-7 [Internet]. 2017. Available from: https://sites.lsa.umich.edu/fastlab/yale-food-addiction-scale. [Accessed: January 25, 2024]

[115] Ifland J, Epstein E. DSM 5 SUD criterion 3: Time spent. In: Ifland J, Marcus M, Preuss H, editors. Processed Food Addiction: Foundations, Assessment, and Recovery. 1st ed. Roca Raton, Florida: CRC Press; 2018. pp. 175-186. ISBN: 978-0367503420

[116] Kessler DA. The End of Overeating: Taking Control of the Insatiable American Appetite. Emmaus, Pennsylvania: Rodale; 2010. p. 352

[117] Meule A, Gearhardt AN. Food addiction in the light of DSM-5. Nutrients. 2014;**6**(9):3653-3671. DOI: 10.3390/nu6093653

[118] Pelchat ML, Johnson A, Chan R, Valdez J, Ragland JD. Images of desire: Food-craving activation during fMRI. NeuroImage. 2004;**23**(4):1486-1493. DOI: 10.1016/j.neuroimage.2004.08.023

[119] Van den Eynde F, Koskina A, Syrad H, Guillaume S, Broadbent H, Campbell IC, et al. State and trait food craving in people with bulimic eating disorders. Eating Behaviors. 2012;**13**(4):414-417. DOI: 10.1016/j.eatbeh.2012.07.007

[120] Burmeister JM, Hinman N, Koball A, Hoffmann DA, Carels RA. Food addiction in adults seeking weight loss treatment. Implications for psychosocial health and weight loss. Appetite. 2013;**60**(1):103-110. DOI: 10.1016/j.appet.2012. 09.013

[121] Forhan M, Gill SV. Obesity, functional mobility and quality of life. Best Practice & Research Clinical Endocrinology and Metabolism. 2013;**27**(2):129-137. DOI: 10.1016/j.beem.2013.01.003

[122] Praxedes DRS, Silva-Júnior AE, Macena ML, Oliveira AD, Cardoso KS, Nunes LO, et al. Prevalence of food addiction determined by the Yale food addiction scale and associated factors: A systematic review with meta-analysis. European Eating Disorders Review. 2022;**30**(2):85-95. DOI: 10.1002/erv.2878

[123] Iflad J, Willey CL. In: Ifland J, Marcus M, Preuss H, editors. Processed Food Addiction: Foundations, Assessment, and Recovery. 1st ed. CRC Press; 2018. pp. 217-230. ISBN:978-0367503420

[124] Schulte E.M., Gearhardt A.N. Yale Food Addiction Scale 2.0, questions 19 & 27 [Internet]. 2017. Available from: https://sites.lsa.umich.edu/fastlab/yale-food-addiction-scale. [Accessed: January 25, 2024]

[125] Anderson K, Rieger E, Caterson I. A comparison of maladaptive schemata in treatment-seeking obese adults and normal-weight control subjects. Journal of Psychosomatic Research. 2006;**60**(3):245-252. DOI: 10.1016/j.jpsychores.2005. 08.002

[126] Fassino S, Leombruni P, Pierò A, Abbate-Daga G, Giacomo RG. Mood, eating attitudes, and anger in obese women with and without binge eating disorder. Journal of Psychosomatic Research. 2003;**54**(6):559-566. DOI: 10.1016/s0022-3999(02)00462-2

[127] Schulte EM, Gearhardt AN. Yale Food Addiction Scale 2.0, questions 9 & 35 [Internet]. 2017. Available from: https://sites.lsa.umich.edu/fastlab/yale-food-addiction-scale. [Accessed: January 25, 2024]

[128] Galasso L, Montaruli A, Jankowski KS, Bruno E, Castelli L, Mulè A, et al. Binge eating disorder: What is the role of physical activity associated with dietary and psychological treatment? Nutrients. 2020;**12**(12):3622. DOI: 10.3390/nu12123622

[129] Laster J, Frame LA. Beyond the calories—Is the problem in the processing? Current Treatments and Options in Gastroenterology. 2019;**17**:577-586. DOI: 10.1007/s11938-019-00246-1

[130] Schulte EM, Gearhardt AN. Yale Food Addiction Scale 2.0, questions 8, 10 & 18 [Internet]. 2017. Available from: https://sites.lsa.umich.edu/fastlab/yale-food-addiction-scale. [Accessed: January 25, 2024]

[131] Alosco ML, Spitznagel MB, Fischer KH, Miller LA, Pillai V, Hughes J, et al. Both texting and eating are associated with impaired simulated driving performance. Traffic Injury Prevention. 2012;**13**(5):468-475. DOI: 10.1080/ 15389588.2012.676697

[132] Stutts J, Feaganes J, Reinfurt D, Rodgman E, Hamlett C, Gish K, et al. Driver's exposure to distractions in their natural driving environment. Accident Analysis and Prevention. 2005;**37**(6):1093-1101. DOI: 10.1016/j.aap.2005.06.007

[133] Young MS, Mahfoud JM, Walker GH, Jenkins DP, Stanton NA. Crash dieting: The effects of eating and drinking on driving performance. Accident Analysis and Prevention. 2008;**40**(1):142-148. DOI: 10.1016/j.aap.2007.04.012

[134] Schulte EM, Gearhardt AN. Yale Food Addiction Scale 2.0, questions 33 & 34 [Internet]. 2017. Available from: https://sites.lsa.umich.edu/fastlab/yale-food-addiction-scale [Accessed: January 25, 2024]

[135] Sami W, Ansari T, Butt NS, Hamid MRA. Effect of diet on type 2 diabetes mellitus: A review. International Journal of Health Sciences (Qassim). 2017;**11**(2):65-71

[136] Vidyapith B, Rajasthan J. Consumption of junk foods and risk of type 2 diabetes: A review Shubhi Mishra research scholar, Department of Food Science and Nutrition. International Journal of Horticulture, Agriculture and Food Science. 2023;7(2):7-9. DOI: 10.22161/ijhaf.7.2. Available online: 06 Apr 2023

[137] Elkins G, Whitfield P, Marcus J, Symmonds R, Rodriguez J, Cook T. Noncompliance with behavioral recommendations following bariatric surgery. Obesity Surgery. 2005;**15**(4):546-551. DOI: 10.1381/0960892053723385

[138] Bertoli S, Spadafranca A, Bes-Rastrollo M, Martinez-Gonzalez MA, Ponissi V, Beggio V, et al. Adherence to the Mediterranean diet is inversely

related to binge eating disorder in patients seeking a weight loss program. Clinical Nutrition. 2015;**34**(1):107-114. DOI: 10.1016/j.clnu.2014.02.001

[139] Corsica JA, Pelchat ML. Food addiction: True or false? Current Opinion in Gastroenterology. 2010;**26**(2):165-169. DOI: 10.1097/MOG.0b013e328336528d

[140] Schulte EM, Gearhardt AN. Yale Food Addiction Scale 2.0, questions 24 & 26 [Internet]. 2017. Available from: https://sites.lsa.umich.edu/fastlab/yale-food-addiction-scale [Accessed: January 25, 2024]

[141] Gordon EL, Ariel-Donges AH, Bauman V, Merlo LJ. What is the evidence for "food addiction?" a systematic review. Nutrients. 2018;**10**(4):477. DOI: 10.3390/nu10040477

[142] Parylak SL, Koob GF, Zorrilla GP. The dark side of food addiction. Physiology and Behavior. 2011;**104**(1):149-156. DOI: 10.1016/j.physbeh. 2011.04.063

[143] Flint AJ, Gearhardt AN, Corbin WR, Brownell KD, Field AE, Rimm EB. Food-addiction scale measurement in 2 cohorts of middle-aged and older women. The American Journal of Clinical Nutrition. 2014;**99**(3):578-586. DOI: 10.3945/ajcn.113.068965

[144] Gearhardt AN, Roberto CA, Seamans MJ, Corbin WR, Brownell KD. Preliminary validation of the Yale food addiction scale for children. Eating Behaviors. 2013;**14**(4):508-512. DOI: 10.1016/j.eatbeh.2013.07.002

[145] Schulte EM, Gearhardt AN. Development of the modified Yale food addiction scale version 2.0. European Eating Disorders Review. 2017;**25**(4):302-308. DOI: 10.1002/erv.2515

[146] Schiestl ET, Gearhardt AN. Preliminary validation of the Yale food addiction scale for children 2.0: A dimensional approach to scoring. European Eating Disorders Review. 2018;**6**:605-617. DOI: 10.1002/erv.2648

[147] Wiss D, Brewerton T. Separating the signal from the noise: How psychiatric diagnoses can help discern food addiction from dietary restraint. Nutrients. 2020;**12**(10):2937. DOI: 10.3390/nu12102937

[148] Meule A. A history of "food addiction.". In: Cottone P, Sabino V, Moore CF, Koob GF, editors. Compulsive Eating Behavior and Food Addiction. Academic Press; 2019. pp. 1-13. DOI: 10.1016/B978-0-12-816207-1.00001-9

[149] Horsager C, Bruun JM, Færk E, Hagstrøm S, Lauritsen MB, Østergaard SD. Food addiction is strongly associated with type 2 diabetes. Clinical Nutrition. 2023;**42**(5):717-721. DOI: 10.1016/j.clnu.2023.03.014

[150] DiLeone RJ, Taylor JR, Picciotto MR. The drive to eat: Comparisons and distinctions between mechanisms of food reward and drug addiction. Nature Neuroscience. 2012t;**15**(10):1330-1335. DOI: 10.1038/nn.3202

[151] SHiFT Recovery by ACORN. P.O. Box 50126. Sarasota, FL 34232-0301. [Internet] 2024. Available from: https://foodaddiction.com/contact-us/ [Accessed: January 25, 2024]

[152] Bitten Johnson. Bitten's Addiction. [Internet] 2024. Available from: https://www.bittensaddiction.com/en/professional-training/sugar/ [Accessed: January 29, 2024]

[153] MFM Food Dependency Recovery. Founded 2006. Reykjavík, Capital Regio. [Internet] 2024. Available from: https://www.matarfikn.is/ [Accessed: January 25, 2024]

[154] Milestones in Recovery. 2525 Embassy Drive, Suite 10, Hollywood, FL 33026. [Internet] 2024. Available from: https://www.milestonesprogram.org/about-milestones-in-recovery/ [Accessed: January 25, 2024]

[155] Turning Point of Tampa. 6227 Sheldon Rd, Tampa, FL 33615. [Internet] 2024. Available from: https://www.tpoftampa.com/ [Accessed: January 25, 2024]

[156] The International School of Food Addiction Counseling and Treatment (INFACT) School; Treatment Center for Food Addiction. [Internet] 2024. Available from: https://www.infactschool.online/ [Accessed: January 25, 2024]

[157] Food Addiction Institute. [Internet] 2024. Available from: https://foodaddictioninstitute.org [Accessed: January 25, 2024]

[158] Food Addicts in Recovery Anonymous (FA). [Internet] 2024. Available from: https://www.foodaddics.org/ [Accessed: January 31, 2024]

[159] Unwin J, Delon C, Giæver H, Kennedy C, Painschab M, Sandin F, et al. Low carbohydrate and psychoeducational programs show promise for the treatment of ultra-processed food addiction. Frontiers in Psychiatry. 2022;**13**:1005523. DOI: 10.3389/fpsyt.2022.1005523

[160] Pepino MY, Stein RI, Eagon JC, Klein S. Bariatric surgery-induced weight loss causes remission of food addiction in extreme obesity. Obesity. 2014;**22**(8):1792-1798. DOI: 10.1002/oby.20797

[161] Sevinçer GM, Konuk N, Bozkurt S, Coşkun H. Food addiction and the outcome of bariatric surgery at 1-year: Prospective observational study. Psychiatry Research. 2016;**244**:159-164. DOI: 10.1016/j.psychres.2016.07.022

[162] Ivezaj V, Wiedemann AA, Grilo CM. Food addiction and bariatric surgery: A systematic review of the literature. Obesity Reviews. 2017;**18**(12):1386-1397. DOI: 10.1111/obr.12600

[163] Noria SF, Shelby RD, Atkins KD, Nguyen NT, Gadde KM. Weight regain after bariatric surgery: Scope of the problem, causes, prevention, and treatment. Current Diabetes Reports. 2023;**23**(3):31-42. DOI: 10.1007/s11892-023-01498-z

[164] Major P, Zarzycki P, Rymarowicz J, Wysocki M, Łabul M, Hady HR, et al. Revisional operations among patients after surgical treatment of obesity: A multicenter polish revision obesity surgery study (PROSS). Wideochir Inne Tech Maloinwazyjne. 2022;**17**(2):372-379. DOI: 10.5114/wiitm. 2022.114525

[165] Science 2023 Breakthrough of the Year [Internet] 2024. Available from: https://www.science.org/content/article/breakthrough-of-the-year-2023 [Accessed: January 31, 2024]

[166] Eren-Yazicioglu CY, Yigit A, Dogruoz RE, Yapici-Eser H. Can GLP-1 Be a target for reward system related disorders? A qualitative synthesis and systematic review analysis of studies on palatable food, drugs of abuse, and alcohol. Frontiers in Behavioral Neuroscience. 2021;**14**:614884. DOI: 10.3389/ fnbeh.2020.614884

[167] Wilding JPH, Batterham RL, Calanna S, Davies M, Van Gaal LF, Lingvay I, et al. STEP 1 study group. Once-weekly Semaglutide in adults with overweight or obesity. New England Journal of Medicine. 2021;**384**(11):989-1002. DOI: 10.1056/NEJMoa2032183

[168] Garvey TW, Batterham RL, Bhatta M, Buscemi S, Christensen LN, Frias JF, et al. The STEP 5 study group.

Two-year effects of semaglutide in adults with overweight or obesity: The STEP 5 trial. Nature Medicine. 2022;**28**:2083-2091. DOI: 10.1038/s41591-022-02026-4

[169] JPH W, Batterham RL, Davies M, Van Gaal LF, Kandler K, Konakli K, et al. STEP 1 study group. Weight regain and cardiometabolic effects after withdrawal of semaglutide: The STEP 1 trial extension. Diabetes, Obesity and Metabolism. 2022;**24**(8):1553-1564. DOI: 10.1111/dom.14725

[170] Guan W, Thaw AK, Grondhuis S, Schaechter A. Evaluation of a commercial telehealth weight loss and management program. Journal of Nutrition and Weight Loss. 2018;**3**(2):114-121. DOI: 10.35248/2593-9793.18.3.114

[171] Guan W, Thompson S, Thaw A. Changes in hunger and craving in an 8-week commercial weight loss program using a food addiction framework. Current Developments in Nutrition. 2020;**4**(Suppl. 2):752. DOI: 10.1093/cdn/nzaa052_021

[172] Thompson SP, Thaw AK, Goetting MG, Guan W. Bright line eating: A two-year follow-up evaluation of a commercial telehealth weight loss program within an abstinence-based food addiction framework. Journal of Nutrition and Weight Loss. 2021;**6**(3):125

[173] Xu J, Xiao X, Li Y, Zheng J, Li W, Zhang Q, et al. The effect of gum chewing on blood GLP-1 concentration in fasted, healthy, non-obese men. Endocrine. 2015;**50**(1):93-98. DOI: 10.1007/s12020-015-0566-1

[174] Slyper A. Oral processing, satiation and obesity: Overview and hypotheses. Diabetes, Metabolic Syndrome and Obesity. 2021;**14**:3399-3415. DOI: 10.2147/DMSO.S314379

[175] Karhunen LJ, Juvonen KR, Flander SM, Liukkonen KH, Lähteenmäki L, Siloaho M, et al. A psyllium Fiber-enriched meal strongly attenuates postprandial gastrointestinal peptide release in healthy Young adults. The Journal of Nutrition. 2010;**140**(4):737-744. DOI: 10.3945/jn.109.115436

[176] Laudenslager M, Chaudhry ZW, Rajagopal S, Clynes S, Gudzune KA. Commercial weight loss programs in the Management of Obesity: An update. Current Obesity Reports. 2021;**10**(2):90-99. DOI: 10.1007/s13679-021-00428-y

[177] Toro-Ramos T, Michaelides A, Anton M, Karim Z, Kang-Oh L, Argyrou C, et al. Mobile delivery of the diabetes prevention program in people with prediabetes: Randomized controlled trial. Journal of Medical Internet Research Mobile Health. 2020;**8**(7):e17842. DOI: 10.2196/17842

[178] Toro-Ramos T, Lee D-H, Kim Y, Michaelides A, Tae Jung O, Kim KM, et al. Effectiveness of a smartphone application for the Management of Metabolic Syndrome Components Focusing on weight loss: A preliminary study. Metabolic Syndrome and Related Disorders. 2017;**15**(9):465-473. DOI: 10.1089/met.2017.0062

[179] Tsai AG, Wadden TA. Systematic review: An evaluation of Major commercial weight loss programs in the United States. Annals of Internal Medicine. 2005;**142**(1):56-66. DOI: 10.7326/0003-4819-142-1-200501040-00012

[180] Jolly K, Lewis A, Beach J, Denley J, Adab P, Deeks JJ, et al. Comparison of range of commercial or primary care led weight reduction programmes with minimal intervention control for weight loss in obesity: Lighten up randomised controlled trial. British Medical Journal. 2011;**343**:d6500. DOI: 10.1136/bmj.d6500

[181] Truby H, Baic S, de Looy A, Fox KR, Livingstone MBE, Logan CM, et al. Randomised controlled trial of four commercial weight loss programmes in the UK: Initial findings from the BBC "diet trials". British Medical Journal. 2006;**332**:1309. DOI: 10.1136/bmj.38833.411204.80

[182] Foster GD, Borradaile KE, Vander Veur SS, Shantz KL, Dilks RJ, Goldbacher EM, et al. The effects of a commercially available weight loss program among obese patients with type 2 diabetes: A randomized study. Postgraduate Medicine. 2009;**121**(5):113-118. DOI: 10.3810/pgm.2009.09.2046

[183] Foster G, Wadden T, LaGrotte C, Vander Veur SS, Hesson LA, Homko CJ, et al. A randomized comparison of a commercially available portion-controlled weight-loss intervention with a diabetes self-management education program. Nutrition and Diabetes. 2013;**3**:e63. DOI: 10.1038/nutd.2013.3

[184] Dansinger ML, Gleason JA, Griffith JL, Selker HP, Schaefer EJ. Comparison of the Atkins, Ornish, weight watchers, and zone diets for weight loss and heart disease risk reduction: A randomized trial. Journal of The American Medical Association. 2005;**293**(1):43-53. DOI: 10.1001/jama.293.1.43

[185] Lembke A. Dopamine Nation: Finding Balance in the Age of Indulgence. New York: Dutton; 2021. p. 50. DOI: 10.1017/S0963180122000032

[186] Briefel RR, Reidy K, Karwe V, Devaney B. Feeding infants and toddlers study: Improvements needed in meeting infant feeding recommendations. Journal of the American Dietetic Association. 2004;**104**(1):31-37. DOI: 10.1016/j.jada.2003.10.020

[187] Herrick KA, Fryar CD, Hamner HC, Park S, Ogden CL. Added sugars intake among US infants and toddlers. Journal of the Academy of Nutrition and Dietetics. 2020;**120**(1):23-32. DOI: 10.1016/j.jand.2019.09.007

[188] Gearhardt AN, DiFeliceantonio AG. Highly processed foods can be considered addictive substances based on established scientific criteria. Addiction. 2023;**118**(4):589-598. DOI: 10.1111/add.16065

[189] Ifland J, Preuss HG, Marcus MT, Rourke KM, Taylor W, Wright HT. Clearing the confusion around processed food addiction. Journal of the American College of Nutrition. 2015;**34**(3):240-243. DOI: 10.1080/07315724.2015.1022466

[190] Hebebrand J, Albayrak Ö, Adan R, Antel J, Dieguez C, De Jong J, et al. "Eating addiction", rather than "food addiction", better captures addictive-like eating behavior. Neuroscience and Biobehavioral Reviews. 2014;**47**:295-306. DOI: 10.1016/j.neubiorev.2014.08.016

[191] Sumithran P, Prendergast LA, Delbridge E, Purcell K, Shulkes A, Kriketos A, et al. Long-term persistence of hormonal adaptations to weight loss. New England Journal of Medicine. 2011;**365**(17):1597-1604. DOI: 10.1056/NEJMoa1105816

[192] Monteiro CA, Cannon G, Levy R, Moubarac JC, Jaime P, Martins AP, et al. Food classification. Public health NOVA. The star shines bright. World Nutrition. 2016;**7**:28-38. Available from: https://worldnutritionjournal.org/index.php/wn/issue/view/1

[193] Braesco V, Souchon I, Sauvant P, Haurogné T, Maillot M, Féart C, et al. Ultra-processed foods: How functional is the NOVA system? European Journal of Clinical Nutrition. 2022;**76**:1245-1253. DOI: 10.1038/s41430-022-01099-1

[194] Barbour JA, Stojanovski E, Moran LJ, Howe PRC, Coates AM. The addition of peanuts to habitual diets is associated with lower consumption of savory non-core snacks by men and sweet non-core snacks by women. Nutrition Research. 2017;**41**:65-72. DOI: 10.1016/j.nutres.2017.04.005

[195] Moss M. Hooked: Food, Free Will, and How the Food Giants Exploit our Addictions. National Geographic. McClelland & Stewart. Random House Publishing Group; 2021. ISBN: 9780771059605. Available from: https://books.google.com/books?id=-_2OEAAAQBAJ

[196] Gill S, Panda S. A smartphone app reveals erratic diurnal eating patterns in humans that can Be modulated for health benefits. Cell Metabolism. 2015;**22**(5):789-798. DOI: 10.1016/j.cmet.2015.09.005

[197] Story M, Neumark-Sztainer D, French S. Individual and environmental influences on adolescent eating behaviors. Journal of the American Dietetic Association. 2002;**102**(3 Supplement):S40-S51. DOI: 10.1016/s0002-8223(02)90421-9

[198] Robinson E, Blissett J, Higgs S. Social influences on eating: Implications for nutritional interventions. Nutrition Research Reviews. 2013;**26**(2):166-176. DOI: 10.1017/S0954422413000127

[199] Westwater ML, Fletcher PC, Ziauddeen H. Sugar addiction: The state of the science. European Journal of Nutrition. 2016;**55**(2):55-69. DOI: 10.1007/s00394-016-1229-6

[200] Ogden J, Quirke-McFarlane S. Sabotage, collusion, and being a feeder: Towards a new model of negative social support and its impact on weight management. Current Obesity Reports. 2023;**12**:183-190. DOI: 10.1007/s13679-023-00504-5

[201] Anderson E. Everyone Eats. NYU Press. Available from: https://www.perlego.com/book/720193/everyone-eats-understanding-food-and-culture-second-edition-pdf; 2014 [Accessed: January 20, 2024]

[202] Fletcher PC, Kenny PJ. Food addiction: A valid concept? Neuropsychopharmacology. 2018;**43**:2506-2513. DOI: 10.1038/s41386-018-0203-9

[203] Filipponi C, Visentini C, Filippini T, Cutino A, Ferri P, Rovesti S, et al. The follow-up of eating disorders from adolescence to early adulthood: A systematic review. International Journal of Environmental Research and Public Health. 2022;**19**(23):16237. DOI: 10.3390/ijerph192316237

[204] Fildes A, Charlton J, Rudisill C, Littlejohns P, Prevost AT, Gulliford MC. Probability of an obese person attaining Normal body weight: Cohort study using electronic health records. American Journal of Public Health. 2015;**105**:e54-e59. DOI: 10.2105/AJPH.2015.302773

Chapter 7

Bariatric Metabolic Surgery

Matej Pekař, Pavol Holéczy and Marek Soltes

Abstract

Obesity belongs to the most serious metabolic diseases affecting human health due to its pandemic character and significant impact on the risk of cardiovascular and other obesity-related health complications. The treatment is complex and requires multidisciplinary approach. Currently, bariatric-metabolic surgery (BMS) represents the most effective therapy with long-term effect, leading to significant changes in body composition. BMS procedures not only assure weight loss but also positively affect various metabolic and cardiovascular illnesses. As such, the patient may benefit from improvement of several concomitant diseases after mini-invasive BMS intervention. Standardized BMS procedures most frequently used in the world nowadays include sleeve gastrectomy, Roux-en-Y gastric bypass, one anastomosis gastric bypass, and single anastomosis duodeno-lileal bypass with sleeve. The innovative concept is represented by single anastomosis sleeve ileal bypass. Multidisciplinary assessment helps to select patients suitable for BMS and determine the best type of surgical intervention. Endoscopic procedures may serve as a bridge to surgery for polymorbid high-risk patients. Provided the postoperative regimen is strictly adhered to, the results of BMS are excellent. Sustainable weight loss followed by the improvement of associated obesity-related comorbidities results in a significant increase in the overall quality of life.

Keywords: obesity, bariatric, metabolic, surgery, sleeve gastrectomy, roux-en-Y gastric bypass, one anastomosis gastric bypass

1. Introduction

Obesity belongs to the most serious metabolic diseases affecting human health. It has pandemic character and significantly increases the risk of cardiovascular and other obesity-related health complications. The treatment is complex and requires a multidisciplinary approach.

Obesity is the second most common preventable cause of death (after smoking). It is associated with a number of serious negative effects on glucose & lipid metabolism, cardiovascular, respiratory, and musculoskeletal systems as well as mental health. Obesity has a negative impact on fertility, leads to a decreased quality of life, increases the incidence of certain cancers, and likelihood of ischemic and hemorrhagic stroke—thus being responsible for decreased overall survival.

Obesity is a serious medical, social, and economic problem with an interdisciplinary overlap, so sustainable long-term therapeutical success is a must. Obesity can be treated by lifestyle interventions, diet, pharmacologically, or surgically. Healthy lifestyle change with increased physical activity and reduced caloric intake usually results in the first 10% weight loss. To strengthen the effect of the lifestyle change, psychological support in the form of behavioral therapy is needed, since obesity is considered a maladaptive syndrome of eating habits and physical activity [1, 2]. The problem is that caloric restriction reduces the body's basal metabolism, which significantly reduces the effect of further reduction of food intake in the context of weight loss. Many patients are unable to maintain such a low caloric intake that would lead to continuing weight loss thus risking the "yo-yo effect" (weight regain). Significant progress has been achieved in the field of pharmacotherapy and the new effective drugs such as GLP-1 peptide analogs with better short and long-term effects have appeared on the market [3]. However, in patients who do not achieve a weight loss of more than 5% after 4 months of pharmacological antiobesity therapy, this medication should be discontinued. Nevertheless, bariatric-metabolic surgery (BMS) that leads to significant changes in the body composition remains the most effective long-term therapy for obesity. BMS procedures not only assure weight loss but also positively affect various metabolic and cardiovascular illnesses. As such, the patient may benefit from improvement of several concomitant diseases after mini-invasive BMS intervention.

2. Research methods

A systematic review of the literature was carried out using the databases PubMed, Web of Science, and EBSCO. The MeSH terms relevant for given subchapters were used and subsequently, identified literature resources were reviewed to select the most relevant references.

3. History of BMS

The first attempt at targeted surgery to reduce weight came in the 10th century when a Jewish doctor stitched the lips of the Spanish king, who lost his throne due to obesity. He was left with a small opening to receive liquids, lost half of his weight, and regained the throne [4].

The modern era of bariatric surgery dates back to the 1950s when Swedish surgeon Hendriksson performed the first targeted malabsorptive procedure—resection of part of the small intestine in 1952 [5]. After experimental research on dogs, surgeons began performing jejunoileal bypass in humans in Minnesota (USA). The weight loss was excellent, but malabsorption had unfortunate consequences and the method was soon abandoned due to related complications (liver failure, vitamin deficiency, malnutrition, kidney stones, and others).

In 1966, gastric bypass was introduced into the clinical practice by Mason, inspired by the observation of weight loss in patients after gastric resection for cancer [6]. This operation combines malabsorption (bypasses the duodenum) with restriction (reduces the volume of the stomach). The procedure is currently performed in the Roux-en-Y modification (RYGB) and belongs to the most frequent BMS methods [7].

Jaw wiring was introduced in bariatrics in 1977. The results were excellent, but there was a huge yo-yo effect after the procedure reversal [4].

In 1979, Scopinaro performed biliopancreatic diversion (BPD) [7], and in 1986, Kuzmak invented the silastic ring, based on which adjustable gastric banding was described [8]. In 1987, Johnston introduced gastric sleeve resection, the operation that is currently performed most frequently [9]. Originally it was a part of BPD-duodenal switch.

In 1993, Wittgrove and Clark performed the first laparoscopic RYGB [10]. In the same year, Fried introduced laparoscopic non-adjustable and Broadbent laparoscopic adjustable gastric banding. With laparoscopic approach, perioperative mortality fell below 0.2% and complications decreased to one-third. The length of hospitalization and the patient's recovery time were significantly shortened.

The shift from bariatric to metabolic surgery originated from MacDonald and Pories, who described the positive effect of RYGB on type II Diabetes Mellitus in 1995 [11]. In 1998, obesity was recognized as a metabolic disease, not just an esthetic issue, and costs of BMS began to be covered by health insurance [12].

4. Indications for BMS

Although BMI does not reflect exact body composition, it is widely used as a crucial indicator for BMS due to its simplicity and universal applicability. Patients with greater BMI based on higher muscular mass without obvious excess of fat may not benefit from BMI. Nevertheless, the following indication criteria for the BMS procedures, based on the recommendations of the international working groups IFSO and ASMBS [13], apply in the current general practice:

- individuals with BMI higher than 35 kg/m^2 are indicated for BMS regardless of the presence, absence, or severity of comorbidities.
- individuals with BMI over 30 kg/m^2 who have failed other methods of weight reduction or whose obesity-related comorbidities cannot be compensated satisfactorily
- regarding the Asian population, the BMI thresholds have been shifted to 27.5 and 25 kg/m^2
- age limit for surgery does not exist anymore, also younger and older individuals can be operated on, taking into consideration the individual balance between the risk and benefit
- in children and adolescents, BMS should be considered if they have a BMI above 120% of their 95th percentile associated with obesity-related comorbidities, or if they have a BMI above 140% of the 95th percentile
- BMS is recommended for patients in whom excess weight loss is desirable in order to undergo other major surgical interventions such as joint arthroplasty, abdominal wall hernia repair, or organ transplantation.

Multidisciplinary assessment of patients on individual basis helps to select those suitable for BMS and determine the best type of BMS procedure. Reoperations due to failure or insufficient effect of the first BMS operation are not an exception. The re-do surgeries can either mean extension of the primary procedure (i.e. distalization of the anastomosis in bypass) or conversion to more aggressive type (i.e. sleeve gastrectomy to RYGB).

5. Current BMS (state of the art procedures)

5.1 Sleeve gastrectomy (SG)

Sleeve gastrectomy (**Figure 1**) currently represents the most widespread BMS operation in the world. It is defined by 80–90% pylorus-preserving vertical resection of the stomach. It evolved from biliopancreatic diversion with duodenal switch when it was adopted as the first stage of the procedure in high-risk patients. Subsequently, it was observed that vast majority of those patients experienced significant weight loss and did not have to undergo the second stage of the operation. This procedure is defined by both restrictive—reducing the volume of the stomach and metabolic effect—reducing the production of the orexigenic hormone ghrelin. It appears to be a relatively safe surgical method with perioperative mortality close to zero and very low morbidity. The most common complications include bleeding from the resection line, leakage, and gastric fistula. Micronutrient depletion occurs postoperatively, but it seems to be less prominent than after RYGB and disappears after 5 years. Nevertheless, laboratory screening for depletion should be carried out once a year to allow for appropriate supplementation of micronutrients.

The biggest advantage of the procedure is long-term excess weight loss (EWL) of up to 80%. Furthermore, metabolic diseases, including hyperlipidemia and diabetes, disorders of coagulation cascade, biochemical parameters, nonalcoholic fatty liver disease (NAFLD), cardiovascular disorders, obstructive sleep apnea, and

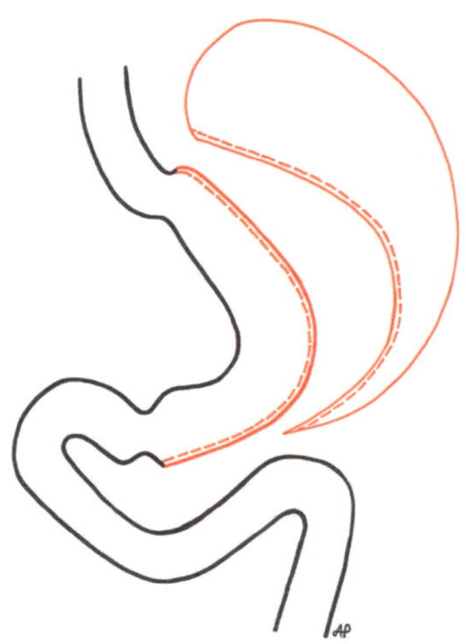

Figure 1.
Sleeve gastrectomy.

hypertension, can be controlled better. Also, non-metabolic diseases, such as musculoskeletal pain, ovarian dysfunction, infertility, incontinence, and the incidence of cancer, are decreased. The procedure is performed laparoscopically, under general anesthesia in the supine position, usually from 5 ports [14–16]. Patients are admitted to the intensive care unit (ICU) for 1 day and in case of uncomplicated postoperative course dismissed on 1st–3rd postoperative day.

Long-term, ideally lifelong follow-up is a necessity. Significant percentage of patients after sleeve gastrectomy report gastroesophageal reflux disease that may progress to Barrett's esophagus. While proton pump inhibitors provide effective therapeutic solution for majority of patients, conversion to RYGB may be necessary in some patients.

5.2 Roux-en-Y gastric bypass (RYGB)

Roux-en-Y gastric bypass (**Figure 2**) means "in the form of a Y" in French. It is the second most spread BMS procedure in the world. This operation consists of several steps. First, a gastric pouch is formed, where a smaller part remains in contact with the esophagus and a larger part is excluded from food intake and remains connected to the duodenum. The goal is to create a small, about 20 ml, gastric reservoir. In the next step, a biliopancreatic limb is formed, which is about 100 cm long (from the ligament of Treitz) and is connected to the alimentary tract about 100 cm aboral from the pylorus by jejunojejunostomy, and after that the continuity of the digestive tube is restored by a gastrojejunostomy [17]. Mesenteric defect is closed with a continuous suture to prevent internal hernia formation after anticipated significant weight loss. Some surgeons close also the Petersen's space. Patient is monitored in the ICU postoperatively, liquids are administered 3–4 hours after the operation through a straw, and mobilization should be started 4–5 hours after the procedure. Nutritional therapist provides education regarding the appropriate food intake and special diet. Hospital stay is usually about 3 days.

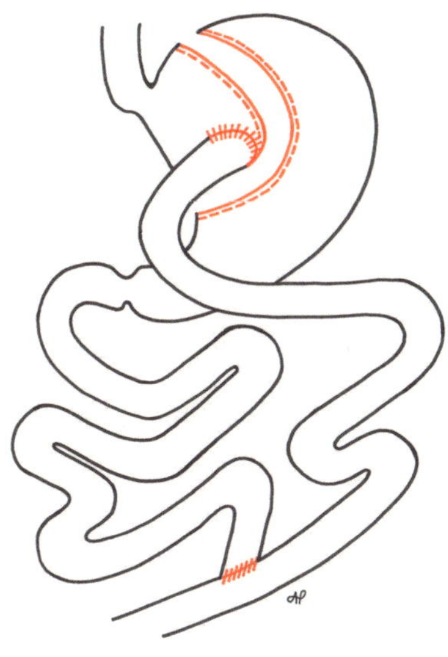

Figure 2.
Roux-en-Y gastric bypass.

The effect of gastric bypass is restrictive, malabsorptive, and metabolic. Reduced volume of the stomach gives a feeling of satiety with less food intake while biliopancreatic loop reduces absorption in the small intestine. Metabolic effect is most pronounced in patients suffering from type 2 diabetes mellitus (DMT2). The operation is also beneficial for patients with gastroesophageal reflux disease. The effect of therapy is long-lasting, and the EWL is around 70–80%. Complications tend to be more frequent after RYGB, and morbidity is doubled compared to that of SG. It is absolutely necessary to pay attention to the supplementation of micronutrients and vitamins, as there is an increased risk of their depletion. Malnutrition with liver cirrhosis is very serious consequence of non-compliance with the regime. The follow-up must be performed at standard intervals, and laboratory control should be scheduled once to twice per year. There is a recommendation of standard ion and vitamin supplementation to all patients with possible modifications depending on the laboratory findings. RYGB may also cause "dumping syndrome," a group of symptoms, including diarrhea, nausea, and feeling of sickness after eating or drinking, especially sweets. The risk of internal hernia after RYGB should not be underestimated. Also of note, tobacco and NSAIDs use considerably increases the risk of peptic ulcerations.

5.3 One anastomosis gastric bypass (OAGB)

OAGB (**Figure 3**) is very similar to RYGB and its effect on weight reduction and metabolic effect is practically identical [18]. Nevertheless, the procedure itself is technically easier. The principle of operation is construction of gastric reservoir, which is longer than in the Roux-en-Y modification, but very narrow. It is created by gastric resection along the 36F probe, similar to sleeve gastrectomy after the stomach is partially cut at a right angle to the lesser curvature at the level of the angular incisure. A simple side-to-side gastroenteroanastomosis is then created at a distance of 200 cm from the Treitz ligament. Some studies confirmed certain degree of biliary reflux but did not demonstrate a higher risk of gastric or esophageal cancer. Nevertheless,

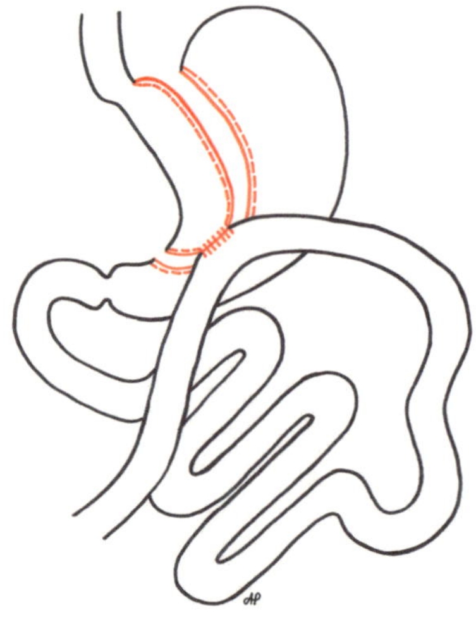

Figure 3.
One anastomosis gastric bypass.

presence of severe gastroesophageal reflux or Barrett's esophagus represents contraindication for OAGB. Postoperative care is identical to RYGB.

5.4 Biliopancreatic diversion with duodenal switch (BPD-DS)

Biliopancreatic diversion (BPD), originally proposed by Scopinaro in 1976, was performed as a 2/3 resection of the stomach and division of the small intestine into alimentary and biliary arm. In the alimentary arm, only carbohydrates and proteins are resorbed while fat resorption takes place in the common channel of the small intestine, 50 cm long, where both arms join. The procedure resembles gastric bypass in the Roux-en-Y modification, but the so-called common channel, that is, the part of the small intestine where all nutrients are resorbed, is significantly shorter than in RYGB (**Figure 4**). This makes the effect of the operation more pronounced, but at the same time, the quality of life is negatively affected and the risk of malnutrition tends to be higher. In an effort to achieve more physiological conditions during the passage of food through the stomach, Hess proposed an operation called "biliopancreatic diversion with duodenal switch." Gastric resection is performed similarly to sleeve gastrectomy but a section of approximately 5 cm of duodenum is left, and duodeno-entero anastomosis is created there. The goal is to reduce acidity at the anastomotic site, achieve a quick feeling of satiety, and preserve antropyloric function. Leaving a short section of the duodenum improves the resorption of iron, calcium, and magnesium. It also eliminates the risk of dumping syndrome and reduces the risk of ulcer formation in the anastomosis.

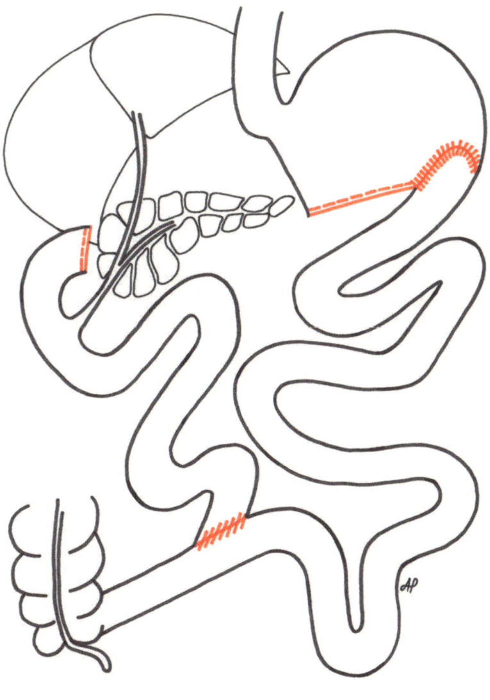

Figure 4.
Biliopancreatic diversion with duodenal switch.

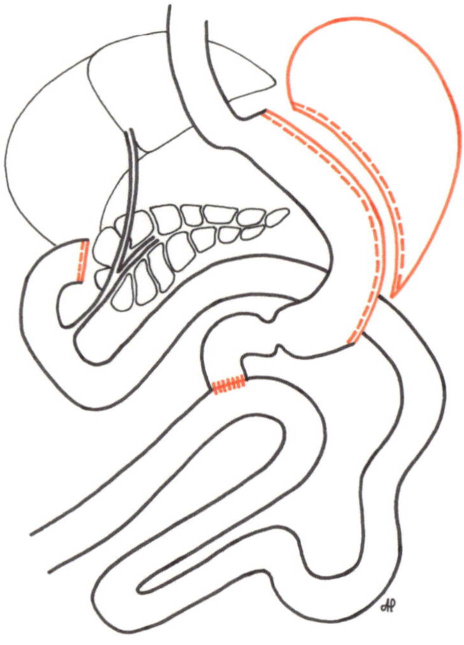

Figure 5.
Single anastomosis duodenoileal bypass with sleeve.

Both modifications—BPD and BPD-DS—are currently performed worldwide only in a minimal number of cases [19].

5.5 Single anastomosis duodenal-ileal bypass with sleeve (SADI-S)

SADI-S represents relatively new approach in BMS. The procedure is technically easier than BPD. The first phase of SADI-S is sleeve gastric resection followed by the transverse incision of the duodenum and creation of duodenoenteroanastomosis. The small bowel suture site is 250–300 cm from the ileocecal junction (**Figure 5**). As such, this operation achieves a combination of food intake restriction and severe malnutrition, which makes this surgery very effective. SADI-S is more frequently used as a re-do procedure after failure of previous sleeve gastrectomy rather than as a primary surgery [20, 21].

5.6 Adjustable gastric banding (AGB)

This BMS procedure gained peak popularity in Europe at the turn of the millennium. In principle, food intake is restricted by application of the silicone ring just below the gastroesophageal junction thus creating a small gastric reservoir (**Figure 6**). The tightness of the band can be adjusted by calibrating the balloon on its inner side by injecting the physiological solution into the calibration chamber (connected with the band by tube) that is subcutaneously implanted into the abdominal wall.

Currently, AGB is practically abandoned because of the fact that other operations are significantly more effective in the long term [22]. At the moment, AGB accounts for less than 1% of bariatric procedures performed worldwide.

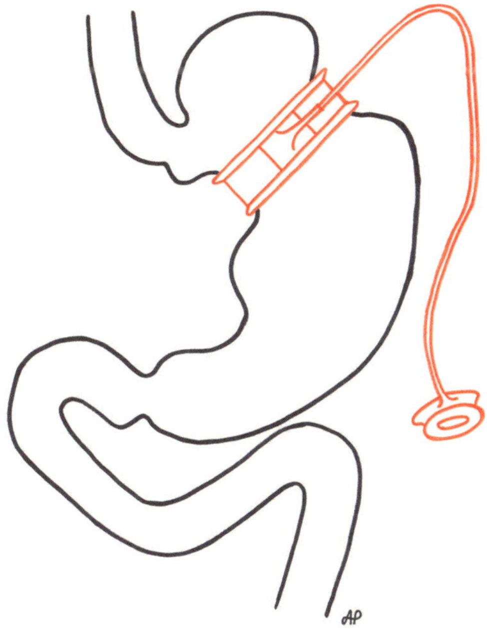

Figure 6.
Adjustable gastric band.

6. Emerging procedures

6.1 Single aastomosis sleeve ileal bypass (SASI)

SASI is the combination of sleeve resection and single side-to-side anastomosis in the region of the gastric antrum and ileum, 250 cm before the ileocecal junction (**Figure 7**). Part of the food passes through the natural pathways and part through the anastomosis, which achieves a certain degree of malnutrition and activates intestinal hormones. The great advantage of this procedure is the preservation of the passage through the pylorus and the duodenum enabling endoscopic access to the papilla of Vater, which can be truly important for the management of the common bile duct stones or other diseases of the extrahepatic bile ducts. This operation, however, has not been recognized yet as standardized BMS approach by the IFSO. SASI offers both excellent weight loss and resolution of comorbidities. Some data suggest the average EWL at 12 months as high as 85.6% and diabetes remission in 95.8% of patients [23]. Nevertheless, more high-quality and large-scale studies are still needed to support the efficacy of SASI.

7. Endoscopic procedures

Endoscopic bariatric metabolic procedures seem optimal in very high-risk patients as a bridge to BMS rather than final solution. There are several endoscopic options that are currently used in clinical practice.

Various types of gastric balloons reducing the effective volume of the stomach have been designed. One of the most up-to-date examples is the Obalon, which can be

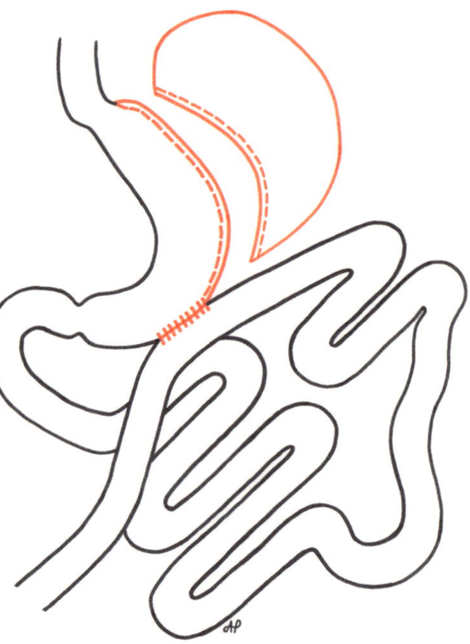

Figure 7.
Single anastomosis sleeve ileal bypass.

swallowed as a small capsule on a connecting tube and then filled with liquid without the aid of endoscopy. It is possible to place up to three balloons in the stomach, which must be removed within 6 months endoscopically. Another interesting concept is represented by the so-called transpyloric shuttle. During this procedure, two interconnected balloons are inserted endoscopically, the larger one in the stomach and smaller one in the duodenum. The gastric part of the shuttle prolongs the evacuation of the stomach (**Figure 8**). This system is indicated for the patients with BMI of 30–40 kg/m^2 and can be left in place for 12 months.

Some endoscopic procedures reduce the volume of the stomach by suturing its wall, thus mimicking SG. The Apollo overstitch system is capable of constructing endoscopic transmural sutures. The disadvantage of the technique is an increased risk of suture line failure compared to SG, which is reflected in the lower efficacy in terms of the weight loss [24].

Another innovative endoscopic option is duodenojejunal sleeve. During the procedure, polyethylene sleeve is anchored in the pyloric area by a metal ring with hooks around its perimeter. The length of the sleeve is 60 cm, so it reaches up to the proximal jejunum. This prevents contact of food with the mucosa of the duodenum (**Figure 9**). As a result, anatomical and pathophysiological effects of the gastric bypass are imitated. Nevertheless, endoscopic sleeve can only be left *in situ* for a maximum of 12 months, after which it must be extracted. Data demonstrates weight gain after sleeve explantation. Also of note, one of the studies had to be discontinued due to unacceptable rate of complications [25].

In general, it can be concluded that endoscopic procedures have not yet been proven effective in the long term. One can appreciate their importance in high-risk patients for whom surgery would be unbearable, or, as a bridge to surgical

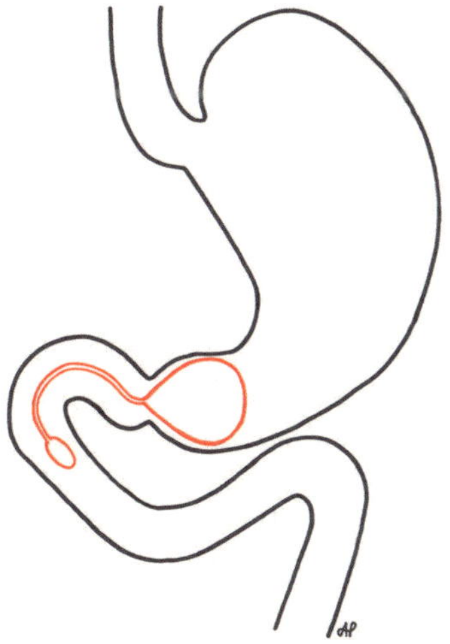

Figure 8.
Transpyloric shuttle.

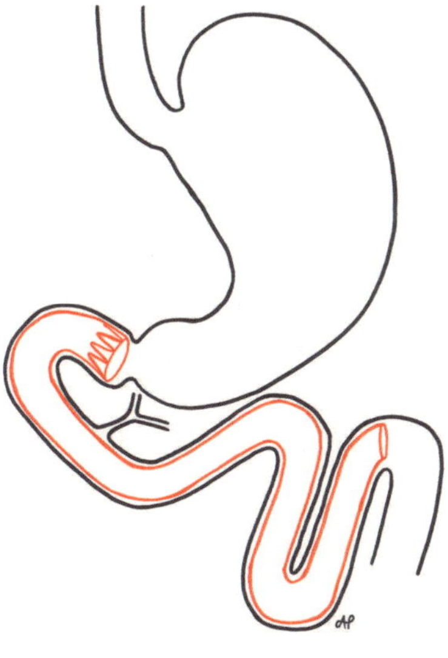

Figure 9.
Duodenojejunal sleeve.

intervention. To evaluate the true potential of endoscopic procedures, future properly designed larger-scale studies with long-term follow-up are necessary.

8. Discussion

Ideal BMS procedure should ensure maximal long-term EWL with minimal complications. Nevertheless, universal single approach does not exist at the moment, so patients require individual assessment and tailored therapy.

In the past, gastric banding was very popular operation among both patients and surgeons due to its relative simplicity, reversibility, and significant weight loss achieved on solely restrictive principle. However, in the long term, EWL did not seem sustainable. Also of note, complications requiring removal of the band lead to almost 100% yo-yo effect [26].

On the contrary, malabsorptive procedures proved to be highly successful in terms of sustainable long-term weight loss, but their results were discredited by metabolic complications and risk of disruption of the internal environment. Nevertheless, RYGB has established itself as a relatively safe and effective option over the time, providing also highly valuable metabolic effects in patients with DM, thus solving very complex condition of obesity with insulin resistance. As such, RYGB began to be widely promoted. However, technical difficulty of the the RYGB was stimulating the search for simpler procedures that could comparably modify metabolic disease while maintaining excellent long-term results. That is why OAGB has been gradually becoming established in clinical practice as a technically simpler and feasible alternative to RYGB. Besides sustainable EWL, OAGB positively affects DMT2, dyslipidemia, and arterial hypertension, as well as the other metabolic and obesity-related diseases [27].

Later on, interesting observation that SG indicated as the first stage of BPD-DS in polymorbid high-risk patients appeared to provide comparable EWL as well as metabolic effect, which led to the acceptance of SG as primary BMS procedure. The two main reasons why SG is currently the preferred operation worldwide include excellent long-term results and very good safety profile with minimal number of complications [28].

It is important to point out that correct timing of BMS is crucial for its success. Although indication for surgery is relatively straightforward, patient must undergo thorough preoperative preparation not only for the procedure itself but also for the life after BMS. Therefore, multidisciplinary approach and assessment is inevitable. The team consists of a surgeon, gastroenterologist, internist, nutritionist, clinical psychologist, endocrinologist, diabetologist, and selectively other specialists if needed. Every patient indicated for BMS should undergo behavioral intervention as soon as possible—setting-up an ideal diet, defining lifestyle changes, and designing regular physical activity program in the patient's routine. The initial effect of this complex behavioral therapy on EWL should subsequently be supported by pharmacotherapy to improve the patient's adherence to therapy. Only the patient who can successfully complete the preprocedural algorithm should be indicated for BMS with the clear consent. If failure of surgical treatment is reported, it is usually caused by failure to comply with the postoperative regimen in poorly prepared patients [29].

Any malnutritive procedure is potentially dangerous due to the risk of ion imbalance and micronutrient and vitamin deficiency. Although this risk is the same for all the patients in the beginning, there is a huge interindividual variability. Therefore, regular laboratory and clinical checks are necessary after RYGB, OAGB, BPD-DS, and SADI-S. The problem is especially pronounced in non-adherent patients who do not follow the regimen and drop out from regular follow-up, but can occur even in those complying with follow-up [30].

Also of note, the indication criteria for BMS have moved toward the lower BMI limits recently. Generally speaking, a decrease of 5 kg/m^2 can be noticed. This means that BMS is now available to wider range of patients at the earlier stage of obesity. As higher BMI is associated with more severe obesity-related comorbidities and disabilities as well as perioperative and postoperative complication rates, it appears logical that shift toward lower BMI indications could be linked with better results and subsequently with better quality of healthcare accessible to wider range of patients.

The indication for BMS also used to be limited to an upper age limit of 65 years. This policy is no longer valid as the age alone should not be considered a prohibitive factor. Therefore, the decision is left to the attending surgeon and multidisciplinary team on an individual basis, after careful assessment of biological age, comorbidities, BMS risks, and benefits as well as patient's preference.

Furthermore, the prevalence of obesity among the population younger than 18 years is increasing. Children and adolescents with severe obesity are at risk of developing and worsening obesity-related comorbidities, especially hypertension, DM, dyslipidemia, and sleep apnea syndrome, as well as facing psychological problems. Lifestyle changes play a crucial role in these patients, but in more severe obesity, those are often insufficient while use of pharmacotherapy is limited in this age group. Therefore, BMS has become indicated for adolescents under 18 years of age with severe obesity. The preferred BMS procedures are SG and RYGB due to their excellent long-term results. However, the indication has to be based on the careful assessment of the multidisciplinary panel, and only after successful preoperative interventions leading to a change in the lifestyle. Also, the compliance of the patients with recommended postoperative regimen and long-term follow-up must be assured as vitamin and mineral supplementation may be necessary. Successful BMS in the pediatric patients with severe obesity improves the overall quality of life, solves the associated comorbidities, and prolongs life expectancy in this subpopulation [31–36].

It is not uncommon for the initial BMS to fail and thus, re-do surgeries are not unusual. The reasons may vary but they are mostly related either to non-compliance with the postoperative regimen by the patient or inadequate choice of the procedure by the surgeon. Most commonly, BMS reoperations are performed after gastric band removal when SG is usually indicated. In case of failed SG due to dilated gastric sleeve, a re-sleeve gastrectomy can be attempted, but higher complication rate can be expected compared to primary procedure. In case of failed SG without dilatation of the gastric sleeve, modification to OAGB, RYGB, or SADI-S is feasible, thus adding malabsorptive effect to the procedure [37].

Currently, progress may be noted in the pharmacotherapy of obesity as well. Significant weight loss can be achieved by using GLP-1 peptide analog (liraglutide), the dual GLP-1/GIP receptor agonist (tirzepatide), and the triple-hormone-receptor agonist (retatrutide). Randomized controlled trials provided support for the use of liraglutide 3.0 mg for weight management in the adults with obesity or overweight [38]. Recent meta-analysis suggested that tirzepatide led to substantial weight, BMI, and waist circumference reduction for the cost of increased frequency of gastrointestinal symptoms (nausea, vomiting, and diarrhea) compared to placebo [39]. The double-blind, randomized, placebo-controlled trial on 338 adults showed that retatrutide treatment for 48 weeks resulted in substantial reduction in body weight [40]. Although the weight loss under these novel medications appears to be comparable to the results of BMS, future randomized trials are needed to assess the true potential of pharmacotherapy to compete with surgical management.

9. Conclusion

BMS is currently the most successful therapeutic approach to obesity. It provides desirable long-term effects and excellent results if patient complies with the postoperative regimen. Besides weight loss, there are also positive effects on associated metabolic diseases, obesity-related diseases, and overall increase in the quality of life that is achieved. Therefore, BMS has an impact not only from medical point of view but also from psychological, social, and economic one. Prevention of complications related to diseases associated with obesity thus significantly reduces the costs that would have to be spent on their treatment in future. Also of note, obese patients often complain about negative experiences in their social life with tendency to depression. Successful BMS significantly improves their postoperative quality of life both from physical and psychological perspectives.

Acknowledgements

Great thanks belong to Mrs. Anna Pekarova MD., PhD. for the figures illustrations. This study was supported by Specific University Research Grant no. MUNI/A/1547/2023 provided by the Ministry of Education, Youth, and Sports of the Czech Republic. We want to acknowledge the Hospital AGEL Czech Republic for the support in writing this chapter.

Conflict of interest

The authors declare no conflict of interest.

Author details

Matej Pekař[1,2*], Pavol Holéczy[3,4] and Marek Soltes[5]

1 Mini-invasive and Vascular Surgery Center, Hospital AGEL, Trinec-Podlesi, Czech Republic

2 Faculty of Medicine, Department of Physiology, Masaryk University, Brno, Czech Republic

3 Bariatric Center, Hospital AGEL, Ostrava-Vitkovice, Czech Republic

4 Faculty of Medicine, Department of Surgical disciplines, University Ostrava, Ostrava, Czech Republic

5 First Department of Surgery, Pavol Jozef Safarik University in Kosice and University Hospital of L. Pasteur, Kosice, Slovak Republic

*Address all correspondence to: matej.pekar@npo.agel.cz

References

[1] Jacob JJ, Isaac R. Behavioral therapy for management of obesity. Indian Journal of Endocrinology and Metabolism. 2012;**16**(1):28-32. DOI: 10.4103/2230-8210.91180

[2] Adachi Y, Sato C, Yamatsu K, Ito S, Adachi K, Yamagami T. A randomized controlled trial on the long-term effects of a 1-month behavioral weight control program assisted by computer tailored advice. Behaviour Research and Therapy. 2007;**45**(3):459-470. DOI: 10.1016/j.brat.2006.03.017

[3] Haluzík M, Müllerová D, Sucharda P, Boženský J, Holéczy P, Fried M, et al. Obesity pharmacotherapy - update 2023. Casopís Lékařů Ceských. 2023;**162**(1):19-31

[4] Faria GR. A brief history of bariatric surgery. Porto Biomedical Journal. 2017;**2**(3):90-92. DOI: 10.1016/j.pbj.2017.01.008

[5] Celio AC, Pories WJ. A history of bariatric surgery: The maturation of a medical discipline. The Surgical Clinics of North America. 2016;**96**(4):655-667. DOI: 10.1016/j.suc.2016.03.001

[6] Mason EE, Ito C. Gastric bypass in obesity. The Surgical Clinics of North America. 1967;**47**(6):1345-1351. DOI: 10.1016/s0039-6109(16)38384-0

[7] Scopinaro N, Gianetta E, Adami GF, Friedman D, Traverso E, Marinari GM, et al. Biliopancreatic diversion for obesity at eighteen years. Surgery. 1996;**119**(3):261-268. DOI: 10.1016/s0039-6060(96)80111-5

[8] Kuzmak LI, Yap IS, McGuire L, Dixon JS, Young MP. Surgery for morbid obesity. Using an inflatable gastric band. AORN Journal. 1990;**51**(5):1307-1324. DOI: 10.1016/s0001-2092(07)70154-0

[9] Johnston D, Dachtler J, Sue-Ling HM, King RF, Martin LG. The magenstrasse and mill operation for morbid obesity. Obesity Surgery. 2003;**13**(1):10-16. DOI: 10.1381/096089203321136520

[10] Wittgrove AC, Clark GW, Tremblay LJ. Laparoscopic gastric bypass, Roux-en-Y: Preliminary report of five cases. Obesity Surgery. 1994;**4**(4):353-357. DOI: 10.1381/096089294765558331

[11] MacDonald KG Jr, Long SD, Swanson MS, Brown BM, Morris P, Dohm GL, et al. The gastric bypass operation reduces the progression and mortality of non-insulin-dependent diabetes mellitus. Journal of Gastrointestinal Surgery. 1997;**1**(3):213-220; discussion 220. DOI: 10.1016/s1091-255x(97)80112-6

[12] Arrieta F, Pedro-Botet J. Recognizing obesity as a disease: A true challenge. Revista Clínica Española (Barc). 2021;**221**(9):544-546. DOI: 10.1016/j.rceng.2020.08.005

[13] Eisenberg D, Shikora SA, Aarts E, Aminian A, Angrisani L, Cohen RV, et al. 2022 American society of metabolic and bariatric surgery (ASMBS) and international federation for the surgery of obesity and metabolic disorders (IFSO) indications for metabolic and bariatric surgery. Obesity Surgery. 2023;**33**(1):3-14. DOI: 10.1007/s11695-022-06332-1

[14] Nguyen NT, Varela JE. Bariatric surgery for obesity and metabolic disorders: State of the art. Nature Reviews. Gastroenterology &

Hepatology. 2017;**14**(3):160-169. DOI: 10.1038/nrgastro.2016.170

[15] Kheirvari M, Dadkhah Nikroo N, Jaafarinejad H, Farsimadan M, Eshghjoo S, Hosseini S, et al. The advantages and disadvantages of sleeve gastrectomy; clinical laboratory to bedside review. Heliyon. 2020;**6**(2):e03496. DOI: 10.1016/j.heliyon.2020.e03496

[16] Coutant R, Bouhours-Nouet N, Donzeau A, Fauchard M, Decrequy A, Malka J, et al. Bariatric surgery in adolescents with severe obesity: Review and state of the art in France. Annales d'endocrinologie. 2017;**78**(5):462-468. DOI: 10.1016/j.ando.2017.03.002

[17] Mitchell BG, Gupta N. Roux-en-Y Gastric Bypass. In: StatPearls. [Internet]. Treasure Island (FL): StatPearls Publishing; 2023 [Accessed: Jul. 25, 2023]

[18] De Luca M, Piatto G, Merola G, Himpens J, Chevallier JM, Carbajo MA, et al. IFSO update position statement on one anastomosis gastric bypass (OAGB). Obesity Surgery. 2021;**31**(7):3251-3278. DOI: 10.1007/s11695-021-05413-x

[19] Conner J, Nottingham JM. Biliopancreatic diversion with duodenal switch. In: StatPearls [Internet]. Treasure Island (FL): StatPearls Publishing; 2023 [Accessed: Sep. 19, 2022]

[20] Torres A, Rubio MA, Ramos-Leví AM, Sánchez-Pernaute A. Cardiovascular risk factors after single anastomosis Duodeno-Ileal bypass with sleeve gastrectomy (SADI-S): A new effective therapeutic approach? Current Atherosclerosis Reports. 2017;**19**(12):58. DOI: 10.1007/s11883-017-0688-4

[21] Sánchez-Pernaute A, Rubio Herrera MA, Pérez-Aguirre E, García Pérez JC, Cabrerizo L, Díez Valladares L, et al. Proximal duodenal-ileal end-to-side bypass with sleeve gastrectomy: Proposed technique. Obesity Surgery. 2007;**17**(12):1614-1618. DOI: 10.1007/s11695-007-9287-8

[22] Angrisani L, Santonicola A, Iovino P, Vitiello A, Higa K, Himpens J, et al. IFSO worldwide survey 2016: Primary, endoluminal, and revisional procedures. Obesity Surgery. 2018;**28**(12):3783-3794. DOI: 10.1007/s11695-018-3450-2

[23] Romero RJ, Colorado-Subizar R, De Uriarte-Lorente M, Barradas-Lagunes M, Bravo-De Ávila P, Romero-Espejo JJ. Single anastomosis sleeve ileal bypass (SASI bypass): Short-term outcomes and concerns. Obesity Surgery. 2021;**31**(5):2339-2343. DOI: 10.1007/s11695-020-05145-4

[24] Jirapinyo P, McCarty TR, Dolan RD, Shah R, Thompson CC. Effect of endoscopic bariatric and metabolic therapies on nonalcoholic fatty liver disease: A systematic review and meta-analysis. Clinical Gastroenterology and Hepatology. 2022;**20**(3):511-524.e1. DOI: 10.1016/j.cgh.2021.03.017

[25] Holéczy P, Pekař M, Bužga M, Evinová E. Current bariatric-metabolic surgery. Casopís Lékařů Ceských. 2022;**161**(3-4):100-106

[26] Aarts EO, Dogan K, Koehestanie P, Janssen IM, Berends FJ. What happens after gastric band removal without additional bariatric surgery? Surgery for Obesity and Related Diseases. 2014;**10**(6):1092-1096. DOI: 10.1016/j.soard.2013.10.014

[27] Affinati AH, Esfandiari NH, Oral EA, Kraftson AT. Bariatric surgery in the treatment of type 2 diabetes. Current Diabetes Reports. 2019;**19**(12):156. DOI: 10.1007/s11892-019-1269-4

[28] Ozsoy Z, Demir E. Which bariatric procedure is the most popular in the world? A bibliometric comparison. Obesity Surgery. 2018;**28**(8):2339-2352. DOI: 10.1007/s11695-018-3163-6

[29] Istfan NW, Lipartia M, Anderson WA, Hess DT, Apovian CM. Approach to the patient: Management of the post-bariatric surgery patient with weight regain. The Journal of Clinical Endocrinology and Metabolism. 2021;**106**(1):251-263. DOI: 10.1210/clinem/dgaa702

[30] Gasmi A, Bjørklund G, Mujawdiya PK, Semenova Y, Peana M, Dosa A, et al. Micronutrients deficiences in patients after bariatric surgery. European Journal of Nutrition. 2022;**61**(1):55-67. DOI: 10.1007/s00394-021-02619-8

[31] Armstrong SC, Bolling CF, Michalsky MP, Reichard KW, Section on Obesity, Section on Surgery. Pediatric metabolic and bariatric surgery: Evidence, barriers, and best practices. Pediatrics. 2019;**144**(6):e20193223. DOI: 10.1542/peds.2019-3223

[32] Steinhart A, Tsao D, Pratt JSA. Pediatric metabolic and bariatric surgery. The Surgical Clinics of North America. 2021;**101**(2):199-212. DOI: 10.1016/j.suc.2020.12.007

[33] Bolling CF, Armstrong SC, Reichard KW, Michalsky MP, Section on Obesity, Section on surgery. Metabolic and bariatric surgery for pediatric patients with severe obesity. Pediatrics. 2019;**144**(6):e20193224. DOI: 10.1542/peds.2019-3224

[34] Lewit RA, Harmon CM, Ricca R, Rich BS, Raval MV, Weatherall YZ. Bariatric surgery practice patterns among pediatric surgeons in the United States. Journal of Pediatric Surgery. 2022;**57**(12):887-891. DOI: 10.1016/j.jpedsurg.2022.07.003

[35] Gonzalez DO, Michalsky MP. Update on pediatric metabolic and bariatric surgery. Pediatric Obesity. 2021;**16**(8):e12794. DOI: 10.1111/ijpo.12794

[36] Pratt JSA, Browne A, Browne NT, Bruzoni M, Cohen M, Desai A, et al. ASMBS pediatric metabolic and bariatric surgery guidelines, 2018. Surgery for Obesity and Related Diseases. 2018;**14**(7):882-901. DOI: 10.1016/j.soard.2018.03.019

[37] Switzer NJ, Karmali S, Gill RS, Sherman V. Revisional bariatric surgery. The Surgical Clinics of North America. 2016;**96**(4):827-842. DOI: 10.1016/j.suc.2016.03.004

[38] Lin Q, Xue Y, Zou H, Ruan Z, Ung COL, Hu H. Efficacy and safety of liraglutide for obesity and people who are overweight: A systematic review and meta-analysis of randomized controlled trials. Expert Review of Clinical Pharmacology. 2022;**15**(12):1461-1469. DOI: 10.1080/17512433.2022.2130760

[39] de Mesquita YLL, Pera Calvi I, Reis Marques I, Almeida Cruz S, Padrao EMH, Carvalho PEP, et al. Efficacy and safety of the dual GIP and GLP-1 receptor agonist tirzepatide for weight loss: A meta-analysis of randomized controlled trials. International Journal of Obesity. 2023;**47**(10):883-892. DOI: 10.1038/s41366-023-01337-x

[40] Jastreboff AM, Kaplan LM, Frías JP, Wu Q, Du Y, Gurbuz S, et al. Retatrutide phase 2 obesity trial investigators. Triple-hormone-receptor agonist retatrutide for obesity - A phase 2 trial. The New England Journal of Medicine. 2023;**389**(6):514-526. DOI: 10.1056/NEJMoa2301972. Epub 2023 Jun 26

Chapter 8

Endoscopic Methods in Obesity Treatment

Anıl Ergin and Cihan Şahan

Abstract

Obesity is a multifactorial, chronic disease that occurs with a pathologic increase in the body fat ratio and significantly increases mortality and morbidity. It has become a global health problem with increasing prevalence day by day. Methods used in the treatment of obesity are classified as diet, exercise, lifestyle changes, medical treatments, surgical treatments and endoscopic treatments. Endoscopic treatments are classified as intragastric balloon, transpyloric shuttle, endoscopic sleeve gastroplasty, gastric aspiration, small bowel procedures, duodenal mucosal resurfacing, intragastric botulinum toxin A injection. Although surgical procedures are known as the most effective methods in the fight against obesity today, the frequency and effectiveness of endoscopic treatments are increasing day by day. Endoscopic methods in obesity treatment are promising. There is a need for new methods with high efficacy and reliability, easy application, low complication rate and low cost in the treatment of obesity.

Keywords: obesity, treatment, endoscopy, intragastric baloon, transpyloric shuttle, endoscopic sleeve gastroplasty, gastric aspiration, duodenal mucosal resurfacing, intragastric botox

1. Introduction

Obesity is a multifactorial, chronic disease that occurs with a pathologic increase in the body fat ratio and significantly increases mortality and morbidity. It has become a global health problem with increasing prevalence day by day [1]. Between 1980 and 2002, the prevalence of obesity doubled in adults (aged over 19 years) and tripled in children and adolescents (aged between 6 and 19 years) [2]. Obesity has complex etiologic causes that cannot be defined as overeating alone. Genetic and environmental interactions, behavioral disorders, metabolic and endocrine disorders play an intertwined role in the etiology of obesity. Most of them occur as a result of a series of vicious cyclical events that can be explained in a cause and effect relationship. Although genetic and neuroendocrine factors are rarely encountered, environmental factors constitute the basis of the etiology of obesity [3].

In the diagnosis and evaluation of obesity, the patient's chronological history of weight gain, the age at which the patient started to gain weight, the presence of overweight people in the family, the ages of pregnancy, child rearing and menopause, which are favorable periods for weight gain for female patients, how overweight affects the patient's health, and the patient's expectations from treatment should be questioned. During physical examination, diseases that may cause obesity and the main accompanying comorbidities; coronary artery disease, peripheral artery disease, type 2 diabetes mellitus, obstructive sleep apnea syndrome should be questioned [4].

Anthropometric measurements are used to define and classify obesity. These include methods such as body mass index, skinfold thickness and circumference measurements [5, 6].

2. Obesity treatment methods

2.1 Diet, exercise, lifestyle changes

First of all, realistic goals should be set. Changes should be made in the person's eating habits and physical activity habits. In addition, activity and diet planning should be increased gradually. Access to food intake should be made difficult and self-control should be ensured. Alternative behaviors against eating stimuli should be tried to be developed. Regular weight checks should be performed and social support should be provided if necessary [7].

Diet therapy is applied to ensure a healthy and balanced diet, taking into account the gender, lifestyle, age and physical activity status of the person. It is very important in diet therapy to regulate the wrong eating habits in the process of becoming obese. After the body weight reaches the desired level in diet therapy, it is also necessary to maintain this level and to maintain eating habits for life. In diet therapy for children as well as adults, diet programs are made to maintain development and growth [8].

Exercise, which is one of the methods and essentials of effective weight loss, is one of the types of physical activity. Exercise, which is effective in the treatment of obesity, should be done at moderate intensity, on average 5 times a week and each exercise should be at least 30 minutes. Exercises that should be done in a disciplined manner can be shaped according to the age, gender, living conditions and sports history of the person [9].

In addition to moderate exercises, the person should also do resistance exercises that will work muscles such as the abdomen, hips, legs, shoulders and back. These exercises, which will help to lose weight and help the body reach the desired index, should be done 2 or 3 times a week. The energy burning of all these exercises is valid not only during the activity but also after the activity [9].

In addition to diet, weekly exercise programs are one of the factors that prevent the person from gaining weight again. Regular exercise should be continued after reaching the desired weight. In addition to weight loss, exercise also makes people feel good about themselves. Loss of confidence during obesity can be regained with exercise and it is effective in preventing many diseases. Exercise reduces the risk of many diseases such as decreased insulin resistance, cardiovascular, hypertension, diabetes [9].

Lifestyle changes supported by healthy nutrition and exercise are indispensable conditions for the treatment of obesity.

2.2 Medical treatment

Drug therapy can be used in the treatment of overweight and obese patients in addition to diet, exercise and lifestyle changes. However, problems such as the efficacy and safety of drugs, slowing and plateauing of weight loss during treatment, and weight regain when the drug is discontinued are the limiting points of drug treatment in obesity. Drug treatment can be used for those with a BMI >30 kg/m^2 and those with a BMI of 27–29.9 kg/m^2 with additional morbidity [10].

The rationality of the targets set is of great importance in the success of treatment. Targeting the ideal normal body weight is not a realistic approach. Therefore, physicians and patients should have a realistic approach to weight loss treatment at the beginning. Success in treatment is measured by the amount of weight lost and improvement in existing risk factors. Weight loss exceeding 2 kg in the first month of drug treatment, losing 5% of the basal weight in the 3rd–6th months and staying at this level can be considered an effective treatment. A 5–10% weight loss significantly reduces the risk for diabetes and cardiovascular disease [10, 11].

Drug treatment does not provide a curative result in obesity. During treatment, weight loss stops after maximal treatment response is achieved. After drug treatment is discontinued, weight gain may occur again. Obese patients with concomitant diabetes, depression and cardiovascular diseases should be advised to choose treatments that have a weight loss effect rather than weight gain when planning drug treatment for these conditions. Currently, the drugs approved by the US Food and Drug Administration (FDA) for the treatment of obesity are phentermine, diethylpropion, phendimetrazine, benzfetamine, orlistat, lorcaserin, phentermine/topiramate-Extended Release (ER) combination. Of these drugs, only orlistat, lorcaserin, phentermine/topiramate-ER are approved by the FDA for long-term use. The others are only approved for short-term (a few weeks) use. All drugs are approved for use in patients with a BMI $\geq$ 30 kg/m^2. Benzfetamine and diethylpropion can also be used in patients with a BMI $\geq$ 27 kg/m^2 and an additional obesity-related comorbidity (hypertension, diabetes). Recently, drugs with the active ingredients semaglutide and liraglutide have also been used in the treatment of obesity and show promise [12].

2.3 Surgical treatment

In 1991, the US National Institutes of Health Consensus Conference decided that surgery should be considered as a treatment in selected patients when it became clear that non-surgical treatments resulted in little weight loss and subsequent weight regain. At the same time, the committee recommended that these patients should be evaluated by a multidisciplinary team before surgery and followed up for life after the operation is performed under appropriate conditions [13–15].

If we look at the historical development of bariatric surgery, the first operations were performed in the 1950s to treat severe hyperlipidemia associated with obesity. These operations were ileocolic bypass operations to limit absorption and caused severe postoperative nutritional complications and liver failure. The jejunoileal bypass was then developed and became popular in the mid-1970s [13, 14].

In 1969, Mason and Ito performed the first gastric bypass, which they described as the connection of a jejunum ring to a transverse proximal gastric pouch. Postoperative bile reflux esophagitis was severe and Griffin et al. described the roux-n-Y modification of the gastric bypass in 1977 [14–17].

In 1980, Mason performed the first VBG. This surgery initially achieved excellent weight loss with low mortality and morbidity and became the most commonly performed bariatric operation in the US in the 1980s. However, from the early 1990s, patients who underwent VBG surgery regained weight. In the long term, weight loss was small and by the 1990s, the roux-n-Y gastirk bypass became the preferred operation of bariatric surgery in the US [18–19].

In Italy, Scopinaro developed biliopancreatic diversion in the 1980s. This operation, together with its modification including duodenal switch, has been the only malabsorptive operation with long-term success. It represents less than 5% of the operations performed in the USA [19, 21].

Laparoscopic bariatric surgery started in the 1990s. Belachew performed the first laparoscopic adjustable gastric band operation in 1994. Wittgrove and Clark performed the first laparoscopic RYGB in the same year. In 2001, the application of LAGB was approved in the USA. Its popularity increased until 2009, but has declined since then. Laparoscopic sleeve gastrectomy (LSG) has enjoyed a rapidly increasing popularity in the US and internationally since 2008 [21].

The most commonly used bariatric surgery methods today are Laparoscopic Sleeve Gastrectomy (LSG), Roux n Y Gastric Bypass (RYGB), Single Anastomosis Gastric Bypass (OAGB), Transit Bipartition (TB), Biliopancreatic diversion and duodenal switch (BPD-DS), Single Anastomosis Duodeno-ileal bypass (SADI-S), Single Anastomosis Sleeve-Ileal Bypass (SASI Bypass) [18–21].

2.4 Endoscopic treatment methods

The advantages of endoscopic methods used in the treatment of obesity are that they are minimally invasive, have a reversible effect, are reproducible, are a cost-effective treatment option, and can be used for bridging before surgical treatment. Endoscopic bariatric procedures are divided into two categories: interventions in the stomach and interventions in the small bowel. Gastric interventions include gastric balloon, transpyloric shuttle, endoscopic sleeve gastroplasty, pose and gastric aspiration. Interventions in the small intestine include duodenojejunal diversion, gastroduodenojejunal bypass, jejunoileal diversion and duodenomucosal resurfacing/remodeling (**Figure 1**) [22].

2.4.1 Intragastric balloon

Intragastric balloon application is one of the most commonly used endoscopic bariatric methods today. In 2015, it received FDA approval for use in the treatment of obesity. While the peripheral effects of intragastric balloon application are known as reducing gastric volume and slowing gastric emptying; central effects can be counted as activation of gastric tension receptors, signal transmission to the hypothalamus via vagal nerve and early satiety. In 2022, indications for use were specified in the Indications for Metabolic and Bariatric Surgery guidelines published by ASMBS and IFSO. In addition, the areas and conditions of use are also specified in the Spanish and Brazilian intragastric balloon application consensus [23–25].

According to the Brazilian intragastric balloon consensus agreement, indications are defined as being over 12 years of age (no upper age limit (signed by both parents)), body mass index over 25 and failure of diet, exercise and lifestyle changes, and bridge treatment before bariatric surgery. Contraindications were defined as the presence of active peptic ulcer, presence of gastric or esophageal varices, presence of hiatal hernia larger than 5 cm, and previous gastric surgery. According to this consensus, the intragastric balloon should be removed in case of intolerance (severe nausea and vomiting attacks, severe pain), recurrent fluid-electrolyte disturbance, balloon deflation (methylene blue—72 hours), gastrointestinal bleeding, moderate to severe pancreatitis and pregnancy (2nd trimester) during treatment [24, 25].

Ideal balloon characteristics are defined as a material with a smooth surface, made of durable material, inflatable with liquid or air, adjustable in volume, with

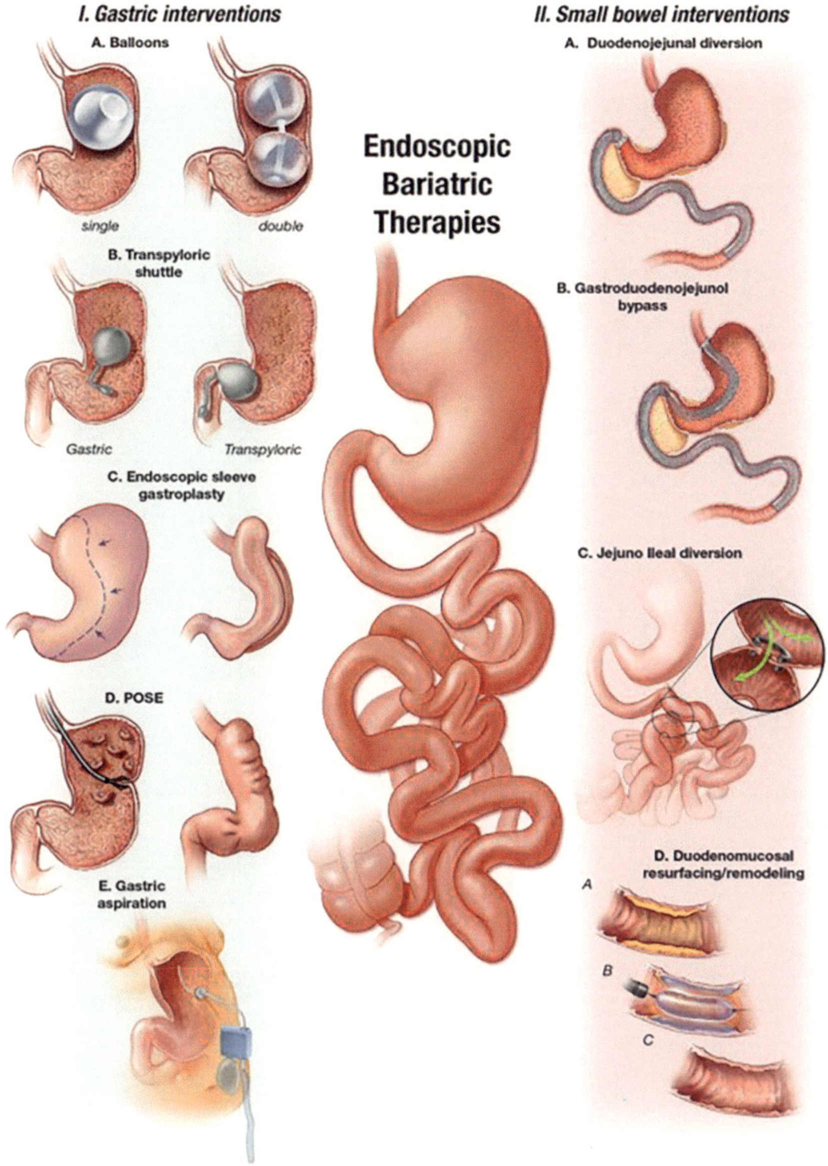

Figure 1.
View of endoscopic treatment methods [22].

a radio-opaque marker to facilitate follow-up [23–25]. The most commonly used intragastric balloon types today are Orbera, ReShape Duo, Obalon, Heliosphere, Spatz and Elipse. Some characteristics of intragastric balloon types are summarized in **Table 1**.

- Obese patients undergoing IGB treatment require concomitant dietary and lifestyle modification.

- PPI prophylaxis should be performed in individuals undergoing IGB therapy.

Summary of Intragastric balloon characteristics						
		FDA/CE approved			CE approved	
Balloon type	**Orbera**	**ReShape Duo**	**Obalon**	**Heliosphere**	**Spatz**	**Elipse**
Manufacturer	Apollo Endosurgery	ReShape Medical	Obalon Therapeutics	Helioscopie Medical Implants	Spatz FGIA	Allurion Technologies
Filled with	Saline	Saline	Nitrogen gas	Air	Saline	Liquid
Capacity (mL)	400-700	450 × 2	250 × 3	900–1000	300–900	550
Number of balloons	1	2	Up to 3	1	1	1
Insertion	Endoscopy	Endoscopy	Swallowed	Endoscopy	Endoscopy	Swallowed
Removal	Endoscopy	Endoscopy	Endoscopy	Endoscopy	Endoscopy	Natural pass
Duration	6	6	6	6	12	4
Adjustable	No	No	No	No	Yes	No

Table 1.
Characteristics of intragastric balloon types [22].

- Intraoperative anesthetics associated with the lowest incidence of nausea should be used during the procedure.
- A planned anti-emetic regimen is recommended for 2 weeks post-procedure.
- Multivitamin supplementation at a daily dose of 1–2 adult doses (**Figure 2**) [23–25].

2.4.2 Trans Pyloric Shuttle

Trans Pyloric Shuttle (TPS) is an endoscopic, minimally invasive method for the treatment of obesity. The TPS is an apparatus that has two ends and is connected to each other with flexible silicone. When the larger part is inflated and filled, it takes the shape of a bulb. The large part of the TPS apparatus, which is delivered to the stomach with an endoscopic application device, is inflated and filled with a coil-like mechanism. After the TPS is endoscopically inserted into the stomach, it remains free in the stomach. Since the small part can easily pass through the pylorus, it passes through the pylorus with peristaltic movements and delays gastric emptying due to the intermittent formation of the large part in the pylorus and at the same time accelerates the filling time of the stomach. This device can stay in the stomach for 12 months and at the end of this period, the internal coil in the large bulb-like part of the TPS is unlocked endoscopically, the part inside the coil is removed first, and the large part is taken out of the stomach after it is narrowed (**Figures 3** and **4**).

After the results of the Endobesity II study were published, TPS received FDA approval in 2019. According to this study, TWL was 9.5% in patients who underwent

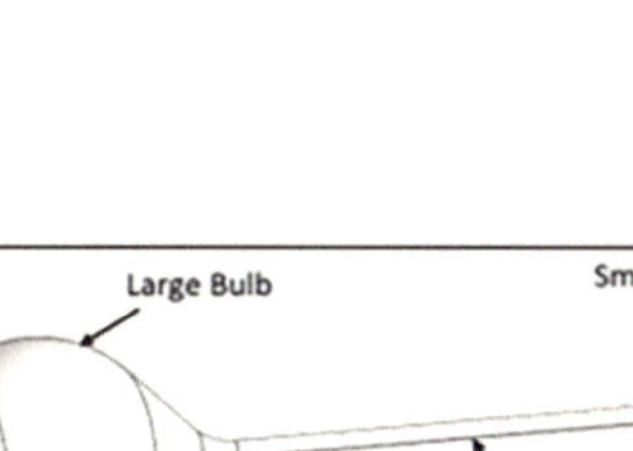

Figure 2.
Intragastric balloon material.

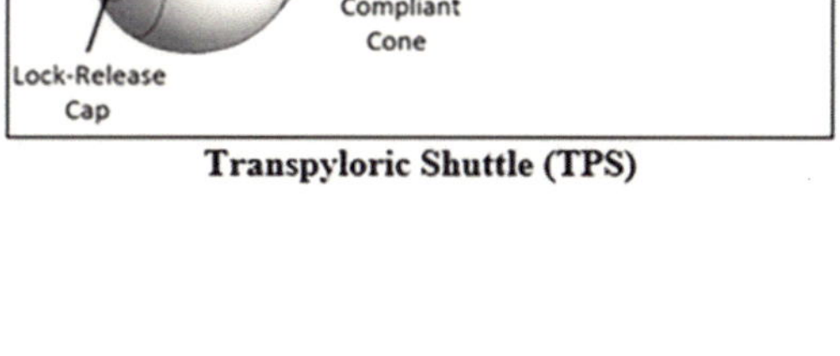

Figure 3.
Transpyloric shuttle [26].

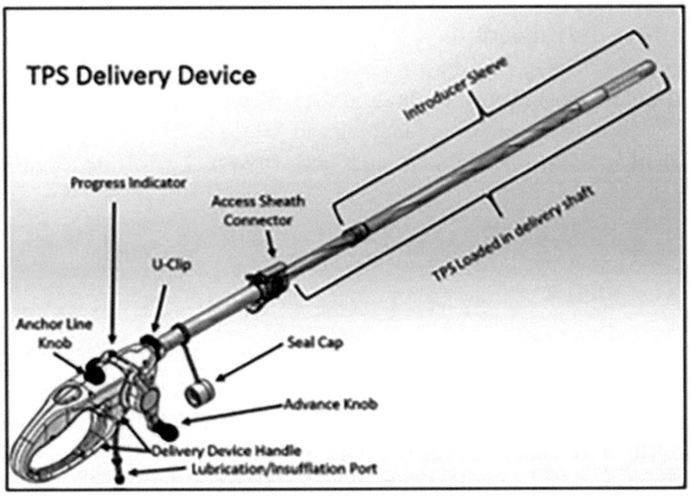

TPS Delivery Device

Figure 4.
Image of the transpyloric shuttle in the stomach [26].

TPS and 2.8% in the control group after 12 months of follow-up. In terms of serious side effects, 4.69% of patients who underwent TPS experienced side effects, while this rate was 1.12% in the control group [26].

2.4.3 Endoscopic sleeve gastroplasty

Endoscopic sleeve gastropilasty (ESG) is a globally accepted method for the treatment of obesity. Although bariatric surgery is the most effective method in the treatment of obesity, many patients avoid surgery because it is perceived as invasive and fear of complications. ESG is a less invasive and organ-sparing option in the treatment of obesity. Endoscopic gastroplasty alters the anatomy and physiology of the stomach by folding the gastric walls and reducing the intragastric volume by up to 75%. Functional exclusion of part of the stomach results in a reduction of both gastric volume and motility [27].

ESG is performed with two types of FDA-approved devices: Overstitch platform (Apollo Endosurgery, Austin, TX), Primary Obesity Surgery Endoluminal (POSE) (USGI Medical, San Clemente, CA).

The Overstitch platform (Apollo Endosurgery, Austin, TX) is used to endoscopically perform gastroplasty with full-thickness suturing and plication of the greater curvature from the inside. This procedure is the most commonly performed endoscopic gastroplasty in recent years. ESG has been shown to be beneficial for weight loss by both reducing gastric volume and gastric emptying [27]. It also has effects on gut hormones and has been shown to reduce ghrelin levels [27]. The most common side effects are nausea and vomiting and abdominal pain. Leakage and free fluid around the stomach, gastric bleeding, some cases of venous thromboembolism and other complications such as pneumotrax, pneumperitnyum have also been seen [27, 28].

Contraindications for ESG, as with other endoscopic options for the treatment of obesity, include large hiatal hernia, gastric ulcer, gastric tumors or intestinal metaplasia, previous surgical procedure, pregnancy, continuous monitoring and anticoagulant use [27, 28].

There are many studies in the literature on this technique. Seven studies including 6775 patients (3413 with ESG and 3362 with LSG) were included in Beran et al. ESG and LSG were compared in the short and long term and significant differences in TBWL% were seen in favor of LSG. The trend towards a lower incidence of adverse events in ESG compared with LSG did not reach statistical significance (RR 0.51, 95% CI 0.23–1.11, P = 0.09). The incidence of new-onset gastroesophageal reflux disease (GERD) was significantly lower after ESG compared to LSG, 1.3% versus 17.9%, respectively (RR 0.10, 95% CI 0.02–0.53, P = 0.006). ESG provided clinically adequate but lower short- and medium-term weight loss and resulted in fewer adverse events, including GERD, compared to LSG. Given the gastroprotective nature of ESG and its acceptable safety profile, it may be considered as an alternative to LSG for patients with mild to moderate obesity [28].

In a study by Lopez-Nava et al. with 248 patients, TBWL was 18.5% after 24 months of follow-up in patients who underwent ESG [29].

In the 91-patient study by Sharaiha et al. TBWL was 17.6% after 1-year follow-up (76% patient follow-up rate). At the same time, the reduction in medical comorbidities, HgA1 C, Blood Pressure, Triglyceride and ALT values were statistically significant [30].

In another study of 148 patients, endolumenal sleeve gastrolasty resulted in a TWBL of 17.53 ± 7.57% at 1 year and 18.5 ± 9% at 18 months. Leptin hormone levels unexpectedly decreased in every patient. As a complication, only 1 patient had a hemorrhage during the passage of the suture helix, which was resolved by sclerotherapy. In this study by Moreles et al., a continuous suture line was created using 4 parallel "Z" suture patterns to minimize the gastric cavity. The suture pattern aimed to eliminate the effect of the distorting force on the suture and to provide a homogeneous distribution between all suture points [31].

Comparison of ESG studies is very difficult due to the difference in technical procedures. However, many studies have been conducted by describing continuous sutures.

Primary obesity surgery endoluminal (POSE) uses an incisionless surgical system to create full-thickness plications in the gastric fundus and body. Many studies have demonstrated the safety and efficacy of the original POSE for the treatment of obesity.

In the meta-analysis by Singh et al. 7 studies were included, 2 of these studies were randmized controlled studies while the others were observational studies. At the end of 12–15 months follow-up, EWL was 48.86% and TWL was 12.68%. Serious adverse events included GI bleeding, extra-gastric bleeding, hepatic abscess, severe pain, severe nausea and severe vomiting; the overall incidence of these serious adverse events was only 2.84% [32] (**Figure 5**).

POSE 1 anatomically reduces the gastric fundus and places a plication line horizontally into the distal gastric body. In POSE 2, by placing plications in the greater curvature of the stomach starting from the level of the incisura and extending proximally to the corpus, the volume of the stomach is reduced so that a small reservoir of food remains in the fundus and the stomach is somewhat reduced and shortened. Both ESG and POSE have shown both gastric volume reduction and hormonal efficacy when compared with other endoscopic procedures. In addition, both ESG and POSE procedures have similar efficacy [33].

2.4.4 Gastric aspiration therapy

The AspireAssist device (Aspire Bariatrics, King of Prussia, PA) is a type of endoscopic gastrostomy tube. It works by partially aspirating ingested food. It is reversible

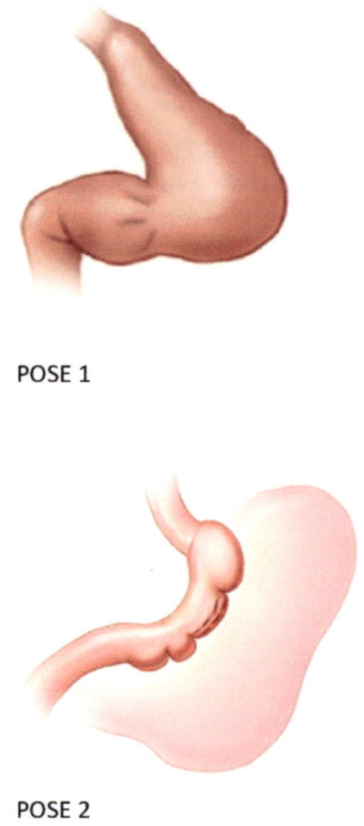

Figure 5.
Illustration showing the differences between the POSE 1 and POSE 2 procedures.

and does not cause significant changes in the anatomy of the stomach. First, the AspireAssist device is inserted. Gastric content is aspirated by feeding water through the part connected to the external apparatus.

In the pilot study conducted by Sullivan et al. in 18 individuals with obesity, 11 patients randomly assigned to aspiration therapy and lifestyle therapy, and 7 patients to lifestyle therapy only. Lifestyle therapy consisted of a 15-session dietary and behavioral education program. After 1 year, TBWL % was 18.6% ± 2.3% in the aspiration therapy group and TWBL % was 5.9% ± 5.0% in the lifestyle therapy group. There was no significant difference between the two groups ($p < 0.4$) (**Figure 6**) [34].

2.4.5 Small bowel procedures

Duodenal bypass sheaths are closed sheaths placed between the mucosa and the GI lumen to block the digestion and absorption of nutrients. Currently, these devices are not FDA approved. Most of the literature mentions the EndoBarrier, a duodenal-jejunal bypass sleeve (DJBS) with a length of 60 cm. During insertion, a self-expanding nitinol anchor is placed inside the duodenal bulb and an impermeable fluoropolymer liner is placed distal to the proximal jejunum. Similarly, the ValenTx is a 120 cm gastro-duodenal-jejunal bypass that is fixed at the gastroesophageal junction and extends into the jejunum. Laparoscopic assistance is required for the placement of this second device [35–38].

A rapid improvement in T2DM and glycemic control, as well as hormonal changes, has been noted after DJBS implantation [39, 40]. Munoz et al. [41] suggest additional weight-independent glycemic control mechanisms. Jirapinyo et al. [42] published a

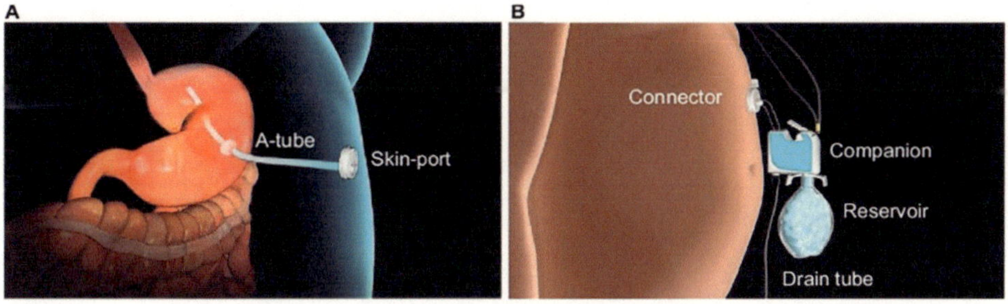

Figure 6.
Aspire Bariatrics AspireAssist. Notes: (A) aspiration tube and skin port in place and (B) external device connected for aspiration [34].

meta-analysis of 4 RCTs showing a 1.3% reduction in HbA1c and a significant reduction of 0.9% compared to control. This reduction was maintained after 6 months. Pooled data from observational and RCTs showed a TWL of 18% that remained significant after 1 year; GLP-1, PYY and ghrelin increased while glucose-dependent insulinotropic polypeptide decreased [41, 42].

There are still safety issues in using these methods that need to be addressed. Betzel et al. [43] published a systematic review of 1057 patients, of whom 33 had serious adverse events, or 3.7%. These included 11 hepatic abscesses, 8 gastrointestinal bleeding, 4 esophageal perforation and 3 acute pancreatitis. 8 patients required surgery but no deaths were reported. Despite these risks, Laubner et al. [44] showed a possible positive risk-benefit ratio in favor of DJBL for the treatment of T2DM.

Currently, bypass procedures are performed laparoscopically with stapler or manual anastomosis. Similarly, performing anastomoses is endoscopically challenging. For the treatment of obesity, type II diabetes and malignant obstructions, a completely endoscopic method of creating a durable reliable bowel bypass is desirable [45–47].

Ryou et al. performed endoscopic jejuno-ileal anastomosis in an animal experiment on 8 pigs. Since the anatomy of the pigs was not suitable, ileal magnets were placed laparoscopically and anastomoses were checked after 3 months in 8 pigs and it was observed that the anastomoses were successful [48]. In the pilot study conducted by Sullivan et al., enteroscopy and colonoscopy were performed in 10 people with obesity and magnets were placed in jejunum and ileum. With the help of laparoscopy, the correct position of the magnets was controlled and adhesion was assisted. Successful anastomoses were performed in normal form. Common side effects were vomiting and diarrhea. At the end of 6 months, TWL was 10.6% (EWL was 28%). HbA1C levels decreased in 4 patients with diabetes [49].

2.4.6 Dudenal mucosal surfacing

Duodenal mucosal resurfacing is performed using specially designed catheters (Fractyl Laboratories) advanced through a guidewire next to the endoscope. Duodenal mucosal resurfacing (DMR) is a single, minimally invasive endoscopic procedure that involves circumferential hydrothermal ablation of the duodenal mucosa followed by regeneration of the mucosa. Before ablation, the mucosa is removed with saline to protect the outer layers of the duodenum. A first-in-human study showed significant improvements in glycemia in T2D patients after DMR and suggested a positive correlation between the length of the ablated segment and efficacy [50].

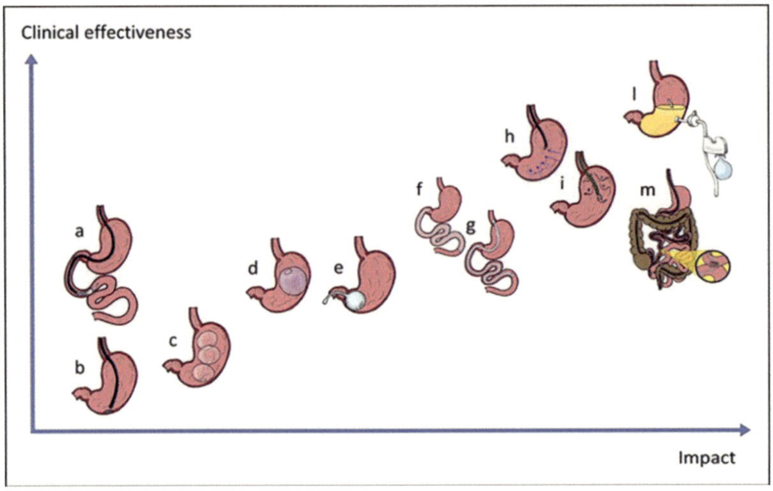

Figure 7.
Endoscopic interventions for obesity and dysmetabolic conditions. Endoscopic interventions: (a) duodenal mucosa resurfacing, (b) intragastric botox injection, (c) gas-filled intragastric balloon, (d) liquid-filled intragastric balloon, (e) transpyloric shuttle, (f) duodenal-jejunal bypass liner, (g) gastro-duodenal-jejunal bypass liner, (h) endoscopic sleeve gastroplasty, (i) primary obesity surgery endoluminal, (l) aspiration therapy, and (m) partial jejunal diversion [36].

Baar et al. evaluated 36 patients and found that DMR is a feasible and safe endoscopic procedure that provides durable glycemic improvement in suboptimally controlled T2D patients on oral glucose-lowering medication regardless of weight loss [51].

2.4.7 Intragastric botulinum toxin a (BTA) injection

Botulinum toxin A (BTA) injection may temporarily inhibit gastric peristalsis by paralyzing the muscular layer of the stomach. This can delay gastric emptying and prolong the duration of satiety. Conflicting evidence on efficacy has been published. Early studies showed weight loss through delayed gastric emptying without side effects [52–54]. In 2015, a meta-analysis of 8 studies concluded that BTA is effective in the treatment of obesity [55]. A recent meta-analysis concluded that intragastric BTA injection is not effective [56]. In another study, intragastric injection of BTX-A does not seem to be an effective method to achieve preoperative weight loss in super obese patients [57]. In a systemic meta-analysis conducted by Yen et al. [58], 192 individuals were evaluated in 6 randomized controlled studies. Intragastric BTA injection was found to be effective in the treatment of obesity, adequate dose (≥200 U), multiple gastric injection sites and combined diet control are very important. However, caution should be exercised due to the small sample size and limited power (**Figure** 7) [58].

3. Conclusion

Although surgical procedures are known as the most effective methods in the fight against obesity today, the frequency and effectiveness of endoscopic treatments are increasing day by day. Endoscopic methods in obesity treatment are promising. There is a need for new methods with high efficacy and reliability, easy application, low complication rate and low cost in the treatment of obesity.

DOI: http://dx.doi.org/10.5772/intechopen.1004427

Author details

Anıl Ergin[1]* and Cihan Şahan[2]

1 Fatih Sultan Mehmet Research and Training Hospital, Istanbul, Turkey

2 Aktif Hospital, Istanbul, Turkey

*Address all correspondence to: dranilergin@gmail.com

References

[1] Babinska Z, Bandosz P, Zdrojewski T, Wyrzykowski B. Epidemiologia otyłosci i otyłosci brzusznej w Polsce, Europie Zachodniej i USA. Kardiologia w Praktyce. 2004;**5**:3-7

[2] Ogden CL, Carroll MD, Curtin LR, McDowell MA, Tabak CJ, Flegal KM. Prevalence of overweight and obesity in the United States, 1999-2004. JAMA. 2006;**295**:1549-1555

[3] Gülay H. Temel ve sistematik cerrahi, Güven Kitabevi, İzmir, Turkey. 2005. ISBN: 9759241285, 9789759241285

[4] Baştürk S. Sleeve gastrektominin orta ve uzun dönem sonuçları, obeziteye eşlik eden komorbiditelere Etkileri. Pamukkale Üniversitesi: Uzmanlık tezi; 2015

[5] James WP. What are health risks? The medical consequences of obesity and its health risks. Experimental and Clinical Endocrinology & Diabetes. 1998;**106**(Suppl. 2):1-6

[6] Kenney WL, Humphrey RH, Bryant CX, Mahler DA. ACSM's Guidelines for Exercise Testing and Prescription. 5th ed. Baltimore: A Waverly Company; 1995. pp. 53-63

[7] Xavier Pi-Sunyer F, Becker DM, Bouchard C, Carleton RA, Colditz GA, William H, et al. Clinical guidelines on the identification, evaluation, and treatment of overweight and obesity in adults. The Evidence Report NIH Publication No. 98-4083. National Institutes Of Health National Heart, Lung, And Blood Institute In Cooperation With The National Institute Of Diabetes And Digestive And Kidney Diseases. Sep 1998

[8] Kaila B, Raman M. Obesity: A review of pathogenesis and management strategies. Canadian Journal of Gastroenterology. 2008;**22**:61-68

[9] Jakicic JM, Otto AD. Physical activity considerations for the treatment and prevention of obesity. The American Journal of Clinical Nutrition. 2005;**82**(suppl):226-229

[10] Knowler WC, Barret-Connor E, Fowler SE. Reduction in the incidence of type 2 diabetes with lifestyle intervention or metformin. The New England Journal of Medicine. 2002;**346**:393. DOI: 10.1056/NEJMoa012512

[11] Douketis JD, Macie C, Thabane L, Williamson DF. Systematic review of long-term weight loss studies in obese adults: Clinical significance and applicability to clinical practice. International Journal of Obesity. 2005;**29**:1153-1167

[12] Yanovski ZS, Yanovski AJ. Long-term drug treatment for obesity: A systematic and clinical review. JAMA. 2014;**311**:74-86

[13] Gastrointestinal surgery for severe obesity: National Institutes of Health consensus development conference statement. American Journal of Clinical Nutrition. 1992;**52**(Suppl. 2):615-619

[14] Schauer PR, Schirmer B. The surgical management of obesity. In: Brunicardi F, Andersen DK, Billiar TR, Dunn DL, Hunter JG, Matthews JB, et al, editors. Schwartz's Principles of Surgery. 10th ed. McGraw-Hill Education; 2015. Available from: https://accessmedicine.mhmedical.com/content.aspx?bookid=980&sectionid=59610869 [Accessed: March 02, 2024]

[15] Richards WO. Sabiston textbook of surgery. The Biological Basis of

Modern Surgical Practice . 21st ed. Morbid Obesity, Chapter 69. Elsevier; Apr 2021. pp. 1160-1187. Hardback ISBN: 9780323640626, eBook ISBN: 9780323640640

[16] Gloy VL, Briel M, Bhatt DL, Kashyap SR, Schauer PR, Mingrone G. Bariatric surgery versus non-surgical treatment for obesity: A systematic review and meta-analysis of randomised controlled trials. British Medical Journal. 2013;**347**:1-16

[17] Pories WJ. Bariatric surgery: Risks and rewards. The Journal of Clinical Endocrinology and Metabolism. 2008;**93**(11):89-96

[18] Buchwald H. Buchwald's Atlas of Metabolic & Bariatric Surgical Techniques and Procedures. Philadelphia, PA: Elsevier/Saunders; 2012. DOI: 10.1016/C2009-0-34090-8

[19] Buchwald H, Buchwald JN. Evolution of operative procedures for the management of morbid obesity 1950- 2000. Obesity Surgery. 2002;**12**(5):705-717

[20] O'Brien P. Bariatric surgery: Mechanisms, indications and outcomes. Journal of Gastroenterology and Hepatology. 2010;**25**(8):1358-1365

[21] Schneider BE, Mun EC. Surgical management of morbid obesity. Diabetes Care. Feb 2005;**28**(2):475-480. DOI: 10.2337/diacare.28.2.475. PMID: 15677820

[22] Dayyeh BKA, Edmundowicz S, Thompson CC. Clinical practice update: Expert review on endoscopic bariatric therapies. Gastroenterology. Mar 2017;**152**(4):716-729

[23] Neto MG, Silva LB, Grecco E, et al. Brazilian intragastric balloon consensus statement (BIBC): Practical guidelines based on experience of over 40,000 cases. Surgery for Obesity and Related Diseases. 2018;**14**(2):151-159

[24] American Society for Metabolic and Bariatric Surgery. Metabolic and Bariatric Surgery: Fact Sheet. 2013. Available from: https://asmbs.org/wp/uploads/2014/05/Metabolic+Bariatric-Surgery.pdf [Accessed: Jul 18, 2016]

[25] Fernandes M, Atallah AN, Soares BGO, et al. Intragastric balloon for obesity. Cochrane Database of Systematic Reviews. 2007;(1):CD004931

[26] Transpyloric Shuttle/Transpyloric Shuttle Delivery Device Instructions for Use. Available from: https://www.clinicaltrials.gov/ct2/show/NCT02518685

[27] Vargas EJ, Rizk M, Gomez-Villa J, Edwards PK, Jaruvongvanich V, Storm AC, et al. Effect of endoscopic sleeve gastroplasty on gastric emptying, motility and hormones: A comparative prospective study. Gut. 2023;**72**(6):1073-1080. DOI: 10.1136/gutjnl-2022-327816. Epub 2022 Oct 14

[28] Beran A, Matar R, Jaruvongvanich V, Rapaka BB, Alalwan A, Portela R, et al. Comparative effectiveness and safety between endoscopic sleeve gastroplasty and laparoscopic sleeve gastrectomy: A meta-analysis of 6775 individuals with obesity. Obesity Surgery. 2022;**32**(11):3504-3512. DOI: 10.1007/s11695-022-06254-y. Epub 2022 Sep 2

[29] Lopez-Nava G, Sharaiha RZ, Vargas EJ, Bazerbachi F, Manoel GN, Bautista-Castaño I, et al. Endoscopic sleeve gastroplasty for obesity: A multicenter study of 248 patients with 24 months follow-up. Obesity Surgery. 2017;**27**(10):2649-2655. DOI: 10.1007/s11695-017-2693-7

[30] Sharaiha RZ, Kumta NA, Saumoy M, Desai AP, Sarkisian AM, Benevenuto A, et al. Endoscopic sleeve gastroplasty significantly reduces body mass index and metabolic complications in obese patients. Clinical Gastroenterology and Hepatology. 2017;**15**(4):504-510. DOI: 10.1016/j.cgh.2016.12.012. Epub 2016 Dec 23

[31] Graus Morales J, Crespo Pérez L, Marques A, Marín Arribas B, Bravo Arribas R, Ramo E, et al. Modified endoscopic gastroplasty for the treatment of obesity. Surgical Endoscopy. 2018;**32**(9):3936-3942. DOI: 10.1007/s00464-018-6133-0. Epub 2018 Feb 28

[32] Singh S, Bazarbashi AN, Khan A, Chowdhry M, Bilal M, de Moura DTH, et al. Primary obesity surgery endoluminal (POSE) for the treatment of obesity: A systematic review and meta-analysis. Surgical Endoscopy. 2022;**36**(1):252-266. DOI: 10.1007/s00464-020-08267-z. Epub 2021 Feb 1

[33] Espinós JC, Turró R, Moragas G, Bronstone A, Buchwald JN, Mearin F, et al. Gastrointestinal physiological changes and their relationship to weight loss following the POSE procedure. Obesity Surgery. 2016;**26**(5):1081-1089. DOI: 10.1007/s11695-015-1863-8

[34] Sullivan S, Stein R, Jonnalagadda S, Mullady D, Edmundowicz S. Aspiration therapy leads to weight loss in obese subjects: A pilot study. Gastroenterology. 2013;**145**(6):1245-52.e1-5. DOI: 10.1053/j.gastro.2013.08.056. Epub 2013 Sep 6

[35] Abu Dayyeh BK, Acosta A, Camilleri M, Mundi MS, Rajan E, Topazian MD, et al. Endoscopic sleeve gastroplasty alters gastric physiology and induces loss of body weight in obese individuals. Clinical Gastroenterology and Hepatology. 2017;**15**(1):37-43.e1. DOI: 10.1016/j.cgh.2015.12.030. Epub 2015 Dec 31

[36] Telese A, Sehgal V, Magee CG, Naik S, Alqahtani SA, Lovat LB, et al. Bariatric and metabolic endoscopy: A new paradigm. Clinical and Translational Gastroenterology. 2021;**12**(6):e00364. DOI: 10.14309/ctg.0000000000000364

[37] Sandler BJ, Rumbaut R, Swain CP, Torres G, Morales L, Gonzales L, et al. Human experience with an endoluminal, endoscopic, gastrojejunal bypass sleeve. Surgical Endoscopy. 2011;**25**(9):3028-3033. DOI: 10.1007/s00464-011-1665-6. Epub 2011 Apr 13

[38] Sandler BJ, Rumbaut R, Swain CP, Torres G, Morales L, Gonzales L, et al. One-year human experience with a novel endoluminal, endoscopic gastric bypass sleeve for morbid obesity. Surgical Endoscopy. 2015;**29**(11):3298-3303. DOI: 10.1007/s00464-015-4081-5. Epub 2015 Jan 29

[39] de Jonge C, Rensen SS, Verdam FJ, Vincent RP, Bloom SR, Buurman WA, et al. Endoscopic duodenal-jejunal bypass liner rapidly improves type 2 diabetes. Obesity Surgery. 2013;**23**(9):1354-1360. DOI: 10.1007/s11695-013-0921-3

[40] Cohen RV, Neto MG, Correa JL, Sakai P, Martins B, Schiavon CA, et al. A pilot study of the duodenal-jejunal bypass liner in low body mass index type 2 diabetes. The Journal of Clinical Endocrinology and Metabolism. 2013;**98**(2):E279-E282. DOI: 10.1210/jc.2012-2814. Epub 2013 Jan 21

[41] Muñoz R, Escalona A. Duodenal-jejunal bypass liner to treat type 2 diabetes mellitus in morbidly obese patients. Current Cardiology Reports. 2014;**16**(3):454. DOI: 10.1007/s11886-013-0454-3

[42] Jirapinyo P, Haas AV, Thompson CC. Effect of the duodenal-jejunal bypass liner on glycemic control in patients with type 2 diabetes with obesity: A meta-analysis with secondary analysis on weight loss and hormonal changes. Diabetes Care. 2018;**41**(5):1106-1115. DOI: 10.2337/dc17-1985

[43] Betzel B, Drenth JPH, Siersema PD. Adverse events of the duodenal-jejunal bypass liner: A systematic review. Obesity Surgery. 2018;**28**(11):3669-3677. DOI: 10.1007/s11695-018-3441-3

[44] Laubner K, Riedel N, Fink K, Holl RW, Welp R, Kempe HP, et al. Comparative efficacy and safety of the duodenal-jejunal bypass liner in obese patients with type 2 diabetes mellitus: A case control study. Diabetes, Obesity & Metabolism. 2018;**20**(8):1868-1877. DOI: 10.1111/dom.13300. Epub 2018 Apr 23

[45] Ly J, O'Grady G, Mittal A, Plank L, Windsor JA. A systematic review of methods to palliate malignant gastric outlet obstruction. Surgical Endoscopy. 2010;**24**:290-297

[46] Gentileschi P, Kini S, Catarci M, Gagner M. Evidence-based medicine: Open and laparoscopic bariatric surgery. Surgical Endoscopy. 2002;**16**:736-744

[47] Duan J, Tan C, Xu H, et al. Side-to-side jejunoileal bypass induces better glucose-lowering effect than end-to-side jejunoileal bypass on nonobese diabetic rats. Obesity Surgery. 2015;**25**:1458-1467

[48] Ryou M, Aihara H, Thompson CC. Minimally invasive entero-enteral dual-path bypass using self-assembling magnets. Surgical Endoscopy. 2016;**30**:4533-4538. DOI: 10.1007/s00464-016-4789-x

[49] Sullivan S, Edmundowicz SA, Thompson CC. Endoscopic bariatric and metabolic therapies: New and emerging technologies. Gastroenterology. 2017;**152**(7):1791-1801. DOI: 10.1053/j.gastro.2017.01.044. Epub 2017 Feb 10

[50] Rajagopalan H, Cherrington AD, Thompson CC, Kaplan LM, Rubino F, Mingrone G, et al. Endoscopic duodenal mucosal resurfacing for the treatment of type 2 diabetes: 6-month interim analysis from the first-in-human proof-of-concept study. Diabetes Care. 2016;**39**(12):2254-2261. DOI: 10.2337/dc16-0383. Epub 2016 Aug 12

[51] Van Baar ACG, Holleman F, Crenier L, Haidry R, Magee C, Hopkins D, et al. Endoscopic duodenal mucosal resurfacing for the treatment of type 2 diabetes mellitus: One year results from the first international, open-label, prospective, multicentre study. Gut. 2020;**69**(2):295-303. DOI: 10.1136/gutjnl-2019-318349.Epub 2019 Jul 22

[52] Foschi D, Corsi F, Lazzaroni M, Sangaletti O, Riva P, La Tartara G, et al. Treatment of morbid obesity by intraparietogastric administration of botulinum toxin: A randomized, double-blind, controlled study. International Journal of Obesity. 2007;**31**(4):707-712. DOI: 10.1038/sj.ijo.0803451. Epub 2006 Sep 26

[53] Foschi D, Lazzaroni M, Sangaletti O, Corsi F, Trabucchi E, Bianchi Porro G. Effects of intramural administration of botulinum toxin A on gastric emptying and eating capacity in obese patients. Digestive and Liver Disease. 2008;**40**(8):667-672. DOI: 10.1016/j.dld.2008.02.040

[54] Topazian M, Camilleri M, De La Mora-Levy J, Enders FB,

Foxx-Orenstein AE, Levy MJ, et al. Endoscopic ultrasound-guided gastric botulinum toxin injections in obese subjects: A pilot study. Obesity Surgery. 2008;**18**(4):401-407. DOI: 10.1007/s11695-008-9442-x. Epub 2008 Feb 20

[55] Bang CS, Baik GH, Shin IS, Kim JB, Suk KT, Yoon JH, et al. Effect of intragastric injection of botulinum toxin A for the treatment of obesity: A meta-analysis and meta-regression. Gastrointestinal Endoscopy. 2015;**81**(5):1141-9.e1-7. DOI: 10.1016/j.gie.2014.12.025. Epub 2015 Mar 9

[56] Bustamante F, Brunaldi VO, Bernardo WM, de Moura DTH, de Moura ETH, Galvão M, et al. Obesity treatment with botulinum toxin-a is not effective: A systematic review and meta-analysis. Obesity Surgery. 2017;**27**(10):2716-2723. DOI: 10.1007/s11695-017-2857-5

[57] de Moura EGH, Ribeiro IB, Frazão MSV, Mestieri LHM, de Moura DTH, Dal Bó CMR, et al. EUS-guided intragastric injection of botulinum toxin a in the preoperative treatment of super-obese patients: A randomized clinical trial. Obesity Surgery. 2019;**29**(1):32-39. DOI: 10.1007/s11695-018-3470-y

[58] Yen YA, Wang CC, Sung WW, Fang KC, Huang SM, Lin CC, et al. Intragastric injection of botulinum toxin A for weight loss: A systematic review and meta-analysis of randomized controlled trials. Journal of Gastroenterology and Hepatology. 2022;**37**(6):983-992. DOI: 10.1111/jgh.15847. Epub 2022 Apr 22

Chapter 9

One Size Does Not Fit All: Complexity of Lifestyle Interventions in Primary Care T2D Prevention – Supporting Weight Loss and Weight Loss Maintenance

Maija Huttunen-Lenz

Abstract

Type 2 Diabetes (T2D) is a growing public health problem with potentially severe consequences for those affected. An unhealthy diet leading to being overweight combined with a sedentary lifestyle is considered a significant risk factor in the development of T2D. Changes in lifestyle, especially in diet and physical activity behaviors enabling sustained weight loss, can support T2D prevention. Changing lifestyle behaviors can, however, be challenging. Many individuals perceive intervention attendance and adherence as challenging. Behavioral interventions in T2D prevention are complex due to multiple interactions between intervention components and participants. This chapter discusses intervention complexity, mechanisms, and social-cognitive characteristics in T2D prevention interventions aiming for sustained weight loss. Social-cognitive factors refer to diverse attributes that may influence the success of behavior change. Here, self-efficacy, goal attainment, and participants' sex and socioeconomic status are discussed. Challenges and potential solutions in designing and delivering T2D prevention interventions in primary care are reflected.

Keywords: Type 2 Diabetes, overweight, public health, sedentary behaviour, lifestyle, risk factors, weight loss, diet, physical activity, social-cognitive factors

1. Introduction

T2D is a significant public health issue that can have severe consequences for those affected [1].

This chapter discusses the complexity of interventions for T2D prevention through lifestyle changes. It explores how the complexity of the interventions can affect their effectiveness. Additionally, this chapter discusses social-cognitive factors that can impact behavior change and intervention outcomes. Social-cognitive factors discussed in this chapter include self-efficacy, goal attainment, and participants' sex and socioeconomic status. Research has shown that lifestyle change interventions can effectively prevent T2D [2, 3]. However, it is essential to note that these interventions may also increase health inequalities [4, 5]. This is because women and individuals with higher socioeconomic status are often overrepresented among participants, even though men, ethnic minorities, and those from lower socioeconomic backgrounds have a higher risk of T2D and would benefit significantly from lifestyle interventions [4, 6–8]. Therefore, it is essential to ensure that T2D prevention programs are accessible to all individuals, regardless of background. Finally, this chapter reflects on the challenges of designing and delivering T2D prevention interventions to achieve sustained weight loss in primary care and potential solutions.

2. T2D and prevention

T2D is a growing public health concern, with an estimated global prevalence of 6.1% [1, 9]. This is expected to double by 2050 [1, 9]. A combination of reduced insulin secretion and increased insulin resistance causes T2D. The development of T2D is preceded by prediabetes, an intermediate stage between normal glucose metabolism and T2D [10, 11]. T2D is a chronic condition that worsens over time, leading to physical damage and poorer health outcomes [12]. Over time, T2D can have serious consequences, including lasting damage to the cardiovascular and nervous systems. Individuals with T2D are at an increased risk of nerve impairments, including loss of feeling in extremities like feet due to nerve damage. They also have an increased risk of cardiovascular incidents such as stroke due to damage to the cardiovascular system [13]. Consequently, T2D is associated with higher societal and individual costs and lower quality of life among those affected [9, 14]. Therefore, prevention of T2D in primary care is essential to improve individual and population-level health [14, 15].

The primary risk factors for developing T2D include being overweight or obese, along with a sedentary lifestyle. In particular, an unhealthy diet that leads to overweight and obesity, combined with a lack of physical activity, is considered to be a key factor that increases the risk of developing T2D [2, 16]. However, the risk of developing and the progression of T2D can be modified through preventive lifestyle interventions. Research has shown that lifestyle interventions can potentially change the course of T2D by slowing, stopping, or even reversing the disease progression [17–20]. Several studies have suggested that sustained weight loss can have potential benefits in preventing T2D. Consequently, lifestyle interventions are commonly recommended in the prevention of T2D. These interventions focus on achieving and maintaining a healthy weight through diet and physical activity changes [2, 21–23]. However, despite the benefits, many people find sustained weight loss challenging [2, 21, 24].

Primary prevention of T2D refers to efforts to prevent the risk factors for developing T2D from emerging, thus reducing the likelihood of developing T2D [25]. This type of prevention is often aimed at the population level, including health education and campaigns targeting the population more widely [25]. Here, prevention is used to refer to secondary and tertiary prevention among high-risk populations such as those with prediabetes (secondary prevention) or those already diagnosed with T2D (tertiary prevention) [25, 26]. Individuals with prediabetes have a high risk of progressing to T2D, while those with diagnosed T2D are at increased risk of adverse health outcomes. Individuals with prediabetes or T2D are vulnerable to disease progression and have a higher likelihood of gradually worsening health outcomes [25, 26]. This chapter discusses lifestyle interventions for those with prediabetes or T2D, encouraging weight loss and maintenance to slow, stop, or reverse the disease progression [17–20].

DOI: http://dx.doi.org/10.5772/intechopen.1004694

Although lifestyle interventions have significant potential in preventing T2D, certain limitations may constrain their efficacy. There are certain limitations that can affect the outcome of an intervention. These limitations arise due to self-selection by attendees and participants leaving the intervention before its completion [21, 27]. However, despite these challenges, complex and multidisciplinary lifestyle interventions have shown promise in supporting sustained weight loss for T2D prevention in primary care and are considered a cost-effective approach [1, 27, 28]. Effective design and delivery of T2D prevention programs based on lifestyle changes requires evidence-based and theory-based information for public and primary healthcare providers [29, 30]. In addition, since the effectiveness of lifestyle interventions in the real world often falls short of the efficacy observed in trial conditions [31], primary care providers require knowledge about intervention pathways, that is, how the intervention produces the desired outcomes and how the characteristics of the target population may interact with the intervention pathways and outcomes [32].

3. Complexity in behavioral lifestyle interventions in T2D prevention

Complexity in behavioral lifestyle interventions refers to the various components of an intervention and the interactions between and within these components, which ultimately shape the outcomes of the intervention [33, 34]. Intervention components include techniques utilized to modify behaviors, the targeted population, the location of the intervention, personal factors, intensity, formats such as individual or group interventions, and time of day [33, 34]. The interactions within and between these intervention components can be either anticipated or unforeseen, but they all play a role in determining the intervention's outcomes [33, 34]. For instance, an anticipated interaction between intervention components could be the relationship between the selected intervention location and the target population. Locations with easy access to public and private transportation will be more accessible to a larger group of individuals within the target population than remote locations that are primarily accessible by private means of transportation. On the other hand, unforeseen interactions may refer to unexpected participant group dynamics that either facilitate or hinder the achievement of the intervention's outcomes. An example of intervention complexity is shown in **Figure 1**.

Developing a healthier and sustainable diet and physical activity habits is crucial in preventing T2D [2]. However, creating new health behaviors can be challenging. Therefore, behavioral intervention for T2D prevention is complex, involving multiple interconnected components that can affect the desired outcomes [30, 34]. Like other complex healthcare interventions, preventive interventions for T2D must consider the complexity within and between the intervention, social structures, and environment in which the behavior change occurs [37–39]. It can be a daunting task trying to make sense of this complexity while designing preventive T2D interventions. Therefore, it has been suggested that identifying and describing effective and adaptable behavior change techniques (BCTs) and intervention mechanisms [40–42] could improve the design and delivery of behavioral interventions for T2D prevention [30, 43]. Intervention mechanisms refer to the processes through which the BCTs deployed in an intervention are expected to impact the targeted behaviors [27]. In other words, intervention mechanisms describe how the selected BCTs (e.g., knowledge) are expected to impact behavioral determinants (e.g., beliefs about ability) that affect the performance of specific behaviors, which, in turn, influence the likelihood of performing a behavior such as physical activity [43].

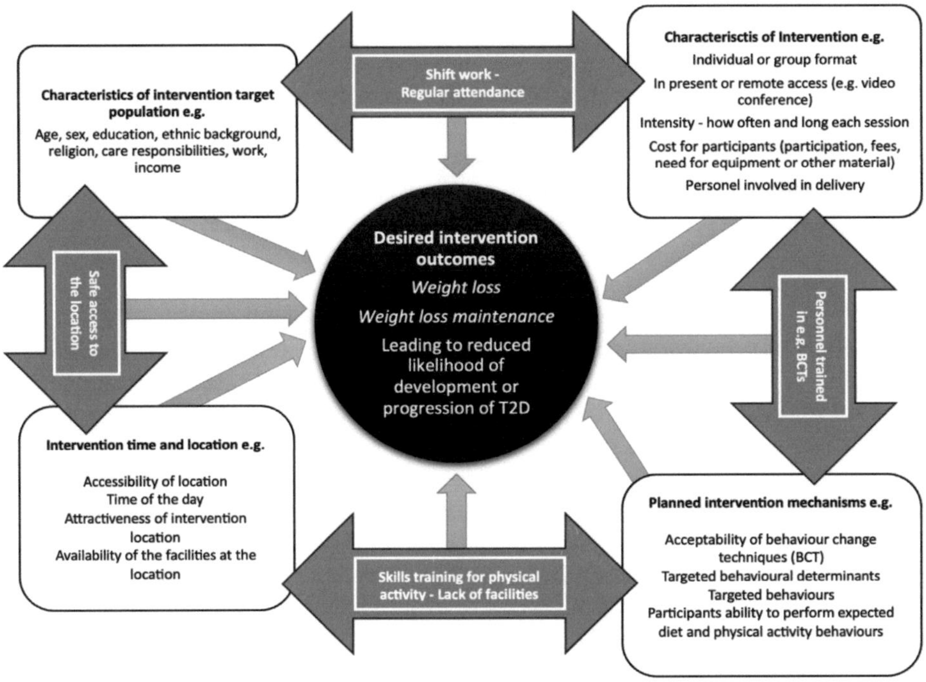

Figure 1.
Example of complexity in behavioral T2D prevention intervention. Adapted from [30, 34–36].

Improved identification of the BCTs that are best suited to impact defined behavioral determinants has facilitated the identification of intervention mechanisms and thus enhanced the design of behavioral interventions [44], including those in the prevention of T2D. As described above, behavioral mechanisms explain how selected BCTs are expected to facilitate changes in behavioral determinants. For example, a BCT, such as increasing skills, can facilitate improved self-efficacy, which, in turn, facilitates changes in behaviors, such as physical activity, that lead to desired outcomes such as sustained weight loss [43]. In behavioral lifestyle interventions, self-efficacy is seen as a central behavioral determinant that describes individuals' beliefs about their ability to perform goal-related behaviors and overcome obstacles [45, 46]. A behavioral mechanism explains how skills training, BCT can improve self-efficacy, increasing the probability of engaging in physical activity. Therefore, improving physical activity skills is expected to increase the likelihood of performing physical activities. This, in turn, supports weight loss in T2D prevention interventions [43, 44]. However, despite carefully planned intervention mechanisms, unexpected interactions between the deployed BCTs and the participating individuals may create unforeseen mechanisms that hinder or facilitate achieving the intended outcomes [43, 47].

In the prevention of T2D, a combination of physical activity and dietary changes that result in sustained weight loss is crucial [48]. Many behavioral interventions for T2D prevention encourage participants to alter their behaviors to promote a healthier diet and physical activity, leading to sustained weight loss [21]. However, despite weight loss benefits, many intervention participants struggle to achieve long-term weight loss [49, 50]. It is suggested that using an intervention theory, which involves planning intervention mechanisms based on behavioral theories, can improve the transparency and effectiveness of interventions [30, 51]. However, even though the existing behavior change theories can provide a framework for theory-based behavioral mechanisms in T2D prevention, a clear theoretical framework is often not articulated at the intervention design stage, which can hinder later evaluation of intervention effectiveness ([32], e.g., [52–54]).

4. Research to practice transfer of preventive T2D lifestyle interventions

T2D prevention often occurs in primary care, where primary care providers are responsible for designing and delivering preventive interventions. However, primary care providers may have limited expertise in adapting complex behavioral intervention research in primary healthcare practice [43, 55]. Researchers are not commonly involved in designing and delivering T2D behavioral interventions within local primary healthcare systems [56]. Primary care practitioners are left to infer research results for practical use. Therefore, it is crucial to have readily available information about effective intervention mechanisms and BCTs that can be efficiently utilized in practice. Without this information, research to practice transfer in T2D prevention may be significantly hindered, as primary care practitioners may struggle to adapt research into practical behavioral interventions within local primary care systems [57–59]. This is why the importance of intervention theory is highlighted, as it can provide clear and easily accessible information about effective intervention features [34]. It is common for behavioral interventions to perform better in experimental settings than when applied in everyday healthcare environments due to the challenges practitioners face in interpreting and replicating research into practice [31].

5. Social-cognitive attributes in preventive T2D lifestyle interventions

Social-cognitive attributes refer to individual characteristics such as age, educational achievement, employment status, family situation, intentions, beliefs about consequences, and self-efficacy. These attributes vary among individuals, over time, and in different situations and can impact the success of T2D prevention interventions [60, 61]. T2D risk is not equally distributed among different demographics. People with male sex, non-Caucasian ethnicity, and lower socioeconomic status are at a higher risk of experiencing adverse consequences from T2D. Unfortunately, these characteristics are associated with a lower likelihood of intervention enrolment and a higher likelihood of intervention cessation in T2D lifestyle interventions [4, 5, 8, 62, 63]. This presents a challenge for designing T2D prevention interventions. It requires addressing cognitive factors like self-efficacy and social support during behavior modification and considering characteristics such as age and sex that can influence behavior modification [54, 61].

Encouraging attendance and adherence to interventions is crucial to ensure the best possible chances of achieving the intended outcomes [35, 46]. Different social-cognitive factors may be involved in individuals' decisions to attend an intervention and later adhere to it. These factors may include fear of T2D consequences and increased self-efficacy to cope with lifestyle changes. Interactions between the diverse factors and intervention components mean that the same social-cognitive factors may directly and indirectly influence intervention success [34, 64, 65]. Intervention design should consider strategies that encourage enrollment and reduce cessation, both influenced by social-cognitive characteristics [8, 35].

Here, the focus is on how social-cognitive factors, BCTs, and behavioral mechanisms influence participants' engagement in T2D lifestyle interventions and success in achieving sustained weight loss. In this regard, factors such as mood and stress, which may also affect the success of the intervention, are not discussed here [65–68]. Furthermore, this chapter does not aim to provide an in-depth analysis of the various social-cognitive factors, BCTs, or intervention mechanisms as described in different behavior change models and theories ([69], e.g., [70–72]). Instead, this chapter discusses social-cognitive variables of self-efficacy, goal achievement, and participants' sex and socioeconomic status.

5.1 Self-efficacy in preventive T2D lifestyle interventions

Self-efficacy is considered one of the key mechanisms in behavior change due to its role in regulating feelings, thinking, and, ultimately, behaviors [69]. In various theoretical models, such as the Theory of Planned Behavior [73], the Social Cognitive Theory [74], or the Transtheoretical Model (TTM) [75], self-efficacy has a central role. Self-efficacy refers to an individual's belief in their ability to overcome obstacles while striving toward their goals [54]. Various studies have shown that self-efficacy plays a significant role in achieving and maintaining weight loss [45]. Higher levels of self-efficacy have been linked to increased physical activity in T2D prevention interventions, leading to better weight loss outcomes [47, 76]. Building new lifestyle habits is easier with strong self-efficacy [22, 74]. Therefore, T2D prevention interventions typically aim to improve self-efficacy to develop and maintain healthier physical activity and diet behaviors, thus increasing the likelihood of successful weight loss outcomes [21, 43]. **Figure 2** presents an intervention mechanism with self-efficacy as an example.

It is important to note that self-efficacy is not a single concept. In lifestyle change interventions, it can be differentiated between action and coping self-efficacy [54]. Action self-efficacy refers to the willingness to initiate new behaviors, while coping self-efficacy pertains to maintaining new behaviors despite challenges and setbacks [54, 77]. During the initial stages of lifestyle interventions, action self-efficacy is more important as it enables individuals to form new behaviors. Conversely, coping self-efficacy is central to maintaining newly formed behaviors despite challenges such as work and family commitments [78].

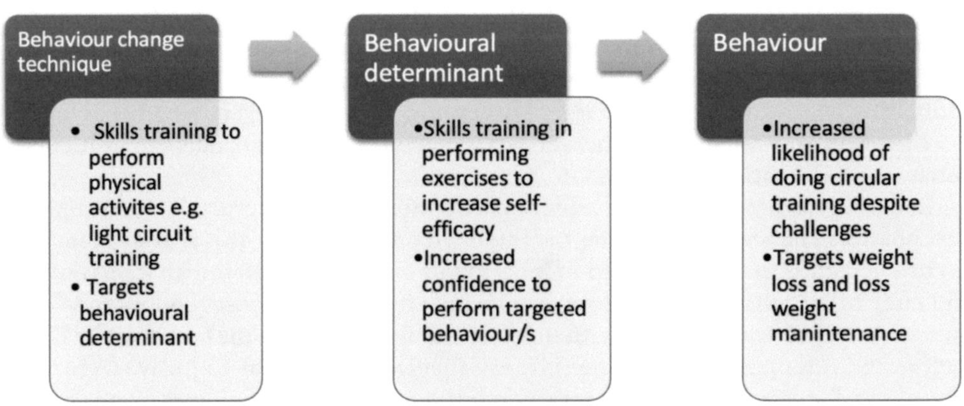
Behaviour change technique
• Skills training to perform physical activites e.g. light circuit training
• Targets behavioural determinant
Behavioural determinant
•Skills training in performing exercises to increase self-efficacy
•Increased confidence to perform targeted behaviour/s
Behaviour
•Increased likelihood of doing circular training despite challenges
•Targets weight loss and loss weight manintenance

Figure 2.
Overview of an intervention mechanism targeting physical activity behaviors. Adapted from [34, 44].

DOI: http://dx.doi.org/10.5772/intechopen.1004694

Many behavioral interventions in T2D prevention face challenges in retaining participants [2, 35, 79], especially those with family and work commitments [78, 80]. This often leads to missed opportunities for individuals to receive support in achieving their intervention goals, such as sustained weight loss [78]. Improving self-efficacy is essential in addressing this issue and ensuring that intervention participants maintain new behaviors despite challenges and barriers until they become habits [80]. However, influencing behaviors through self-efficacy may be challenging as research has suggested that for many intervention participants, self-efficacy is already high initially, leaving limited room for improvement [76, 81].

Moreover, high self-efficacy at the start of an intervention does not necessarily translate to success in achieving behavioral goals, such as weight loss [47, 76]. Instead, accessing the support offered by an intervention appears to moderate success in weight loss and weight loss maintenance. Regular intervention attendance has been linked to better weight loss outcomes, not necessarily by increasing self-efficacy [78, 82, 83], but by taking advantage of the support provided by the intervention [76].

5.2 Goal achievement in preventive T2D lifestyle interventions

Personal goals, such as achieving sustained weight loss, can be beneficial in increasing intervention attendance and achieving intervention objectives. Unrealistic goals can cause psychological distress and hinder progress [71]. Successful participation in a behavioral T2D prevention intervention that supports weight loss and weight loss maintenance necessitates accepting these intervention goals [84]. While goal setting is an effective BCT, unattainable goals can be distressing [44, 71, 85]. The distress caused by unattainable goals can lead to disengagement from goals, resulting in worse weight loss outcomes [71]. Engaging and disengaging from goals is called the adaptive self-regulation of goal adjustment, which enables lessening the impacts of unattainable goals [86, 87]. In the first phase, individuals disengage from an unattainable goal by withdrawing their efforts and commitment. In the second phase, individuals re-engage their efforts toward goal attainment elsewhere, such as in work or family pursuits [86].

Individuals often start a T2D prevention intervention with the personal goal of achieving weight loss and weight maintenance targets as specified in the intervention. However, failing to achieve these goals is not uncommon [11, 88]. In such cases, the ability to disengage from unattainable goals is self-protective and lessens emotional distress [86, 87]. However, this can hinder weight loss and weight maintenance efforts. Primary care professionals delivering the interventions must consider whether weight loss and weight maintenance goals are realistically achievable for the individuals. Instead of disengaging, adapting goals may be more beneficial, even if the magnitude of the goals is lesser than initially aimed.

While the ability for goal adjustment has been associated with improved health outcomes, ceasing efforts toward a goal without re-engaging with a new goal can lead to lower mental well-being [71, 87]. This situation can cause unfavorable health consequences [67, 88], whether for individuals' physical or psychological health. Tendency to goal adjustment does not appear to be associated with an individual's sex. However, those with higher Body Mass Index (BMI) at the start of a T2D prevention intervention, as well as those from ethnic minority backgrounds, may be at greater risk of disengaging from goals when unsure of their ability to achieve the intervention goals [89].

The examples of self-efficacy [69] and goal adjustment [71] demonstrate the complex interconnectivity of mechanisms of behavior change in the prevention of T2D. Therefore, it is essential to carefully consider the target populations, aims, and intervention mechanisms when designing and delivering preventive interventions in primary care to optimize weight loss outcomes [90]. While it may not be practical to create separate weight loss and maintenance interventions for every individual, interventions should still be designed to anticipate and respond to the needs of individuals, particularly those at higher risk of struggling with the demands of the intervention [91, 92].

5.3 Socioeconomic status and sex in preventive T2D lifestyle interventions

A self-selection bias may influence the decision to participate in a lifestyle-based T2D prevention intervention. In other words, those with higher self-efficacy regarding the expected lifestyle changes are more likely to enroll. Despite the expected ability to cope with the intervention challenges, many participants who have decided to enroll still require support to complete the intervention [54, 93]. Numerous studies have investigated how factors such as socioeconomic status and participants' sex impact decisions to participate in type 2 prevention interventions. For instance, individuals belonging to an ethnic minority group and those having a lower socioeconomic background are at a higher risk of developing T2D. However, they may be underrepresented in preventive interventions [5, 35, 94]. Those who are younger have a lower degree of education, higher BMI, lower self-efficacy, or are unemployed are likelier to stop attending lifestyle interventions [35, 62, 95, 96]. This suggests that lifestyle interventions may need to focus on promoting attendance and adherence, particularly for individuals with the characteristics identified above, as part of diabetes type 2 prevention efforts. It appears important to consider ways to support participation among at-risk populations, especially those with lower socioeconomic status, when designing and implementing T2D prevention interventions [97–99].

It is recognized that attributes such as socioeconomic status can be estimated using different methodologies (e.g., [100]). However, the highest degree attained is often used to measure an individual's socioeconomic status [101–103]. Socioeconomic status is a multidimensional concept encompassing occupation, education, and lifetime income [103, 104]. Education level is important to social and health inequalities in T2D prevention [8, 99]. It is essential that individuals from at-risk populations with lower socioeconomic status can benefit just as much from T2D prevention interventions as those with higher socioeconomic status. However, individuals with lower SES may face more limited resources that make it challenging to participate in preventive interventions [99, 103, 104]. Limited resources can include time, money, and health literacy. Health literacy refers to the knowledge and understanding of the role of lifestyle changes in the prevention of T2D. Therefore, the design and delivery of preventive interventions should ensure that individuals with lower socioeconomic status will not be excluded, potentially increasing their risk of experiencing worse health outcomes [63, 103, 105].

While women with higher educational attainment, that is, higher socioeconomic status, tend to be overrepresented in T2D lifestyle interventions, it is important to note that participant's sex may not be associated with intervention attrition after a decision to participate is reached [8, 27]. Being a man with a lower degree of education is considered a risk factor for less favorable intervention outcomes in T2D prevention [4, 106, 107]. However, studies have also implied that women with a higher degree of education may also experience less favorable intervention outcomes [47, 78]. Overall, the degree of education and sex can moderate the relationship between individual participants and intervention outcomes, but the pathways are complex [4, 63]. Although women with higher socioeconomic status may be overrepresented in lifestyle interventions to prevent T2D, there are indications that higher socioeconomic status may be counterproductive for women. In particular, women with a university education and family responsibilities may be at risk for suboptimal intervention outcomes [8, 78]. This is especially true when women experience insufficient family support for their weight loss efforts [78].

6. Discussion

Preventive interventions have demonstrated potential in improving health outcomes among individuals with prediabetes or T2D [3]. However, despite the benefits of lifestyle changes in T2D prevention, interventions may experience challenges in attracting and retaining participants [35]. The design and delivery of primary care interventions are often challenging due to difficulties in adapting experimental intervention designs into primary care practice [57, 58], impacting the intervention's effectiveness in everyday practice. The adaptation process can be further hindered by the complexity of the intervention when there is a lack of clarity on how the intervention causes the observed outcomes, that is, what the intervention mechanisms are [30, 34]. Without a well-founded understanding of intervention components and pathways, primary care providers may encounter difficulties in adapting experimental intervention designs to local primary care systems. These challenges may arise from interactions with different intervention components [30]. Different intervention components can, for example, unexpectedly interact with participants and ultimately affect the outcomes.

Furthermore, clearly formulated intervention mechanisms are needed to lessen challenges in designing and delivering behavioral interventions. A lack of clearly formulated intervention mechanisms may lead to uncertainty about how desired outcomes should be achieved [34, 44]. This also hinders the replication of the intervention into other contexts [34]. Primary care providers may have limited resources to interpret various intervention mechanisms from research studies. This places the responsibility on researchers to provide a clear presentation of intervention mechanisms, which is crucial for effectively adapting complex behavioral interventions for practice [108].

Designing and delivering weight loss interventions for T2D prevention could be improved by enhancing the multidisciplinary approach and partnerships between primary healthcare practice and research [109, 110]. Partnerships between primary care and research institutions may cover research initiatives and research to practice transfer collaborations [57, 110]. Additionally, as sustained weight loss in T2D prevention can be difficult, participants may benefit from involvement in and access to a multidisciplinary team of healthcare professionals during intervention delivery.

To ensure that as many as possible may benefit from lifestyle T2D intervention, it may be necessary to use different approaches to encourage at-risk groups to participate and encourage continuing participation. Individual attributes like the participant's sex and socioeconomic status can affect the success of weight loss and weight loss maintenance for T2D prevention. However, by considering the mechanisms of behavior change and intervention and participant characteristics, it is possible to design interventions that are more likely to attract participation and encourage successful outcomes. Decisions to participate result from complex interactions between intervention components, individuals, and context variables [30, 111]. In other words, effective intervention design in primary healthcare requires considering which intervention is appropriate for whom and under what circumstances [112].

Author details

Maija Huttunen-Lenz
Institute of Nursing Science, University of Education Schwäbisch Gmünd, Oberbettringerstrasse, Schwäbisch Gmünd, Germany

*Address all correspondence to: maija.huttunen-lenz@ph-gmuend.de

References

[1] Khan MAB, Hashim MJ, King JK, Govender RD, Mustafa H, Al KJ. Epidemiology of type 2 diabetes - Global burden of disease and forecasted trends. Journal of Epidemiology and Global Health. 2020;**10**(1):107-111

[2] Raben A, Vestentoft PS, Brand-Miller J, Jalo E, Drummen M, Simpson L, et al. The PREVIEW intervention study: Results from a 3-year randomized 2 x 2 factorial multinational trial investigating the role of protein, glycaemic index and physical activity for prevention of type 2 diabetes. Diabetes, Obesity & Metabolism [Internet]. 2021;**23**(2):324-337. Available from: https://www.scopus.com/inward/record.uri?eid=2-s2.0-85096964555&doi=10.1111%2fdom.14219&partnerID=40&md5=09f6e250b14d2cfd4c07b10678d2fca0

[3] Howells L, Musaddaq B, McKay AJ, Majeed A. Clinical impact of lifestyle interventions for the prevention of diabetes: An overview of systematic reviews. BMJ Open. 2016;**6**(12):1-17

[4] Harreiter J, Kautzky-Willer A. Sex and gender differences in prevention of type 2 diabetes. Frontiers in Endocrinology (Lausanne). 2018;**9**(May):1-15

[5] Kautzky-Willer A, Harreiter J, Pacini G. Sex and gender differences in risk, pathophysiology and complications of type 2 diabetes mellitus. Endocrine Reviews [Internet]. 2016;**37**(3):278-316. Available from: https://www.ncbi.nlm.nih.gov/pubmed/27159875 [Accessed: May 09, 2016]

[6] Sortsø C, Lauridsen J, Emneus M, Green A, Jensen PB. Social inequality in diabetes patients' morbidity patterns from diagnosis to death – A Danish register-based investigation. Scandinavian Journal of Public Health. 2018;**46**(1):92-101

[7] Siegel KR, McKeever Bullard K, Imperatore G, Ali MK, Albright A, Mercado CI, et al. Prevalence of major behavioral risk factors for type 2 diabetes. Diabetes Care. 2018;**41**(5):1032-1039

[8] Gavarkovs AG, Burke SM, Petrella RJ. Engaging men in chronic disease prevention and management programs: A scoping review. American Journal of Men's Health [Internet]. 2016;**10**(6):NP145-NP154. DOI: 10.1177/1557988315587549

[9] Ong KL, Stafford LK, McLaughlin SA, Boyko EJ, Vollset SE, Smith AE, et al. Global, regional, and national burden of diabetes from 1990 to 2021, with projections of prevalence to 2050: A systematic analysis for the global burden of disease study 2021. The Lancet [Internet]. 2023;**402**(10397):203-234. Available from: https://linkinghub.elsevier.com/retrieve/pii/S0140673623013016

[10] Tamayo T, Rosenbauer J, Wild SH, Spijkerman AMW, Baan C, Forouhi NG, et al. Diabetes in Europe: An update. Diabetes Research and Clinical Practice. 2014;**103**(2):206-217

[11] Wareham NJ, Herman WH. The clinical and public health challenges of diabetes prevention: A search for sustainable solutions. PLoS Medicine. 2016;**13**(7):5-7

[12] American Diabetes Association. How Type 2 Diabetes Progresses. ADA [Internet]; 2024. Available from: https://diabetes.org/living-with-diabetes/type-2/how-type-2-diabetes-progresses [Accessed: Jan 8, 2024]

[13] National Health Service. NHS Health A to Z. Health Problems Type 2 Diabetes; 2023. Available from: https://www.nhs.uk/conditions/type-2-diabetes/health-problems/ [cited 2024 Mar 12]

[14] Janssen LMM, Hiligsmann M, Elissen AMJ, Joore MA, Schaper NC, Bosma JHA, et al. Burden of disease of type 2 diabetes mellitus: Cost of illness and quality of life estimated using the Maastricht study. Diabetic Medicine. 2020;**37**(10):1759-1765

[15] Messina J, Campbell S, Morris R, Eyles E, Sanders C. A narrative systematic review of factors affecting diabetes prevention in primary care settings. PLoS One. 2017;**12**(5)

[16] Chan JCN, Luk AOY. Diabetes: A Cinderella subject we Can't afford to ignore. PLoS Medicine. 2016;**13**(7):e1002068

[17] Petit Francis L, Spaulding E, Turkson-Ocran RA, Allen J. Randomized trials of nurse-delivered interventions in weight management research: A systematic review. Western Journal of Nursing Research. 2017;**39**(8):1120-1150 [Accessed: 2017 Jan, 08]

[18] Semlitsch T, Stigler FL, Jeitler K, Horvath K, Siebenhofer A. Management of overweight and obesity in primary care—A systematic overview of international evidence-based guidelines. Obesity Reviews. 2019;**20**(9):1218-1230

[19] Aziz Z, Absetz P, Oldroyd J, Pronk NP, Oldenburg B. A systematic review of real-world diabetes prevention programs: Learnings from the last 15 years. Implementation Science. 2015;**10**(1):172

[20] Alouki K, Delisle H, Bermúdez-Tamayo C, Johri M. Lifestyle interventions to prevent type 2 diabetes: A systematic review of economic evaluation studies. Journal Diabetes Research. 2016;**2016**:2159890

[21] Lindström J, Louheranta A, Mannelin M, Rastas M, Salminen V, Eriksson J, et al. The Finnish diabetes prevention study (DPS): Lifestyle intervention and 3-year results on diet and physical activity. Diabetes Care. 2003;**26**(12):3230-3236

[22] Miller CK, Weinhold KR, Nagaraja HN. Impact of a worksite diabetes prevention intervention on diet quality and social cognitive influences of health behavior: A randomized controlled trial. Journal of Nutrition Education and Behavior. 2016;**48**(3):160-169.e1

[23] Diabetes Prevention Program (DPP) Research Group. The diabetes prevention program (DPP): description of lifestyle intervention. Diabetes Care [Internet]. Dec 2002;**25**(12):2165-2171. Available from: https://pubmed.ncbi.nlm.nih.gov/12453955

[24] Rockette-Wagner B, Kriska AM, Storti KL, Dabelea D, Edelstein S, Florez H, et al. Activity and sedentary time 10 years after a successful lifestyle intervention: The diabetes prevention program. American Journal of Preventive Medicine. 2017;**52**(3):292-299

[25] Berry D, Urban A, Grey M. Understanding the development and prevention of type 2 diabetes in youth (part 1). Journal of Pediatric Health Care [Internet]. 2006;**20**(1):3-10. DOI: 10.1016/j.pedhc.2005.08.009

[26] American Diabetes Association. 3. Prevention or delay of type 2 diabetes and associated comorbidities: Standards of medical Care in Diabetes—2022. Diabetes Care [Internet]. 2021;**45** (Suppl. 1):S39-S45. DOI: 10.2337/dc22-S003

[27] Huttunen-Lenz M, Raben A, Meinert-Larsen T, Drummen M, Macdonald I, Martínez JA, et al. Sociocognitive factors associated with lifestyle intervention attrition after successful weight loss among participants with prediabetes—The PREVIEW study. Public Health Nursing. 2020;**37**(3):1-12

[28] The Look AHEAD Research Group. Eight-year weight losses with an intensive lifestyle intervention: The look AHEAD study. Obesity [Internet]. 2014;**22**(1):5-13. DOI: 10.1002/oby.20662

[29] Brownson RC, Fielding JE, Maylahn CM. Frontiers in public health services and systems research evidence-based decision making to improve public health practice evidence-based decision making to improve public health practice. Frontiers in Public Health Services and Systems Research. 2013;**2**(2):1-9

[30] Skivington K, Matthews L, Simpson SA, Craig P, Baird J, Blazeby JM, et al. A new framework for developing and evaluating complex interventions: Update of Medical Research Council guidance. The BMJ. 2021;**374**(2018):1-11

[31] Wareham NJ. Mind the gap: Efficacy versus effectiveness of lifestyle interventions to prevent diabetes. The Lancet Diabetes and Endocrinology [Internet]. 2015;**3**(3):160-161. DOI: 10.1016/S2213-8587(15)70015-X

[32] Skivington K, Matthews L, Simpson SA, Craig P, Baird J, Blazeby J. A new framework for developing and evaluating complex interventions: Update of Medical Research Council guidance. 2021;**374**:n2061

[33] Craig P, Dieppe P, Macintyre S, Michie S, Nazareth I, Petticrew M. Developing and Evaluating Complex Interventions. London: Medical Research Council; 2006

[34] Craig P, Dieppe P, Macintyre S, Michie S, Nazareth I, Petticrew M. Developing and evaluating complex interventions: The new Medical Research Council guidance. BMJ [Internet]. 2008;**337**. Available from: https://www.bmj.com/content/337/bmj.a1655

[35] Burgess E, Hassmén P, Pumpa KL. Determinants of adherence to lifestyle intervention in adults with obesity: A systematic review. Clinical Obesity. 2017;**7**(3):123-135

[36] Fogelholm M, Larsen T, Westerterp-Plantenga M, Macdonald I, Martinez J, Boyadjieva N, et al. Preview: Prevention of diabetes through lifestyle intervention and population studies in Europe and around the world. Design, methods, and baseline participant description of an adult cohort enrolled into a three-year randomised clinical trial. Nutrients. 2017;**9**(6):632

[37] Moore GF, Evans RE, Hawkins J, Littlecott H, Melendez-Torres GJ, Bonell C, et al. From complex social interventions to interventions in complex social systems: Future directions and unresolved questions for intervention development and evaluation. Evaluation [Internet]. 31 Jan 2019;**25**(1):23-45

[38] Shiell A, Hawe P, Gold L. Complex interventions or complex systems? Implications for health economic evaluation. BMJ. 2008;**336**(7656):1281-1283

[39] Norris SL, Rehfuess EA, Smith H, Tunçalp Ö, Grimshaw JM, Ford NP, et al. Complex health interventions in complex systems: Improving the process and methods for evidence-informed health decisions. BMJ

Glob Health [Internet]. Jan 2019;**4**(Suppl 1):e000963

[40] Upsher R, Onabajo D, Stahl D, Ismail K, Winkley K. The effectiveness of behavior change techniques underpinning psychological interventions to improve Glycemic levels for adults with type 2 diabetes: A meta-analysis. Frontiers in Clinical Diabetes and Healthcare. 2021;**2**

[41] Noyes J, Gough D, Lewin S, Mayhew A, Michie S, Pantoja T, et al. A research and development agenda for systematic reviews that ask complex questions about complex interventions. Journal of Clinical Epidemiology. Nov 2013;**66**(11):1262-1270

[42] Michie S, Richardson M, Johnston M, Abraham C, Francis J, Hardeman W, et al. The behavior change technique taxonomy (v1) of 93 hierarchically clustered techniques: Building an international consensus for the reporting of behavior change interventions. Annals of Behavioral Medicine. 2013;**46**(1):81-95

[43] Kahlert D, Unyi-Reicherz A, Stratton G, Meinert Larsen T, Fogelholm M, Raben A, et al. PREVIEW behavior modification intervention toolbox (PREMIT): A study protocol for a psychological element of a multicenter project. Frontiers in Psychology [Internet]. 2016;7:1136. DOI: 10.3389/fpsyg.2016.01136

[44] Michie S, Johnston M, Francis J, Hardeman W, Eccles M. From theory to intervention: Mapping theoretically derived behavioural determinants to behaviour change techniques. Applied Psychology. 2008;**57**(4):660-680

[45] Delahanty LM, Conroy MB, Nathan DM, Group DPPR. Psychological predictors of physical activity in the diabetes prevention program. Journal of the American Dietetic Association [Internet]. 2006;**106**(5):698-705. Available from: https://pubmed.ncbi.nlm.nih.gov/16647327

[46] Schwarzer R, Luszczynska A, Ziegelmann JP, Scholz U, Lippke S. Social-cognitive predictors of physical exercise adherence: Three longitudinal studies in rehabilitation. Health Psychology. 2008;**27**(Suppl. 1):54-63

[47] Hansen S, Huttunen-Lenz M, Sluik D, Brand-Miller J, Drummen M, Fogelholm M, et al. Demographic and social-cognitive factors associated with weight loss in overweight, pre-diabetic participants of the preview study. International Journal of Behavioral Medicine. 2018;**25**(6)

[48] Uusitupa M, Khan TA, Viguiliouk E, Kahleova H, Rivellese AA, Hermansen K, et al. Prevention of type 2 diabetes by lifestyle changes: A systematic review and meta-analysis. Nutrients [Internet]. 2019;**11**(11):2611. Available from: https://pubmed.ncbi.nlm.nih.gov/31683759

[49] Vanderwood KK, Hall TO, Harwell TS, Arave D, Butcher MK, Helgerson SD. Factors associated with the maintenance or achievement of the weight loss goal at follow-up among participants completing an adapted diabetes prevention program. Diabetes Research and Clinical Practice [Internet]. 2011;**91**(2):141-147. Available from: https://www.sciencedirect.com/science/article/pii/S0168822710005917

[50] Dombrowski SU, Knittle K, Avenell A, Araújo-Soares V, Sniehotta FF. Long term maintenance of weight loss with non-surgical interventions in obese adults: Systematic review and meta-analyses of randomised controlled trials. BMJ (Online) [Internet]. 2014;**348**(May):1-12. DOI: 10.1136/bmj.g2646

[51] French SD, Green SE, O'Connor DA, McKenzie JE, Francis JJ, Michie S. Developing theory-informed behaviour change interventions to implement evidence into practice: A systematic approach using the theoretical domains framework. Implementation Science [Internet]. 2012;**7**:38. DOI: 10.1186/1748-5908-7-38

[52] Ryan R, Patrick H, Deci E, Williams G. Facilitating health behaviour change and its maintenance: Interventions based on self-determination theory. The European Health Psychologist. 2008;**10**:2-5

[53] Schwarzer R, Luszczynska A. How to overcome health-compromising Behaviors. European Psychologist [Internet]. 2008;**13**(2):141-151. DOI: 10.1027/1016-9040.13.2.141

[54] Schwarzer R, Renner B. Social-cognitive predictors of health behavior: Action self-efficacy and coping self-efficacy. Health Psychology. 2000;**19**(5):487-495. DOI: 10.1037/0278-6133.19.5.487

[55] Kuhlmann E, Groenewegen PP, Bond C, Burau V, Hunter DJ. Primary care workforce development in Europe: An overview of health system responses and stakeholder views. Health Policy (New York) [Internet]. 2018;**122**(10):1055-1062. Available from: https://www.sciencedirect.com/science/article/pii/S0168851018303233

[56] Semahegn A, Manyazewal T, Hanlon C, Getachew E, Fekadu B, Assefa E, et al. Challenges for research uptake for health policymaking and practice in low- and middle-income countries: A scoping review. Health Research Policy and Systems [Internet]. 2023;**21**(1):131. DOI: 10.1186/s12961-023-01084-5

[57] Damschroder LJ, Aron DC, Keith RE, Kirsh SR, Alexander JA, Lowery JC. Fostering implementation of health services research findings into practice: A consolidated framework for advancing implementation science. Implementation Science [Internet]. 2009;**4**:50. DOI: 10.1186/1748-5908-4-50

[58] Kessler R, Glasgow RE. A proposal to speed translation of healthcare research into practice: Dramatic change is needed. Americal Journal of Preventive Medicine [Internet]. 2011;**40**:637-644. DOI: 10.1016/j.amepre.2011.02.023

[59] Kelly MP, Speller V, Meyrick J. Getting Evidence into Practice in Public Health. London: NHS Health Development Agency; 2004

[60] Rieger S, Göllner R, Spengler M, Trautwein U, Nagengast B, Roberts BW. Social cognitive constructs are just as stable as the big five between grades 5 and 8. AERA Open. [Internet]. 2017;**3**(3):2332858417717691. DOI: 10.1177/2332858417717691

[61] Schwarzer R. Social-cognitive factors in changing health-related Behaviors. Current Directions in Psychological Science. 2001;**10**(2):47-51

[62] Haughton CF, Silfee VJ, Wang ML, Lopez-cepero AC, Estabrook DP, Frisard C, et al. Racial/ethnic representation in lifestyle weight loss intervention studies in the United States: A systematic review. Preventive Medical Reports [Internet]. 2018;**9**:131-137. DOI: 10.1016/j.pmedr.2018.01.012

[63] Walker J, Halbesma N, Lone N, McAllister D, Weir CJ, Wild SH. Socioeconomic status, comorbidity and mortality in patients with type 2 diabetes mellitus in Scotland 2004-2011: A cohort study. Journal of Epidemiology and Community Health. 2016;**70**(6):596-601

[64] Mouchacca J, Abbott GR, Ball K. Associations between psychological stress, eating, physical activity, sedentary behaviours and body weight among women: A longitudinal study. BMC Public Health. 2013;**13**(1):828

[65] Torres SJ, Nowson CA. Relationship between stress, eating behavior, and obesity. Nutrition. 2007;**23**(11-12):887-894

[66] Lazarus RS, Folkman S. Stress, Appraisal, and Coping. New York, NY: Springer; 1984

[67] Kim KH-C, Bursac Z, Dilillo V, Brown White D, Smith West D. Stress, race, and body weight. Health Pschology. 2016;**28**(1):131-135

[68] Langer SL, Flood AP, Welsh EM, Levy RL, Jaeb MA, Laqua PS, et al. Mood, weight, and physical activity among obese individuals enrolled in a long-term weight-loss program: Trajectories and associations with gender. Journal of Mental Health [Internet]. 2009;**6**(1)

[69] Bandura A. Self-efficacy. In: Ramachaudran VS, editor. Encyclopedia of human behavior. New York: Academic Press; 1994. pp. 71-78

[70] Ajzen I. Perceived behavioral control, self-efficacy, locus of control, and the theory of planned behavior. Journal of Applied Social Psychology [Internet]. 2002;**32**(4):665-683. DOI: 10.1111/j.1559-1816.2002.tb00236.x

[71] Wrosch C, Scheier MF, Carver CS, Schulz R. The importance of goal disengagement in adaptive self-regulation: When giving up is beneficial. Self and Identity. 2003;**2**:1-20

[72] Prochaska JO, DiClemente CC. Stages of change in the modification of problem behaviors. In: Hersen M, Eisler RM, Miller P, editors. Progress on Behavior Modification. Sycamore, IL: Sycamore Press; 1992. pp. 184-214

[73] Ajzen I. The theory of planned behavior. Organizational Behavior and Human Decision Processes. 1991;**50**(2):178-211

[74] Bandura A. Social cognitive theory of human development. In: Husen T, Postlethwaite TN, editors. International Encyclopedia of Education. 2nd ed. Oxford: Pergamon Press; 1996. pp. 5513-5518

[75] Prochaska JO, Velicer WF. The transtheoretical change model of health behavior. American Journal of Health Promotion. 1997;**12**(1):38-48

[76] Huttunen-Lenz M, Hansen S, Christensen P, Larsen TM, Sandø-Pedersen F, Drummen M, et al. PREVIEW study—Influence of a behavior modification intervention (PREMIT) in over 2300 people with pre-diabetes: Intention, self-efficacy and outcome expectancies during the early phase of a lifestyle intervention. Psychology Research and Behavior Management. 2018;**11**

[77] Chesney MA, Neilands TB, Chambers DB, Taylor JM, Folkman S. A validity and reliability study of the coping self-efficacy scale. British Journal of Health Psychology. 2006;**11**:421-437

[78] Huttunen-Lenz M, Raben A, Adam T, Macdonald I, Taylor MA, Stratton G, et al. Socio-economic factors, mood, primary care utilization, and quality of life as predictors of intervention cessation and chronic stress in a type 2 diabetes prevention intervention (preview study). BMC Public Health [Internet]. 2023;**23**(1):1666. DOI: 10.1186/s12889-023-16569-9

[79] Roumen C, Feskens EJM, Corpeleijn E, Mensink M, Saris WHM, Blaak EE. Predictors of lifestyle intervention outcome and dropout: The SLIM study. European Journal of Clinical Nutrition. 2011;**65**(10):1141-1147

[80] Huttunen-Lenz M, Hansen S, Raben A, Westerterp-Plantenga M, Macdonald I, Stratton G, et al. Forming new health behavior habits during weight loss maintenance—The preview study. Health Psychology [Internet]. 2022;**41**(8):549-558. DOI: 10.1037/hea0001182Title

[81] Kreausukon P, Gellert P, Lippke S, Schwarzer R. Planning and self-efficacy can increase fruit and vegetable consumption: A randomized controlled trial. Journal of Behavioral Medicine. 2012;**35**(4):443-451

[82] Westland H, Sluiter J, te Dorsthorst S, Schröder CD, Trappenburg JCA, Vervoort SCJM, et al. Patients' experiences with a behaviour change intervention to enhance physical activity in primary care: A mixed methods study. PLoS One [Internet]. 2019;**14**(2):e0212169. DOI: 10.1371/journal.pone.0212169

[83] Michael EL, Brosnahan N, Leslie WS, Thom G, Barnes AC. Primary care weight-management for type 2 diabetes: The cluster-randomised diabetes remission clinical trial (DiRECT). The Lancet [Internet]. 2018;**391**(10120):541-551. Available from: http://nrl.northumbria.ac.uk/1019/1/Frequency conversion based on three-wave parametric solitons.pdf

[84] Wrosch C, Scheier MF, Carver CS, Gables C, Schulz R. The Importance of Goal Disengagement in Adaptive Self-Regulation: When Giving Up is Beneficial. 2003;**2**(1):1-20

[85] Ryan R, Deci E. Self-determination theory and the facilitation of intrinsic motivation, social development, and well-being. The American Psychologist. 2000;**55**(1):68-78

[86] Wrosch C, Miller GE, Scheier MF, Brun de Pontet S. Giving up on unattainable goals: Benefits for health? Personality and Social Psychology Bulletin. 2007;**22**(2):251-265

[87] Wrosch C, Scheier MF, Miller GE. Goal adjustment capacities, subjective well-being, and physical health. Social and Personality Psychology Compass. 2013;**7**(12):847-860

[88] Toft UN, Kristoffersen LH, Aadahl M, Von Huth SL, Pisinger C, Jørgensen T. Diet and exercise intervention in a general population - mediators of participation and adherence: The Inter99 study. European Journal of Public Health. 2007;**17**(5):455-463

[89] Huttunen-Lenz M, Hansen S, Vestentoft PS, Meinert Larsen T, Westerterp-Plantenga M, Drummen M, et al. Goal achievement and adaptive goal adjustment in a behavioral intervention for participants with prediabetes. Journal of Health Psychology. 2020

[90] Pfadenhauer LM, Gerhardus A, Mozygemba K, Lysdahl KB, Booth A, Hofmann B. Making sense of complexity in context and implementation: The context and implementation of complex interventions (CICI) framework. Implementation Science [Internet]. 2017;**12**:21. DOI: 10.1186/s13012-017-0552-5

[91] Fitzpatrick SL, Appel LJ, Bray B, Brooks N, Stevens VJ. Predictors of long-term adherence to multiple health behavior recommendations for weight

management. Health Education and Behavior. 2018;**45**(6):997-1007

[92] Middleton KR, Anton SD, Perri MG. Long-term adherence to health behavior change. American Journal of Lifestyle Medicine. 2013;7(6):395-404

[93] Krauss A. Why all randomised controlled trials produce biased results. Annals of Medicine [Internet]. 2018;**50**(4):312-322. DOI: 10.1080/07853890.2018.1453233

[94] Americal Diabetes Association. Good to know: Race and type 2 diabetes. Clinical Diabetes [Internet]. 2020;**38**(4):403-404. DOI: 10.2337/cd20-pe04

[95] Leung AWY, Chan RSM, Sea MMM, Woo J. An overview of factors associated with adherence to lifestyle modification programs for weight Management in Adults. International Journal of Environmental Research and Public Health. 2017;**14**(9):922

[96] Goode RW, Ye L, Sereika SM, Zheng Y, Mattos M, Acharya SD, et al. Socio-demographic, anthropometric, and psychosocial predictors of attrition across Behavioral weight-loss trials. Eating Behaviors. 2016;**20**:27-33

[97] Gonzalez-Zacarias AA, Mavarez-Martinez A, Arias-Morales CE, Stoicea N, Rogers B. Impact of demographic, socioeconomic, and psychological factors on glycemic self-management in adults with type 2 diabetes mellitus. Frontiers in Public Health [Internet]. 2016;**4**(September):1-8 Available from: http://journal.frontiersin.org/Article/10.3389/fpubh.2016.00195/abstract

[98] Nutakor JA, Zhou L, Larnyo E, Addai-Danso S, Tripura D. Socioeconomic status and quality of life: An assessment of the mediating effect of social capital. Healthcare (Basel). 2023;**11**(5)

[99] Safieddine B, Sperlich S, Beller J, Lange K, Epping J, Tetzlaff J, et al. Socioeconomic inequalities in type 2 diabetes among different population subgroups. European Journal of Public Health[Internet]. 2020;**30**(Suppl. 5): ckaa165.1044. DOI: 10.1093/eurpub/ckaa165.1044

[100] Pourfarzi F, Rezaei S, Malekzadeh R, Etemadi A, Zahirian Moghadam T, Zandian H. Socio-economic inequality in prevalence of type 2 diabetes among adults in north-west of Iran: A blinder-Oaxaca decomposition. Journal of Diabetes and Metabolic Disorders. 2022;**21**(2):1519-1529

[101] Galobardes B, Shaw M, Lawlor DA, Lynch JW, Davey SG. Indicators of socioeconomic position (part 1). Journal of Epidemiology and Community Health. 2006;**60**(1):7-12

[102] American Psychological Association. Resources - Socioeconomic Status. 2023. Education and Socioeconomic Status. Available from: https://www.apa.org/pi/ses/resources/publications/education

[103] Stringhini S, Dugravot A, Shipley M, Goldberg M, Zins M, Kivimäki M, et al. Health behaviours, socioeconomic status, and mortality: Further analyses of the British Whitehall II and the French GAZEL prospective cohorts. PLoS Medicine. 2011;**8**(2):e1000419

[104] Stringhini S, Batty GD, Bovet P, Shipley MJ, Marmot MG, Kumari M, et al. Association of lifecourse socioeconomic status with chronic inflammation and type 2 diabetes risk: The Whitehall II prospective cohort study. PLoS Medicine [Internet].

2013;**10**(7):e1001479. DOI: 10.1371/journal.pmed.1001479

[105] Poulsen K, Cleal B, Willaing I. Diabetes and work: 12-year national follow-up study of the association of diabetes incidence with socioeconomic group, age, gender and country of origin. Scandinavian Journal of Public Health. 2014;**42**(8):728-733

[106] Adam TC, Drummen M, Macdonald I, Jalo E, Siig-Vestentoft P, Martinez JA, et al. Association of psychobehavioral variables with HOMA-IR and BMI differs for men and women with prediabetes in the preview lifestyle intervention. Diabetes Care. 2021;**44**(July):dc210059

[107] Volz K, Wyckoff E, Medina TH, Denmat Z, Field C, LaRose J, et al. Impact of income and perceived stress on engagement and weight loss outcomes in an online behavioral weight loss program. Journal of Behavioral Medicine. 2021;**44**(6):853-859

[108] Villeval M, Bidault E, Shoveller J, Alias F, Basson JC, Frasse C. Enabling the transferability of complex interventions: Exploring the combination of an intervention's key functions and implementation [Internet]. International Journal of Public Health. 2016;**61**:1031-1038. DOI: 10.1007/s00038-016-0809-9

[109] Sibbald SL, Kang H, Graham ID. Collaborative health research partnerships: A survey of researcher and knowledge-user attitudes and perceptions. Health Research Policy and Systems [Internet]. 2019;**17**(1):92. DOI: 10.1186/s12961-019-0485-3

[110] Nyström ME, Karltun J, Keller C, Andersson GB. Collaborative and partnership research for improvement of health and social services: researcher's experiences from 20 projects. Health Research Policy and Systems [Internet]. 2018;**16**(1):46. DOI: 10.1186/s12961-018-0322-0

[111] Sevild CH. The complexity of lifestyle change, motivation, and health among participants in a healthy life [PhD thesis UiS, no. 591] [Internet]. Stavanger: University of Stavanger; 2021. Available from: https://hdl.handle.net/11250/2757479

[112] King AC. Theory's role in shaping behavioral health research for population health. International Journal of Behavioral Nutrition and Physical Activity [Internet]. 2015;**12**(1):146. DOI: 10.1186/s12966-015-0307-0

Chapter 10

The Interplay of Sarcopenic Obesity and Mental Health: A Complex Relationship

Lin Jia Cheah and Khang Jin Cheah

Abstract

Obesity and mental health issues are two pressing concerns in today's society. This chapter delves into the intriguing and multifaceted relationship between these two seemingly disparate areas of health—sarcopenic obesity and mental well-being. Sarcopenic obesity, characterised by the simultaneous presence of obesity and muscle wasting, has garnered increasing attention in recent years. Its implications go beyond physical health and extend into the realm of mental well-being as the chapter reveals. The chapter begins by offering an in-depth exploration of sarcopenic obesity, outlining its definition, prevalence and associated health risks. It explores the physiological mechanisms underpinning this condition, shedding light on how it affects the body's composition and metabolism. Through the latest research findings, the reader gains an understanding of the intricate interplay between fat mass, muscle mass and the implications for overall health. The narrative then transitions into the critical components of comprehensive treatment and management, encompassing dietetics, medical intervention and psychological approaches.

Keywords: sarcopenic obesity, mental health, nutrition, psychological, obesity, older adults

1. Introduction

1.1 Background of sarcopenic obesity and mental disorder

Obesity and mental health issues are two pressing concerns today across the entire population in this planet. The World Obesity Atlas 2023 estimates that the global overweight and obesity (BMI $\geq$ 25 kg/m^2) prevalence will increase from 38% in 2020 to over 50% of the world's population by 2035 [1]. On the other hand, the prevalence of obesity alone (BMI $\geq$30 kg/m^2) is expected to rise from 14–24%, affecting nearly 2 billion individuals, including adults, adolescents and children [1]. A growing number of high- and middle-income countries are presently facing severe obesity epidemic, while among low-income countries, steeper increase in the prevalence of obesity is observed [2]. The high prevalence of obesity will put economic in burden in terms of healthcare costs, economic productivity, as well as premature retirement or death [1].

Besides the rise in obesity prevalence, attention should be paid to the global prevalence of mental illness. A large-scale epidemiology study conducted in 29 nations revealed the risk for any mental illness by age 75 years to be around one in two people [3] suggesting by age 75 years, approximately half the population can be expected to develop one or more mental illnesses. This is a concerning issue as the predicted prevalence was a significant increase from data available from WHO just a few years back in 2019, whereby, one in every eight people, or 970 million people around the world were living with a mental illness [4]. Mental illnesses are associated with poor health outcomes in the affected individuals [5]. Mental illnesses encompass substantial disruptions in thinking, emotional regulation or behaviour [4], which may additionally impact individuals experiencing comorbidities such as obesity, including specific conditions, such as sarcopenic obesity.

Sarcopenic obesity is a condition, whereby there is coexistence of sarcopenia and obesity and is characterised by decreased muscle mass, strength and performance along with abnormally excessive fat mass [6]. There have been varying definitions and criteria for sarcopenic obesity. It is worthy to note that in 2022, a consensus on definition and diagnostic criteria has been reached jointly by the European Society for Clinical Nutrition and Metabolism (ESPEN) and the European Association for the Study of Obesity (EASO), as shown in **Figure 1** [6].

Based on the consensus, the evaluation of sarcopenic obesity is divided into two stages: screening and diagnosis [6]. At the screening stage, patients will be assessed based on:

a. Body mass index (BMI) or waist circumference using ethnicity-specific cut points, and;

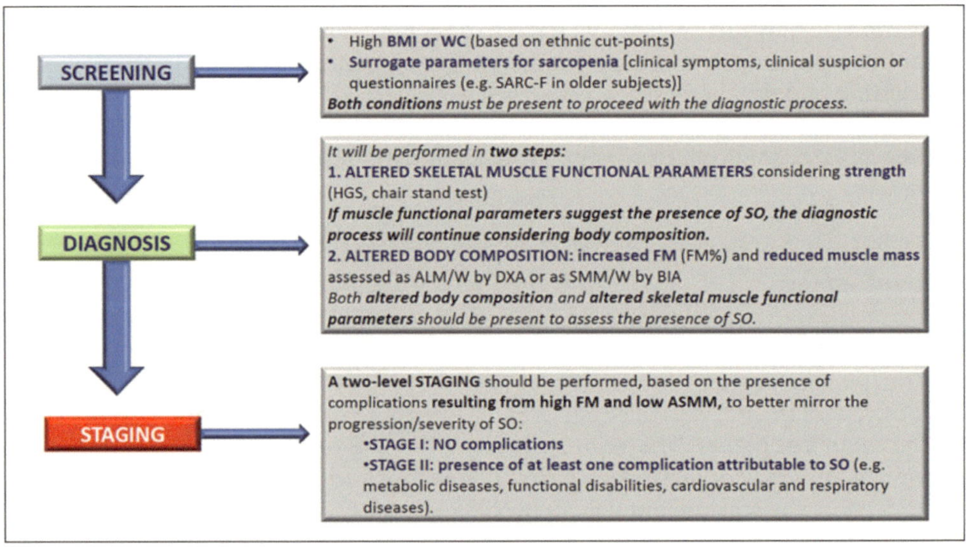

Figure 1.
Diagnostic procedure for sarcopenic obesity. ALM/W, appendicular lean mass adjusted to body weight; ASMM, absolute skeletal muscle mass; BIA, bioelectrical impedance analysis; BMI, body mass index; DXA, dual X-ray absorptiometry; FM, fat mass; HGS, hand-grip strength; SMM/W, total skeletal muscle mass adjusted by weight; SO, sarcopenic obesity; WC, waist circumference; SARC-F, strength, assistance with walking, rising from a chair, climbing stairs and falls. Note. This figure was produced by previous article. From Ref. [6]. Reprint with permission from Elsevier.

b. Indicators for sarcopenia, which can include clinical evaluation or validated questionnaires.

If the patient has positive screening of both the condition of obesity and sarcopenia, the evaluation will move on to the diagnosis phase, which will be performed in the order of two steps:

a. Assess for altered skeletal muscle functional parameters, for example, hand-grip strength and chair stand test, if the finding is positive, proceed to the following step.

b. Assess for altered body composition, aiming to look for increased fat mass and reduced muscle mass. Assessment techniques can be dual-energy X-ray absorptiometry (DXA) or bioelectrical impedance analysis (BIA).

Computerised tomography (CT) imaging is not usually needed unless clinically indicated for additional diagnostic reasons in specific cases.

This approach demonstrates a comprehensive evaluation combining both functional and compositional aspects for an accurate diagnosis of sarcopenic obesity.

As for mental illness, the diagnosis is usually made based on the below three available diagnostic manuals, namely the eleventh revision of the International Classification of Diseases (ICD) by WHO in 2018 [7], the fifth edition of the Diagnostic and Statistical Manual of Mental Disorders (DSM), published by the American Psychiatric Association (APA) in 2013 [8] and the Research Domain Criteria (RDoC) project initiated by the U.S. National Institute of Mental Health (NIMH) in 2009 [9]. The DSM-5 and the ICD Classification of Mental and Behavioural Disorders are the most widely recognised frameworks for both classifying and making psychiatric diagnoses. With a standardised framework and set of criteria that the clinicians can follow, they promote uniformity and accuracy in the identification and classification of mental health conditions.

Evidence shows that sarcopenic obesity in adults is associated with adverse mental health and a lower quality of life compared to body mass index-based general obesity [10]. Among all the mental illnesses, depressive symptoms are the most commonly studied conditions within the sarcopenic obesity population, particularly among older adults [11, 12]. The evidence indicates that sarcopenia and obesity appear to exert a synergistic impact on the risk of mental health compared to obesity alone. However, it is acknowledged that younger populations are also susceptible to developing sarcopenic obesity [13], as well as experiencing mental illness [14].

Therefore, we should raise awareness of the potential development of both mental health conditions and sarcopenic obesity as they can manifest in individuals of any age. The interrelated relationship between sarcopenic obesity and mental health highlights the importance of recognising and addressing these conditions comprehensively. By promoting awareness and understanding of the potential coexistence of mental health challenges and sarcopenic obesity across all age groups, we can foster early detection, intervention and holistic care strategies for individuals facing these interconnected health concerns.

1.2 Pathogenesis of sarcopenic obesity

As sarcopenic obesity is a syndrome consisting of two multifactorial and overlapping mechanisms of clinical condition (i.e., sarcopenia and obesity), it is difficult to pinpoint one clear disease mechanism [15]. However, there are a few proposed theories to explain the pathogenesis of sarcopenic obesity.

1.2.1 Inflammation of adipose tissue

In obesity, adipocytes in the adipose tissue undergo the abnormal cellular process of hypertrophy, hyperplasia and activation. The adipocytes, together with the macrophages infiltrated within the adipose tissue, induce the production of a range of pro-inflammatory cytokines, such as interleukin-6 (IL-6), tumour necrosis and factor-alpha (TNF-α). It leads to chronic systemic low-grade inflammatory response, which will then inhibit protein synthesis and contribute to muscle catabolism and sarcopenia [16–18]. It is worth noting that IL-6 and TNF-α are known to be associated with declining muscle mass and strengths in sarcopenic obesity [16]. The whole inflammatory process will also result in insulin resistance [19]. The relevant effect will be further discussed below.

1.2.2 Lipotoxicity

When the level of fatty acids becomes excessively high, they are distributed to skeletal muscle as intermuscular adipose tissue (IMAT), intramuscular adipose tissue and intramyocellular lipids (IMCLs) [15]. IMCLs impair muscle fibre contractility and lower muscle strength [17]. IMCLs found at the mitochondria level impair β-oxidation of fatty acids, raising reactive oxygen species and causing destruction of muscle cells [15, 20]. The process also results in insulin resistance, which is associated with muscle anabolic resistance [15, 16]. Anabolic resistance indicates lower rates of muscle protein synthesis, higher rate of muscle protein degradation [19] and subsequent reduced muscle mass and muscle atrophy [16].

1.2.3 Resistance to leptin

Leptin is a peptide hormone released by adipose tissue. Leptin is responsible for energy homeostasis by regulating appetite [21], as well as acting as a drive for myoblast proliferation [16]. The higher level of leptin in patients with sarcopenic obesity is believed to be an upregulation, resulting from leptin resistance [16]. Leptin resistance not only blunt the positive effect of leptin has on muscles but also causes increased uptake and accumulation of lipids, and subsequent insulin resistance [22].

1.2.4 Other hormonal changes

Obesity is associated with decreased testosterone level. Lower testosterone level alters metabolism of muscle and mitochondrial function, reducing muscle mass [23]. For women, the decline in oestrogen level is the contributing factor [12]. Other hormonal changes related to ageing itself that could contribute to sarcopenic obesity are insulin resistance, lower thyroid hormone level and higher cortisol level [19].

1.2.5 Ageing and lifestyle factors

With ageing, it is common to observe reduced physical activities and inadequate dietary intake of protein, which could cause sarcopenic obesity [19]. Not to mention ageing itself is associated with reduced resting metabolic rate, reduced muscle mass, increased visceral fat and ectopic fat accumulation [12].

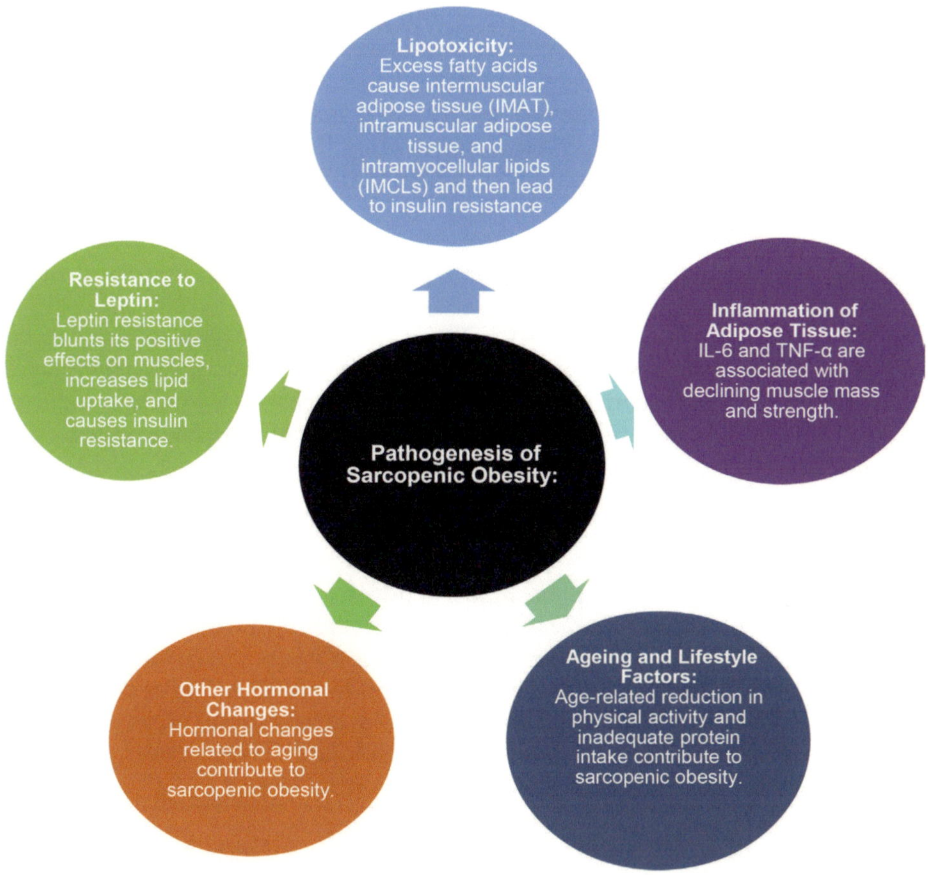
Lipotoxicity:
Excess fatty acids cause intermuscular adipose tissue (IMAT), intramuscular adipose tissue, and intramyocellular lipids (IMCLs) and then lead to insulin resistance
Resistance to Leptin:
Leptin resistance blunts its positive effects on muscles, increases lipid uptake, and causes insulin resistance.
Inflammation of Adipose Tissue:
IL-6 and TNF-α are associated with declining muscle mass and strength.
Pathogenesis of Sarcopenic Obesity:
Other Hormonal Changes:
Hormonal changes related to aging contribute to sarcopenic obesity.
Ageing and Lifestyle Factors:
Age-related reduction in physical activity and inadequate protein intake contribute to sarcopenic obesity.

Figure 2.
Pathogenesis of sarcopenic obesity.

The pathogenesis of sarcopenic obesity is summarised in **Figure 2**. Collectively, the typical physiological changes associated with ageing, coupled with environmental factors, such as sedentary lifestyle and an unhealthy diet, create a foundation for the development of sarcopenic obesity. The intricate interplay of these elements sets the stage for interacting and overlapping mechanisms, including inflammation, oxidative stress and insulin resistance. Increased awareness of these interconnected mechanisms is essential for developing targeted interventions that address both the physiological aspects of ageing and the lifestyle factors that contribute to the complex landscape of sarcopenic obesity.

2. Physical health impacts of sarcopenic obesity (SO)

2.1 Sarcopenic obesity and its impact to physical health

Sarcopenic obesity is related to several physical health consequences:

a. Increased ADL disability, increased frailty, increased fall risk, reduced grip strength and poor functional outcomes [12, 24, 25].

b. Higher risk of cardiovascular disease (CVD) and mortality [18]. Pro-inflammatory state in sarcopenic obesity as depicted under *pathogenesis* induces vascular endothelium damage and leads to atherosclerosis—a common pathological culprit for many cardiovascular diseases. It also exacerbates insulin resistance, which also triggers endothelial dysfunction [18], forming a vicious cycle, which is a phenomenon commonly observed in the complex disease mechanism of sarcopenic obesity.

c. Positive correlation to diabetes, hypertension, dyslipidaemia and non-alcoholic fatty liver disease [12, 26, 27].

d. Higher risk of knee osteoarthritis and osteoporosis [12], and poorer therapeutic outcomes for osteoarthritis with increased surgical risk post-joint arthroplasty [28]. Therapeutic outcomes for osteoarthritis and surgical risk and recovery after joint arthroplasty.

e. Higher CVD-related and all-cause mortality [12, 29].

In a broader context, the complex clinical syndrome of sarcopenic obesity demonstrates more pronounced adverse effects on physical health when compared to obesity alone [30]. Overall, sarcopenic obesity is associated with various adverse physical health outcomes, including increased disability in activities of daily living, heightened frailty, elevated fall risk, diminished grip strength and poorer functional outcomes. It also contributes greater effect on metabolic disorders driven by a pro-inflammatory state, inducing vascular damage and atherosclerosis.

2.2 Sarcopenic obesity (SO) and its relationship to mental health

From the previous epidemiological, cross-sectional and longitudinal studies, there is an established association between obesity and mental health disorders, most commonly mood disorders [10]. Several studies have also shown relation between sarcopenia and depression [31–33]. But when the focus is zoomed into the specific clinical syndrome of sarcopenic obesity, there are less studies available. Furthermore, mixed findings have been reported with some studies found no signification correlation between the complex clinical syndrome and mental health impact. One example is a cross-sectional study, involving over 7000 patients conducted in Korea from 2010 to 2011 [34].

The unclear relation warranting more reliable studies with larger sample size and consistent criteria to be done is supported by a systemic review by Pilati et al. published in 2021, with conflicting results among a few of the cross-sectional studies included [35, 36]. Nonetheless, the heterogenous results are not surprising given the inconsistent definition and measurement criteria of sarcopenic obesity [37]. When the measurement is based on muscle strength, there is a great association with depressive symptoms [34, 35]. Having said that, and with the challenge of sarcopenic obesity being a relatively newly recognised clinical syndrome, we managed to collate some evidence that exhibits positive correlation between sarcopenic obesity and negative mental health impacts:

2.2.1 Higher stress level and depressive symptoms

- A cross-sectional study involving over 10,000 patients conducted in Korea investigated the correlation between sarcopenic obesity and negative mental health impact by using self-reporting questionnaire. It found that sarcopenic obesity is associated with higher perceived stress and suicidal ideations, as compared to both general population and population with general obesity [10].

- This finding is supported by a recent study conducted among elderly Japanese females, where sarcopenic obesity combined with lower physical function was found to worsen depressive symptoms [38]. Similar result was demonstrated even among functionally independent Japanese women at similar age group [11].

- In a longitudinal 16-year period study involving over 1000 female patients in Australia, with the assessment based on DSM-IV-TR, higher rates of major depressive disorders were reported in patients with sarcopenic obesity, especially when it is metabolically unhealthy with high inflammatory markers [36].

- In a systemic review conducted up to year 2019 supported that sarcopenic obesity is a predictor of depressive symptoms [35]. Among patients with known depression, sarcopenic obesity is a predictor of non-remission of depression. This finding is supported by a 2-year cohort study conducted in the Netherland with the involvement of 378 elderly patients [39].

There are several theories explaining the association between sarcopenic obesity and mental health. One theory focuses on metabolic disturbances, such as leptin resistance and chronic inflammation, which can negatively impact mental well-being [11, 30, 36]. Another theory suggests that the chronic inflammatory state associated with sarcopenic obesity can dysregulate the hypothalamic-pituitary-adrenal (HPA) axis, and HPA overactivity is known to be linked with depressed mood and cognitive dysfunction [30, 36, 40]. Additionally, insulin resistance and dyslipidemia observed in sarcopenic obesity show a positive association with the severity and chronicity of major depressive disorder [41].

The latest research proposes that DNA methylation serves as the epigenetic mechanism, underlying the development of obesity and other metabolic disorders [42, 43]. Concurrently, DNA methylation exhibits a significant association with an increased risk of depression [44]. This suggests a complex interplay between epigenetic modifications and the risk of both metabolic and mental health disorders. Moreover, the relationship between sarcopenic obesity and depressive disorders may be bidirectional. It is postulated that individuals with depression may experience reduced physical activity, leading to a subsequent decline in muscle mass and strength, ultimately resulting in sarcopenia [45, 46].

2.2.2 Cognitive impairment

- A cross-sectional study done in 2012 with over 1000 elderly patients suggested both sarcopenia and sarcopenic obesity are linked to cognitive impairment [47].

- The finding is supported by another cross-sectional study of 353 elderly female white patients with the evaluation based on clinic visits and Montreal Cognitive Assessment (MoCA) [48]. The effect of cognitive impairment is found to be more profound on orientation and executive function and the association is greater in patients with lower muscle mass [48].

- Using Moca and Mini-mental State Examination (MMSE) as assessment tool, another study conducted in Japan in 2022 portrayed independent association between sarcopenic obesity and mild cognitive impairment and dementia [49].

- The association could be explained by the shared pathophysiology of chronic inflammation in sarcopenic obesity and dementia and brain atrophy associated with high body mass index [49].

In summary, the existing body of research on sarcopenic obesity and its impact on mental health reveals a complex and multifaceted relationship. While some studies present conflicting findings, there is accumulating evidence supporting a positive correlation between sarcopenic obesity and negative mental health outcomes, particularly in terms of higher stress levels, depressive symptoms and cognitive impairment. The association is, further, nuanced by factors such as metabolic disturbances, chronic inflammation and dysregulation of key physiological pathways. The bidirectional perspective suggests that not only does sarcopenic obesity contribute to mental health disorders but individuals with depression may also experience physical decline, reinforcing the intricate nature of this relationship. Recognising the interplay between genetic, epigenetic and lifestyle factors is crucial for developing comprehensive interventions tailored to address the intricate connections between sarcopenic obesity and depressive disorders. This understanding lays the foundation for targeted strategies aimed at mitigating the risk and managing the complexities associated with these interconnected health conditions.

3. Relationship between eating disorders and sarcopenic obesity

This section is dedicated to exploring the link between eating disorders and sarcopenic obesity. The most common eating disorders associated with obesity itself include bulimia nervosa, binge-eating disorder and night-eating syndrome [50, 51].

For an overview, the following key definitions for the above-mentioned eating disorders are taken from DSM-5, not including the respective full diagnostic criteria [8]:

3.1 Bulimia nervosa

Recurrent episodes of binge eating in a discrete period of time, involving a large amount of food and a sense of lack of control, with inappropriate compensatory behaviours, which have occurred for at least once weekly for 3 months.

3.2 Binge-eating disorder

Recurrent episodes of binge eating as described above, with the features of eating more quickly than usual, eating until feeling uncomfortably full, eating large amount of food despite not feeling hungry, eating alone because of embarrassment, feeling of guilt and disgust and depression after the episodes, which have occurred for at least once weekly for 3 months.

3.3 Night-eating syndrome (listed under "other unspecified eating disorders" in DSM-5)

Recurrent episodes of night eating, usually characterised by eating after waking up from sleep, or by excessive food intake after evening meal, which causes marked distress or functional impairment.

The prevalence of binge-eating disorder, night-eating disorder, and bulimia nervosa increases with increasing BMI [50, 51]. For example, individuals with binge-eating disorders are at three to six times risks suffering from obesity than general population, apart from having higher prevalence of obesity-associated physical comorbidities [50]. Data from a study conducted in the United States involving over a thousand of patients showed that among patients with binge-eating disorder and bulimia nervosa, 87 and 33% of the respective group also experienced obesity [52].

The bidirectional relationship between eating disorders and obesity has been well-studied. The factors contributing to that include genetic predisposition and personality risk factors, whereby mood dysregulation and negative evaluation of self and body image contribute to the vicious cycle of binge eating and poor weight control, dysregulated hypothalamic-pituitary-adrenal axis, which is associated with both obesity and eating disorders, disrupted gut microbiota, which has recently raised academic interest in regards to its association with metabolic disorders and the link between gut microbiota and eating disorder has been demonstrated to affecting up to 10% of the population [53].

Focusing specifically on sarcopenic obesity, to date, there is no established evidence of its correlation with eating disorders in general. Eating disorders are prevalent among adolescents and young adults, particularly among females. A large sample study conducted in Austria showed that as high as 31% of females aged 10–18 years old are at risk of developing eating disorder [54], and that is associated with risk factors of vulnerable self-image and body image dissatisfaction as supported by a systemic review in 2015 and a Swedish study [55, 56]. In contrast, sarcopenia is an age-related clinical condition and is more commonly found among elderly patients with multiple comorbidities [57].

Having said that, eating disorders do occur among elderly age group. Such evidence has been available from a systemic review conducted 10 years ago, looking into reported cases of eating disorders among those who are over the age of 50 [58]. The reported age of onset ranged from 50 to 94 years old, with 88% of them being females. While more than half of the reported cases were anorexia nervosa, 10% of the cases were bulimia nervosa [58]. An epidemiological study focusing on 342 females with age of 65–94 years in Portugal demonstrated binge-eating episodes among around 6% of the females, and 18.9% prevalence of picking/nibbling, which is associated with increased BMI [59].

Although eating disorder is rarely considered among elderly patients in day-to-day clinical practice, the above information is valuable to remind us not to overlook the possibility of eating disorder in older age groups. In these cases, especially among patients with comorbid mental health conditions, such as depressive disorders, sarcopenia can become another possible comorbid clinical condition. The mechanisms are as discussed in previous section. With that predisposition, elderly patients, particularly those with eating disorders, can be at risk of developing sarcopenic obesity. However, in a practical clinical setting, it can be challenging to pinpoint this specific condition as elderly patients with complex medical conditions often do not present with only one specific issue. There might be other more pressing medical issues that need prioritisation compared to sarcopenic obesity itself. In an ideal circumstance where there is a realistic capacity to deal with a patient holistically, managing both the eating disorder and sarcopenic obesity can evidently improve the quality of life of the patient.

4. Multidisciplinary management of sarcopenic obesity: medical, dietetics and psychological approach

There is no definitive treatment for sarcopenic obesity. The mainstay of management is lifestyle intervention with the aim to improve quality of life [16]. In the first line of management for sarcopenic obesity, an exercise programme serves as a foundational approach. As a second-line strategy, interventions include micronutrient supplementation, weight management through dietary, medical or surgical means, and hormonal replacement if deemed necessary. In severe cases of sarcopenic obesity, where patients experience immobilisation, palliative care becomes a viable option [16].

4.1 First-line management: exercise programme

Resistance exercise is presently recognised as the most effective exercise programme for sarcopenic obesity, having demonstrated its ability to enhance and preserve muscle mass, improve muscle function [60], and increase both muscle strength and overall physical performance [61]. Additionally, resistance exercises play a crucial role in mitigating the pathological progression of sarcopenic obesity by downregulating inflammatory cytokines, reducing oxidative stress and enhancing mitochondrial function [62].

Aerobic exercise is recommended as a strategy to address sarcopenic obesity given its known benefits of enhancing insulin sensitivity [63] and reducing oxidative stress [64]. Although there is limited evidence available regarding the specific effects of aerobic exercise on sarcopenic obesity, it appears to be an effective approach for reducing excess fat mass and enhancing muscle performance in this population [65]. Despite the limited evidence, aerobic exercise is recognised as a valuable therapeutic intervention for weight control management.

Recent meta-analysis evidence indicates that BMI decreases only in the group that undergoes combined resistance and aerobic training. While per cent body fat decreases with both resistance and aerobic training, the most significant reduction occurs in the group that engaged in both exercise types. Notably, muscle strength shows substantial improvement with resistance exercise [66]. Implementing an exercise programme that combines both resistance and aerobic exercises appears to offer additional benefits to individuals with sarcopenic obesity. However, it is crucial to acknowledge that there is no one-size-fits-all approach, the key lies in determining the specific needs of each individual with sarcopenic obesity to tailor a beneficial exercise regime [67].

4.2 Weight management: dietary therapy

Hypocaloric diet with the restriction of energy intake has been proposed as a weight loss strategy for sarcopenic obesity. The optimal and safe range of energy restriction is an energy deficit of about 200–700 kcal per day [68] or prescription of 1200–1800 kcal/day calorie-restricted diet for sarcopenic obese older adults [69]. However, in obese older adults, an energy-restricted diet designed for weight loss often results in the simultaneous loss of both fat mass and skeletal muscle mass. This is particularly concerning for sarcopenic obese older adults as the loss of skeletal muscle mass significantly impacts their ability to walk or climb stairs, highlighting the potential negative consequences of calories restriction weight loss interventions in this population [65].

Studies suggest that a high protein intake may enhance muscle mass and strength during calorie restriction for sarcopenic obesity [70]. Therefore, a weight loss diet in this population should prioritise the preservation of muscle mass and could benefit from incorporating a high protein diet and/or protein supplementation [71]. Generally, the recommended protein intake for sarcopenic obesity individuals falls within the range of 1.0 to 1.8 g/kg BW/day [71]. Some literature suggests a more conservative protein intake recommendation, ranging from 1.0 to 1.2 g/kg BW, with an even higher intake (1.2–1.5 g/kg BW), especially for individuals dealing with chronic diseases [65]. However, caution is advised for a protein intake of 1.4 g/kg BW in individuals with kidney disease [71].

According to the latest evidence, the most promising approach to sarcopenic obesity involves a combination of exercise training, especially resistance training, and an increased protein intake using protein supplements [71]. Regarding sarcopenia, protein supplementation, with or without exercise, has been shown to positively improve muscle mass, strength and physical function in older adults with sarcopenia [72]. A recent systematic review identifies whey protein supplementation as effective for individuals in the sarcopenic obesity population [60, 71]. Simultaneously, it is also acknowledged that a proper diet and exercise are crucial components in the prevention of sarcopenic obesity [60]. Recognising the varied presentations of sarcopenic obesity, such as constraints in performing resistance exercises for certain patients, a patient-centred approach tailored to the individual's lifestyle is essential in the treatment of both sarcopenic obesity and mental health. Additionally, micronutrient supplementation should be considered in the event of deficiencies occurring during the weight loss intervention period.

4.3 Weight management: medical/surgical

Medication option for weight loss in sarcopenic obesity could be glucagon-like peptide-1 receptor agonist (GLP-1RA) [18]. GLP-1 agonist is a drug commonly used in obesity and diabetes mellitus with reasonable safety profile [73]. Apart from anti-diabetic function, GLP-1 analogues or agonists result in weight loss by decreasing appetite and delaying gastric emptying. Most critically, it reduces fat mass as opposed to lean muscle mass [74].

Semaglutide is a GLP-1 agonist known for its substantial impact on weight loss and is among the FDA-approved drugs for treating obesity, along with liraglutide [75]. However, its potential influence on muscle improvement is a relatively recent consideration. In a recent animal study, semaglutide and liraglutide are shown to be able to decrease excessive lipid deposition and improve obesity-induced muscle atrophy at the same time [76]. The findings support a previous animal study in 2022, which reported the effect of muscle protein synthesis in obesity from semgalutide [75].

Bariatric surgery is an effective surgical procedure to help with weight loss in sarcopenic patients, but the outcome in improvement of daily living activities is elusive [77]. A 2-year follow-up study in 2021 observed early loss of fat-free mass in patients with sarcopenic obesity post-bariatric surgery [78]. However, it is essential to highlight that the study lacks a control group for comparison. Further, research is warranted to thoroughly investigate the suitability of bariatric surgery for individuals with sarcopenic obesity. On a positive note, there is a potential solution to address or prevent sarcopenia postoperatively implementing an exercise intervention programme to counteract muscle mass loss following bariatric surgery [79].

4.4 Hormonal replacement

While testosterone replacement may appear to be a plausible treatment from a physiological perspective, it is currently not recommended for addressing obesity or sarcopenia [18]. Looking ahead, selective androgen receptor modulators (SARMs) emerge as a potential future hormonal treatment given their selective binding to androgen receptors in muscles and bones, promoting anabolic processes without exerting systemic effects [18, 80]. However, due to potential side effects, further clinical studies are necessary before their clinical use can be approved [80].

4.5 Management of comorbid mental illness

The connection between sarcopenic obesity and mental illness remains unclear, with evidence suggesting a potential link between sarcopenic obesity and depressive disorders [12]. However, a systematic review has indicated that the results are heterogeneous due to significant variability in assessment methods and outcome measurements for sarcopenic obesity and depressive disorders [81]. Notably, patterns of comorbidity between sarcopenic obesity and the prevalence of depression have been observed, as highlighted in a recent systematic review and meta-analysis reporting a high prevalence of depression in patients with sarcopenia across nineteen included articles [82]. Research focusing on other mental health conditions is relatively scarce.

Selective serotonin reuptake inhibitors (SSRIs), namely escitalopram, sertraline, paroxetine, fluvoxamine, vortioxetine and fluoxetine, are widely prescribed as a first-choice treatment for various mental health conditions [83]. While SSRIs are popular, it is important to note their contraindication with concurrent use of MAOIs (e.g., linezolid), which can elevate serotonin levels and pose a risk of life-threatening serotonin syndrome [84]. Clinical responses to SSRIs may take several weeks (e.g., 6 weeks) as adaptive processes require time to take effect [85]. During the treatment process, it is imperative to closely monitor any adverse metabolic changes and vital signs, especially considering that sarcopenic obesity is associated with several clinical complications.

The treatment model combining a selective serotonin reuptake inhibitor (SSRI) with psychotherapy, such as cognitive behavioural therapy (CBT), has proven to be more effective. A meta-analysis of randomised trials utilising regression analyses to test the relationship between continuous variables and effect size concluded that monotherapy with medication may not be optimal for common mental illness. The combined treatment approach was found to be more effective than medication alone, particularly for mental illness, such as depression [86]. These findings are, further, supported by recent meta-analysis review papers, focusing on adults with depression [86].

Another treatment model, known as the sequential model treatment, involves the sequential combination of pharmacotherapy and psychotherapy and has been investigated in patients with major depressive disorder (MDD). The findings from this comprehensive examination and meta-analysis suggest that the sequential incorporation of psychotherapeutic treatment following a positive response to acute-phase drug therapy, either independently or in conjunction with antidepressant medication, is correlated with a reduced likelihood of relapse and recurrence in MDD patients [87].

In the case of eating disorders, multidisciplinary approach is essential to ensure input from medical, mental health and dietetics team. The framework of management will only be discussed briefly here for an overview understanding as eating disorder is a broad topic with different management plan depending on the specific type of diagnosis. According to Clinical Practice Guidelines in Australia, the first-line treatment for bulimia nervosa and binge-eating disorders is psychological therapy, that is, CBT. Behavioural weight loss can be initiated for weight management. Tricyclic antidepressants have shown to be of use to patients with bulimia nervosa, but this class of medication is notorious for their wide range of side effects. High-dose fluoxetine up to 60 mg per day can be effective in controlling bulimia nervosa. Other SSRIs can be considered for both bulimia nervosa and binge-eating disorder. Topiramate, an antiepileptic medication, is useful for both the conditions as well and is associated with weight loss, but there are side effects of taste changes and paraesthesia [88]. It is important to keep in mind the criteria for medical admission if there is significant physical deterioration from eating disorders; otherwise, the management is generally outpatient-based [88].

In summary, a multidisciplinary management approach tailored to each patient should be adopted for sarcopenic obesity with mental disorders. **Figure 3** above summarises the multidisciplinary management for sarcopenic obesity with mental disorders discussed earlier. First-line management includes foundational exercise programmes, while second-line strategies encompass high protein intake or micronutrient supplementation. We do not recommend weight loss diets for this population.

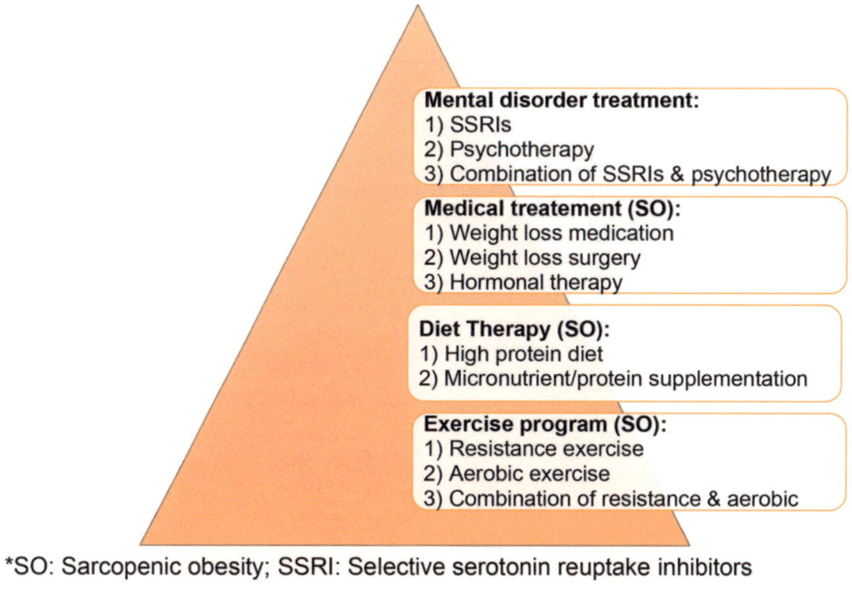

Figure 3.
*Multidisciplinary management for sarcopenic obesity with mental disorder. *SO: Sarcopenic obesity; SSRI: Selective serotonin reuptake inhibitors.*

If necessary, hormonal replacement therapy may be considered. In cases of sarcopenic obesity with mental illnesses, the patients should be referred to the psychiatric or mental health team as appropriate for further evaluation and consideration of the adoption of SSRIs and psychotherapy.

4.6 Multidisciplinary management: final consideration/challenges

Sarcopenic obesity treatment is a comprehensive undertaking that involves a combination of muscle training exercises and dietary therapy. However, if mental illness coexists with sarcopenic obesity, the treatment process becomes even more complex. An essential aspect of the treatment approach is to assess the patient's readiness to accept the proposed treatment plan. On the other hand, the socio-economic status of the individual can influence access to resources, affordability of specialised treatments and overall healthcare engagement. Additionally, understanding the patient's eating behaviours, nutritional preferences and lifestyle choices becomes crucial in tailoring an effective and sustainable treatment regimen.

Depending on the priority and severity of each condition, whether to focus on addressing the mental disorder first, sarcopenic obesity or both concurrently, requires careful planning. Given the lack of specific evidence guiding this specific decision making process, clinical judgement plays a significant role in guiding the direction of management. Early referral and involvement of multidisciplinary and interdepartmental team would evidently be beneficial in dealing with the complex clinical syndrome. For example, in patients with co-existing sarcopenic obesity and depressive disorders, involvement of medical team for physical assessment and addressing further underlying medical issues would be essential. Involvement of dietetics and physiotherapy team is valuable to offer input on dietary or nutritional advice and appropriate exercise programme to address the sarcopenic obesity. If the disordered mood is suspected, mental health team should be referred for further assessment and specialised management. This is a significant step as depressive mood can cause lack of motivation for patients to take part in a comprehensive plan in managing this complex clinical syndrome and cause further deterioration in physical health, contributing to the vicious cycle of the bidirectional relationship between sarcopenic obesity and depressive disorders. Eating disorders are rarely directly related to sarcopenic obesity, but if found to be the case, should be dealt with as well. But as discussed prior, the management would depend on the clinical priority and multidisciplinary team discussion as those patients often have complex chronic medical conditions.

Additionally, considerations of the cost of treatment and the potential economic burden on the country should not be overlooked, adding another layer of complexity to the overall treatment strategy. Balancing these various factors is crucial for developing a tailored and effective treatment plan for individuals dealing with both mental disorders and sarcopenic obesity. This broader perspective ensures a more nuanced and personalised treatment strategy that addresses the complex interplay between mental health, sarcopenic obesity and the broader contextual factors influencing the patient's well-being.

5. Summary

This chapter contributes insights on understanding between sarcopenic obesity and mental health. Both sarcopenia condition and obesity not only will provide synergy effect on metabolic disorders but also mental health conditions. This chapter brings together several existing interventions for such conditions, including dietary management, medical treatment, as well as mental health treatment. While the evidence on lifestyle management approach, which is combination of exercise and nutrition seems promising, there is still no concrete evidence to guide medical treatment specific for sarcopenia obesity. This could also indicates that lifestyle management is the most important aspect in managing sarcopenic obesity, while medications could be used as an adjuvant treatment if clinically indicated. Sarcopenic obesity can evidently become more complicated if affected individual have comorbid mental illness, therefore individualised approach and involvement of multidisciplinary and interdepartmental team is mandatory for this population.

Acknowledgements

We would like to thank the Library of North West Regional Hospital and Universiti Tunku Abdul Rahman for providing the online database resource.

Conflict of interest

The authors declare no conflict of interest.

Author details

Lin Jia Cheah[1] and Khang Jin Cheah[2*]

1 Mental Health Registrar, Mental Health and Specialised Services, Sunshine Coast Hospital and Health Service, Queensland, Australia

2 Department of Allied Health Sciences, Universiti Tunku Abdul Rahman (UTAR), Kampar, Malaysia

*Address all correspondence to: cheahkj@utar.edu.my

References

[1] Lobstein T, Powis J, Brinsden H, MJLR G. World Obesity Atlas 2023. UK: World Obesity Federation; 2023. Available from: https://data.worldobesity.org/publications/?cat=19

[2] Koliaki C, Dalamaga M, Liatis S. Update on the obesity epidemic: After the sudden rise, is the upward trajectory beginning to flatten? Current Obesity Reports. 2023;**12**(4):514-527. DOI: 10.1007/s13679-023-00527-y

[3] McGrath JJ, Al-Hamzawi A, Alonso J, et al. Age of onset and cumulative risk of mental disorders: A cross-national analysis of population surveys from 29 countries. Lancet Psychiatry. 2023;**10**(9):668-681. DOI: 10.1016/S2215-0366(23)00193-1

[4] World Health Organization (WHO). Mental Disorders. Gevena: WHO; 2022

[5] Vaingankar JA, Chong SA, Abdin E, et al. Understanding the relationships between mental disorders, self-reported health outcomes and positive mental health: Findings from a national survey. Health and Quality of Life Outcomes. 2020;**18**(1):55. DOI: 10.1186/s12955-020-01308-0

[6] Donini LM, Busetto L, Bischoff SC, et al. Definition and diagnostic criteria for sarcopenic obesity: ESPEN and EASO consensus statement. Obesity Facts. 2022;**15**(3):321-335. DOI: 10.1159/000521241

[7] World Health Organization (WHO). ICD-11 International Classification of Diseases 11th Revision. Gevena: WHO; 2018

[8] American Psychiatric Association (APA). Diagnostic and Statistical Manual of Mental Disorders. 5th ed. Arlington, VA: APA; 2013

[9] Clark LA, Cuthbert B, Lewis-Fernández R, Narrow WE, Reed GM. Three approaches to understanding and classifying mental disorder: ICD-11, DSM-5, and the National Institute of Mental Health's research domain criteria (RDoC). Psychological Science in the Public Interest. 2017;**18**(2):72-145. DOI: 10.1177/1529100617727266

[10] Cho Y, Shin SY, Shin MJ. Sarcopenic obesity is associated with lower indicators of psychological health and quality of life in Koreans. Nutrition Research. 2015;**35**(5):384-392. DOI: 10.1016/j.nutres.2015.04.002

[11] Ishii S, Chang C, Tanaka T, et al. The association between sarcopenic obesity and depressive symptoms in older Japanese adults. PLoS One. 2016;**11**(9):e0162898. DOI: 10.1371/journal.pone.0162898

[12] Roh E, Choi KM, Front E. Health consequences of sarcopenic obesity: A narrative review. Frontiers in Endocrinology (Lausanne). 2020;**11**:332. DOI: 10.3389/fendo.2020.00332

[13] Wagenaar CA, Dekker LH, Navis GJ. Prevalence of sarcopenic obesity and sarcopenic overweight in the general population: The lifelines cohort study. Clinical Nutrition. 2021;**40**(6):4422-4429. DOI: 10.1016/j.clnu.2021.01.005

[14] Schlack R, Peerenboom N, Neuperdt L, Junker S, Beyer AK, Monit JH. The effects of mental health problems in childhood and adolescence in young adults: Results of the KiGGS cohort. Journal of Health Monitoring. 2021;**6**(4):3-9. DOI: 10.25646/8863

[15] Wei LC, Yu K, Shyh-Chang N, et al. Pathogenesis of sarcopenia and the relationship with fat mass: Descriptive review. Journal of Cachexia, Sarcopenia and Muscle. 2022;**13**(2):781-794. DOI: 10.1002/jcsm.12901

[16] Axelrod CL, Dantas WS, Kirwan JP. Sarcopenic obesity: Emerging mechanisms and therapeutic potential. Metabolism. 2023;**146**:155639. DOI: 10.1016/j.metabol.2023.155639

[17] Kalinkovich A, Livshits G. Sarcopenic obesity or obese sarcopenia: A cross talk between age-associated adipose tissue and skeletal muscle inflammation as a main mechanism of the pathogenesis. Ageing Research Reviews. 2017;**35**:200-221. DOI: 10.1016/j.arr.2016.09.008

[18] Wei S, Nguyen TT, Zhang Y, Ryu D, Gariani K. Sarcopenic obesity: Epidemiology, pathophysiology, cardiovascular disease, mortality, and management. Frontiers in Endocrinology (Lausanne). 2023;**14**:1185221. DOI: 10.3389/fendo.2023.1185221

[19] Ji T, Li Y, Ma L. Sarcopenic obesity: An emerging public health problem. Aging and Disease. 2022;**13**(2):379-388. DOI: 10.14336/AD.2021.1006

[20] Al Saedi A, Debruin DA, Hayes A, Hamrick M. Lipid metabolism in sarcopenia. Bone. 2022;**164**:116539. DOI: 10.1016/j.bone.2022.116539

[21] Obradovic M, Sudar-Milovanovic E, Soskic S, et al. Leptin and obesity: Role and clinical implication. Frontiers in Endocrinology (Lausanne). 2021;**12**:585887. DOI: 10.3389/fendo.2021.585887

[22] Dyck DJ. Leptin sensitivity in skeletal muscle is modulated by diet and exercise. Exercise and Sport Sciences Reviews. 2005;**33**:189-194. Available from: www.acsm-essr.org

[23] Venkatesh VS, Grossmann M, Zajac JD, Davey RA. The role of the androgen receptor in the pathogenesis of obesity and its utility as a target for obesity treatments. Obesity Reviews. 2022;**23**(6):e13429. DOI: 10.1111/obr.13429

[24] Hirani V, Naganathan V, Blyth F, et al. Longitudinal associations between body composition, sarcopenic obesity and outcomes of frailty, disability, institutionalisation and mortality in community-dwelling older men: The Concord health and ageing in men project. Age and Ageing. 2017;**46**(3):413-420. DOI: 10.1093/ageing/afw214

[25] Agarwal K, Chorsiya V, Kaushik D, Yadav A. Impact of sarcopenic obesity on body composition, physical performance and fall risk in community dwelling older adults. Science Talks. 2022;**4**:100074. DOI: 10.1016/j.sctalk.2022.100074

[26] Yin T, Zhang JX, Wang FX, et al. The association between sarcopenic obesity and hypertension, diabetes, and abnormal lipid metabolism in Chinese adults. Diabetes, Metabolic Syndrome and Obesity. 2021;**14**:1963-1973. DOI: 10.2147/DMSO.S308387

[27] Nishikawa H, Asai A, Fukunishi S, Nishiguchi S, Higuchi K. Metabolic syndrome and sarcopenia. Nutrients. 2021;**13**:10. DOI: 10.3390/nu13103519

[28] Godziuk K, Prado CM, Woodhouse LJ, Forhan M. The impact of sarcopenic obesity on knee and hip osteoarthritis: A scoping review. BMC Musculoskeletal Disorders. 2018;**19**(1):271. DOI: 10.1186/s12891-018-2175-7

[29] Zhang X, Xie X, Dou Q, et al. Association of sarcopenic obesity with the risk of all-cause mortality among adults over a broad range of different settings: A updated meta-analysis. BMC Geriatrics. 2019;**19**(1):183. DOI: 10.1186/s12877-019-1195-y

[30] Khatoon BS, Saravanan D, Ganamurali N, Sabarathinam S. A narrative review on the impact of sarcopenic obesity and its psychological consequence in quality of life. Diabetes and Metabolic Syndrome: Clinical Research and Reviews. 2023;**17**(9):102846. DOI: 10.1016/j.dsx.2023.102846

[31] Lee JSW, Auyeung TW, Kwok T, Lau EMC, Leung PC, Woo J. Associated factors and health impact of sarcopenia in older Chinese men and women: A cross-sectional study. Gerontology. 2007;**53**(6):404-410. DOI: 10.1159/000107355

[32] Hsu Y, Liang C, Chou M, et al. Association of cognitive impairment, depressive symptoms and sarcopenia among healthy older men in the veterans retirement community in southern Taiwan: A cross-sectional study. Geriatrics & Gerontology International. 2014;**14**(S1):102-108. DOI: 10.1111/ggi.12221

[33] Kim NH, Kim HS, Eun CR, et al. Depression is associated with sarcopenia, not central obesity, in elderly Korean men. Journal of the American Geriatrics Society. 2011;**59**(11):2062-2068. DOI: 10.1111/j.1532-5415.2011.03664.x

[34] Byeon CH, Kang KY, Kang SH, Kim HK, Bae EJ. Sarcopenia is not associated with depression in Korean adults: Results from the 2010-2011 Korean National Health and nutrition examination survey. Korean Journal of Family Medicine. 2016;**37**(1):37. DOI: 10.4082/kjfm.2016.37.1.37

[35] Pilati I, Slee A, Frost R. Sarcopenic obesity and depression: A systematic review. The Journal of Frailty & Aging. 2021;**11**:1-8. DOI: 10.14283/jfa.2021.39

[36] Pasco JA, Berk M, Penninx B, et al. Obesity and sarcopenic obesity characterized by low-grade inflammation are associated with increased risk for major depression in women. Frontiers in Nutrition. 2023;**10**:1222019. DOI: 10.3389/fnut.2023.1222019

[37] Barazzoni R, Bischoff SC, Boirie Y, et al. Sarcopenic obesity: Time to meet the challenge. Clinical Nutrition. 2018;**37**(6):1787-1793. DOI: 10.1016/j.clnu.2018.04.018

[38] Osugi Y, Imai A, Kurihara T, Kishigami K, Higashida K, Sanada K. Interaction between sarcopenic obesity and nonlocomotive physical activity on the risk of depressive symptoms in community-dwelling older adult Japanese women. Journal of Aging and Physical Activity. 2023;**31**(4):541-547. DOI: 10.1123/japa.2022-0142

[39] Kokkeler KJE, van den Berg KS, Comijs HC, Oude Voshaar RC, Marijnissen RM. Sarcopenic obesity predicts nonremission of late-life depression. International Journal of Geriatric Psychiatry. 2019;**34**(8):1226-1234. DOI: 10.1002/gps.5121

[40] Mikulska J, Juszczyk G, Gawrońska-Grzywacz M, Herbet M. HPA Axis in the pathomechanism of depression and schizophrenia: New therapeutic strategies based on its participation. Brain Sciences. 2021;**11**(10):1298. DOI: 10.3390/brainsci11101298

[41] Watson KT, Simard JF, Henderson VW, et al. Association of insulin resistance with depression severity and remission status. JAMA Psychiatry. 2021;**78**(4):439. DOI: 10.1001/jamapsychiatry.2020.3669

[42] McAllan L, Baranasic D, Villicaña S, et al. Integrative genomic analyses in adipocytes implicate DNA methylation in human obesity and diabetes. Nature Communications. 2023;**14**(1):2784. DOI: 10.1038/s41467-023-38439-z

[43] Wu FY, Yin RX. Recent progress in epigenetics of obesity. Diabetology and Metabolic Syndrome. 2022;**14**(1):171. DOI: 10.1186/s13098-022-00947-1

[44] Zhu JH, Bo HH, Liu BP, Jia CX. The associations between DNA methylation and depression: A systematic review and meta-analysis. Journal of Affective Disorders. 2023;**327**:439-450. DOI: 10.1016/j.jad.2023.01.079

[45] Venant V, Pouget M, Lahaye C, et al. Depression severity as a risk factor of sarcopenic obesity in morbidly obese patients. The Journal of Nutrition, Health & Aging. 2019;**23**(8):761-767. DOI: 10.1007/s12603-019-1218-6

[46] Wang DK, Li YH, Guo XM. Depression and sarcopenia-related traits: A Mendelian randomization study. World Journal of Psychiatry. 2023;**13**(11):929-936. DOI: 10.5498/wjp.v13.i11.929

[47] Levine ME, Crimmins EM. Sarcopenic obesity and cognitive functioning: The mediating roles of insulin resistance and inflammation? Current Gerontology and Geriatrics Research. 2012;**2012**:826398. DOI: 10.1155/2012/826398

[48] Tolea MI, Chrisphonte S, Galvin JE. Sarcopenic obesity and cognitive performance. Clinical Interventions in Aging. 2018;**13**:1111-1119. DOI: 10.2147/CIA.S164113

[49] Someya Y, Tamura Y, Kaga H, et al. Sarcopenic obesity is associated with cognitive impairment in community-dwelling older adults: The Bunkyo health study. Clinical Nutrition. 2022;**41**(5):1046-1051. DOI: 10.1016/j.clnu.2022.03.017

[50] McCuen-Wurst C, Ruggieri M, Allison KC. Disordered eating and obesity: Associations between binge-eating disorder, night-eating syndrome, and weight-related comorbidities. Annals of the New York Academy of Sciences. 2018;**1411**(1):96-105. DOI: 10.1111/nyas.13467

[51] da Luz F, Hay P, Touyz S, Sainsbury A. Obesity with comorbid eating disorders: Associated health risks and treatment approaches. Nutrients. 2018;**10**(7):829. DOI: 10.3390/nu10070829

[52] Villarejo C, Fernández-Aranda F, Jiménez-Murcia S, et al. Lifetime obesity in patients with eating disorders: Increasing prevalence, clinical and personality correlates. European Eating Disorders Review. 2012;**20**(3):250-254. DOI: 10.1002/erv.2166

[53] Stabouli S, Erdine S, Suurorg L, Jankauskienė A, Lurbe E. Obesity and eating disorders in children and adolescents: The bidirectional link. Nutrients. 2021;**13**(12):4321. DOI: 10.3390/nu13124321

[54] Sander J, Moessner M, Bauer S. Depression, anxiety and eating disorder-related impairment: Moderators in female adolescents and young adults. International Journal of Environmental Research and Public Health. 2021;**18**(5):2779. DOI: 10.3390/ijerph18052779

[55] Jones BA, Griffiths KM. Self-objectification and depression: An integrative systematic review. Journal of Affective Disorders. 2015;**171**:22-32. DOI: 10.1016/j.jad.2014.09.011

[56] Ivarsson T, Svalander P, Litlere O, Nevonen L. Weight concerns, body image, depression and anxiety in Swedish adolescents. Eating Behaviors. 2006;**7**(2):161-175. DOI: 10.1016/j.eatbeh.2005.08.005

[57] Pacifico J, Geerlings MAJ, Reijnierse EM, Phassouliotis C, Lim WK, Maier AB. Prevalence of sarcopenia as a comorbid disease: A systematic review and meta-analysis. Experimental Gerontology. 2020;**131**:110801. DOI: 10.1016/j.exger.2019.110801

[58] Lapid MI, Prom MC, Burton MC, McAlpine DE, Sutor B, Rummans TA. Eating disorders in the elderly. International Psychogeriatrics. 2010;**22**(4):523-536. DOI: 10.1017/S1041610210000104

[59] Conceição EM, Gomes FVS, Vaz AR, Pinto-Bastos A, Machado PPP. Prevalence of eating disorders and picking/nibbling in elderly women. International Journal of Eating Disorders. 2017;**50**(7):793-800. DOI: 10.1002/eat.22700

[60] Kim YJ, Moon S, Yu JM, Chung HS. Implication of diet and exercise on the management of age-related sarcopenic obesity in Asians. Geriatrics & Gerontology International. 2022;**22**(9):695-704. DOI: 10.1111/ggi.14442

[61] Hita-Contreras F, Bueno-Notivol J, Martínez-Amat A, Cruz-Díaz D, Hernandez AV, Pérez-López FR. Effect of exercise alone or combined with dietary supplements on anthropometric and physical performance measures in community-dwelling elderly people with sarcopenic obesity: A meta-analysis of randomized controlled trials. Maturitas. 2018;**116**:24-35. DOI: 10.1016/j.maturitas.2018.07.007

[62] Chen HT, Chung YC, Chen YJ, Ho SY, Wu HJ. Effects of different types of exercise on body composition, muscle strength, and IGF-1 in the elderly with sarcopenic obesity. Journal of the American Geriatrics Society. 2017;**65**(4):827-832. DOI: 10.1111/jgs.14722

[63] Lin Y, Fan R, Hao Z, et al. The association between physical activity and insulin level under different levels of lipid indices and serum uric acid. Frontiers in Physiology. 2022;**13**:809669. Available from: https://www.frontiersin.org/articles/10.3389/fphys.2022.809669

[64] Powers SK, Deminice R, Ozdemir M, Yoshihara T, Bomkamp MP, Hyatt H. Exercise-induced oxidative stress: Friend or foe? Journal of Sport and Health Science. 2020;**9**(5):415-425. DOI: 10.1016/j.jshs.2020.04.001

[65] Trouwborst I, Verreijen A, Memelink R, et al. Exercise and nutrition strategies to counteract sarcopenic obesity. Nutrients. 2018;**10**(5):605. DOI: 10.3390/nu10050605

[66] Eglseer D, Traxler M, Schoufour JD, et al. Nutritional and exercise interventions in individuals with sarcopenic obesity around retirement age: A systematic review and meta-analysis. Nutrition Reviews. 2023;**81**(9):1077-1090. DOI: 10.1093/nutrit/nuad007

[67] Hershberger D, Bollinger L. Sarcopenic obesity: Background and exercise training strategies. Strength & Conditioning Journal. 2015;**37**:78-83. DOI: 10.1519/SSC.0000000000000170

[68] Mathus-Vliegen EM, Obes F. Prevalence, pathophysiology, health consequences and treatment options of obesity in the elderly: A guideline. Obesity Facts. 2012;**5**(3):460-483. DOI: 10.1159/000341193

[69] Sartorio A, Lafortuna CL, Agosti F, Proietti M, Maffiuletti NA. Elderly obese women display the greatest improvement in stair climbing performance after a 3-week body mass reduction program. International Journal of Obesity. 2004;**28**(9):1097-1104. DOI: 10.1038/sj.ijo.0802702

[70] Li Z, Heber D. Sarcopenic obesity in the elderly and strategies for weight management. Nutrition Reviews. 2012;**70**(1):57-64. DOI: 10.1111/j.1753-4887.2011.00453.x

[71] Cheah KJ, Cheah LJ. Benefits and side effects of protein supplementation and exercise in sarcopenic obesity: A scoping review. Nutrition Journal. 2023;**22**(1):52. DOI: 10.1186/s12937-023-00880-7

[72] Hou V, Madden K, Can GJ. Assessing the effects of dietary protein supplementation on sarcopenia in community-dwelling older adults. Canadian Geriatrics Journal. 2022;**25**(4):390-403. DOI: 10.5770/cgj.25.608

[73] Keeping the weight off. Nature Medicine. 2023;**29**(10):2377-2378. DOI: 10.1038/s41591-023-02614-y

[74] Zhang X, Zhao Y, Chen S, Shao H. Anti-diabetic drugs and sarcopenia: Emerging links, mechanistic insights, and clinical implications. Journal of Cachexia, Sarcopenia and Muscle. 2021;**12**(6):1368-1379. DOI: 10.1002/jcsm.12838

[75] Ren Q, Chen S, Chen X, et al. An effective glucagon-like peptide-1 receptor agonists, semaglutide, improves sarcopenic obesity in obese mice by modulating skeletal muscle metabolism. Drug Design, Development and Therapy. 2022;**16**:3723-3735. DOI: 10.2147/DDDT.S381546

[76] Xiang J, Qin L, Zhong J, Xia N, Liang Y. GLP-1RA liraglutide and semaglutide improves obesity-induced muscle atrophy via SIRT1 pathway. Diabetes, Metabolic Syndrome and Obesity. 2023;**16**:2433-2446. DOI: 10.2147/DMSO.S425642

[77] Mastino D, Robert M, Betry C, Laville M, Gouillat C, Disse E. Bariatric surgery outcomes in sarcopenic obesity. Obesity Surgery. 2016;**26**(10):2355-2362. DOI: 10.1007/s11695-016-2102-7

[78] Martínez MC, Meli EF, Candia FP, et al. The impact of bariatric surgery on the muscle mass in patients with obesity: 2-year follow-up. Obesity Surgery. 2022;**32**(3):625-633. DOI: 10.1007/s11695-021-05815-x

[79] Amaro Santos C, Cinza AM, Laranjeira Â, et al. The impact of exercise on prevention of sarcopenia after bariatric surgery: The study protocol of the EXPOBAR randomized controlled trial. Contemporary Clinical Trials Communications. 2023;**31**:101048. DOI: 10.1016/j.conctc.2022.101048

[80] Solomon ZJ, Mirabal JR, Mazur DJ, Kohn TP, Lipshultz LI, Pastuszak AW. Selective androgen receptor modulators: Current knowledge and clinical applications. Sexual Medicine Reviews. 2019;**7**(1):84-94. DOI: 10.1016/j.sxmr.2018.09.006

[81] Pilati I, Fau SA, Frost R, Frost R, Aging JF. Sarcopenic obesity and depression: A systematic review. The Journal of Frailty & Aging.

2022;**11**(1):51-58. DOI: 10.14283/jfa.2021.39

[82] Li Z, Tong X, Ma Y, Bao T, Yue J. Prevalence of depression in patients with sarcopenia and correlation between the two diseases: Systematic review and meta-analysis. Journal of Cachexia, Sarcopenia and Muscle. 2022;**13**(1):128-144. DOI: 10.1002/jcsm.12908

[83] Golder S, Medaglio D, O'Connor K, Hennessy S, Gross R, Gonzalez HG. Reasons for discontinuation or change of selective serotonin reuptake inhibitors in online drug reviews. JAMA Network Open. 2023;**6**(7):e2323746. DOI: 10.1001/jamanetworkopen.2023.23746

[84] Chu AWR. Selective Serotonin Reuptake Inhibitors. Treasure Island (FL): StatPearls Publishing; 2022. Available from: https://pubmed.ncbi.nlm.nih.gov/32119293/

[85] Malhi GS, Bell E, Morris G, Hamilton A. The delay in response to antidepressant therapy: A window of opportunity? Australian & New Zealand Journal of Psychiatry. 2020;**54**(2):127-129. DOI: 10.1177/0004867419900313

[86] Cuijpers Sijbrandij M, Koole SL, Andersson G, Beekman AT, Reynolds CF 3rd. Adding psychotherapy to antidepressant medication in depression and anxiety disorders: A meta-analysis. World Psychiatry. 2014;**13**:56-67. DOI: 10.1002/wps.20089

[87] Guidi J, Fava GA. Sequential combination of pharmacotherapy and psychotherapy in major depressive disorder. JAMA Psychiatry. 2021;**78**(3):261. DOI: 10.1001/jamapsychiatry.2020.3650

[88] Hay P, Chinn D, Forbes D, et al. Royal Australian and New Zealand College of psychiatrists clinical practice guidelines for the treatment of eating disorders. Australian & New Zealand Journal of Psychiatry. 2014;**48**(11):977-1008. DOI: 10.1177/0004867414555814

Section 3

Eating Disorders

Chapter 11

A Collaborative and Therapeutic Approach for Measuring the Correct Body Weight in People with Anorexia Nervosa

Marie Hehl, Gemma Peachey, Ivana Picek, Camilla Day, Georgia Faulkner, Alexandra Harvey, Janet Treasure and Hubertus Himmerich

Abstract

Diagnostic criteria for anorexia nervosa (AN) include significantly low body weight, fear of weight gain, and body image disturbance. Being severely underweight is associated with physical health risks, for example, electrolyte disturbances, epileptic seizures, cardiac arrhythmias, organ failure, and sudden death. It is also a perpetuating factor of AN. Therefore, the correct measurement of body weight is necessary for safe clinical management of AN. In clinical practice, there may be a requirement to attain a certain target weight before discharge from inpatient treatment or to prevent hospital admission. Schools, universities, and employers sometimes require a minimum body weight depending on the physical demands of the tasks at hand. Understandably, people with AN are therefore tempted to falsify their weight, for example, by water loading or using weights, to circumvent these restrictions and avoid disadvantages resulting from their mental health condition. In this chapter, we consider how to obtain an accurate assessment of body weight in the best possible collaborative, therapeutic, and motivating way.

Keywords: anorexia nervosa, body weight, weight falsification, therapeutic relationship, risk management

1. Introduction

According to the 5th edition of the Diagnostic and Statistical Manual of Mental Disorders (DSM-5), anorexia nervosa (AN) is an eating disorder characterized by a restricted energy intake and a significantly low body weight, an intense fear of gaining weight, and a disturbed body image. DSM-5 distinguishes two subtypes, the restrictive and the binge-purge type. The restrictive type is defined by excessive dieting and physical exercise, whereas the binge-purge type describes periods of binge eating followed by self-induced vomiting or the use of laxatives [1].

The 11th edition of the International Classifications of Diseases (ICD-11) specifies the criteria of significantly low body weight as a body mass index (BMI) <18.5 kg/m^2 [2].

DSM-5 and ICD-11 use the BMI to rate the severity of AN. According to DSM-5, a BMI below 15 kg/m^2 indicates extreme, a BMI between 15 and 15.99 kg/m^2 severe, a BMI between 16 and 16.99 kg/m^2 moderate, and a BMI above 17 kg/m^2 mild AN.

In ICD-11, a BMI below 14 kg/m^2 indicates dangerously low body weight and a BMI between 14 and 18 kg/m^2 indicates a significantly low body weight. A BMI higher than 18.5 kg/m^2 is normal. In children, a BMI under the fifth percentile indicates AN according to ICD-11.

Being seriously underweight can have various harmful effects on the body, for example, electrolyte disturbances, osteoporosis, bone fractures, hypothermia, epileptic seizures, weak immunity, or even cardiac arrest and sudden death. In addition, starvation due to AN can lead to psychiatric symptoms such as memory problems, decreased cognitive flexibility, depression, and anxiety [3, 4].

Treatment of AN involves weight gain to manage the health risks that are linked to starvation. Weight gain is key in supporting other psychological, physical, and quality of life changes that are needed for improvement or recovery [5].

Therefore, treatment includes regular weighing (usually weekly for outpatients and twice weekly for inpatients) to document the therapeutic process and risk management. Exposure to weight gain needs to be carefully managed as it is associated with high levels of anxiety. In individual cases, where weighing is unbearable for a patient because of an overvaluation of the number on the scale, a collaborative decision to weigh the patient without sharing the body weight with them might be considered.

For the transition from inpatient treatment to outpatient treatment, there are often weight requirements alongside therapeutic milestones that are desirable for such a transition, for example, a regular eating pattern and the ability to attend psychotherapeutic groups and individual therapy and maintaining or increasing weight while on leave from inpatients.

For this chapter, we reviewed the literature on weight falsification in AN and performed internet searches. However, as there is little evidence published about weight falsification in AN, we have formed a team of authors that consists of professional peer support workers with lived experience of AN and clinicians with experience in the treatment of AN to fill the gaps in the literature with personal experience. We have tried to make suggestions on how the measurement of weight can be performed correctly but at the same time in a collaborative and therapeutically meaningful way.

2. Challenges of measuring the correct body weight

As fear of weight gain is a core diagnostic criterium of AN [1, 2], the falsification of weight is a frequently associated problem. In total, 30–50% of people with AN reported weight falsification during therapeutic weigh-ins in a web-based survey [6]. However, the underlying motivation may vary.

2.1 The potentially undesirable consequences of the correct body weight

Depending on the treatment setting, the correct body weight might have negative consequences for people with AN. A significantly low body weight might lead to the clinical recommendation of inpatient admission. For the person with AN, this means restricted freedom and an inflexible therapy and activity schedule on an inpatient ward. Therefore, patients with AN who anticipate such a recommendation might try to change the displayed weight on the scale without real weight gain [7].

For inpatients, a reason to manipulate weight could be the desire to be discharged to gain more independence, to be reunited with their family, and to meet friends which might all not be possible during inpatient treatment.

The daily routine and the food intake are often very controlled for inpatients in an eating disorders ward. However, progress in therapy, which is reflected by weight gain, might prompt an increase in daily leave from the ward and more options for food choices and meals outside the ward. Weight loss, however, might result in leave restrictions and bigger portion sizes. Therefore, weight falsification is a comprehensible effort to regain control.

As AN comes with an intense fear of gaining weight [1, 2], patients with AN falsify their weight to appear as if they were gaining weight because they are so scared of a weight increase. Thus, the scale might indicate an increasing body weight, while they are losing weight or maintaining their current significantly low weight. Some patients set themselves a maximum body weight, that does not align with suggestions made by the therapists.

Despite knowing that they do not make progress during therapy, some patients do not want to disappoint their therapists and their family members.

Another reason could be that people want to normalize their life (e.g., go to university, keep their driver's license), for which a certain BMI is needed. A too-low BMI will not allow these "normal" things, as the risks included are too high.

2.2 Methods of weight falsification

The main methods of falsification are an increase in the body's water content, the consumption of food with very few calories, and attaching weight to the body [6–9]:

- Increasing the body's water content
    - Water loading: Drinking large amounts of water or other liquids.
    - Going to the toilet less often to retain feces or urine.
    - Consuming high amounts of salt to increase water retention.
- Consuming food with very few calories
    - Eating high-fiber, low-caloric food, for example., cucumbers, sauerkraut.
- Using weights
    - Wearing weights under sweaters or around ankles.
    - Stuffing coins/weights in pockets or underwear.
    - Sewing weights into the seams of clothing.

- Wearing heavy hair accessories or jewelry as well as adding weights in the hair/ponytail.
- Stuffing weights in their cheeks.
- Wearing padded clothing (bras, sweaters…).
- Internal weights: Putting weights inside the anus or vagina.

2.3 Consequences of weight falsification

The falsification of weight can have various consequences for the patient and their health. Drinking large amounts of water, for example, can decrease sodium plasma concentrations, which can lead to fatigue, other electrolyte disturbances or seizures, and cardiac arrhythmias [10]. Putting weights internally or swallowing them might harm the internal organs.

Other potential consequences can be an erroneously early discharge from services with the consequent risks to their health and life.

Furthermore, others could be at risk as a result, for example, if a person with a very low BMI drives a car while they are unwell. Due to dizziness, extreme fatigue, blurred vision, and poor concentration, they may cause a car accident [11].

Premature discharge from inpatient treatment might limit further improvement or trigger a relapse into AN. Patients who are too unwell to manage their AN in the community might get rejected by outpatient therapists and dietitians.

3. Measures to prevent weight falsification

3.1 Additional physical examinations

Therapeutic weighing of people with AN is a continuous process of systematic desensitization toward acceptance of a higher and healthier body weight. However, it is also part of medical risk management and an assessment of a person's strength or frailty. Additional physical examinations that can inform the management of undernourishment include:

- Mid-upper arm circumference measurement (MUAC): Measuring the circumference of the arm between the tip of the elbow and the shoulder on the upper arm.
- Grip strength: Static force measured by gripping a dynamometer as hard as possible.

Both parameters improve as nutritional intake improves and weight restores. Additional instrument-based examinations are the determination of starvation markers, such as the leukocyte count or thyroid hormones [12].

3.2 Specific methods of weight falsification and countermeasures

If the body weight of a person with AN seems implausible, the weigh-in should be repeated. This can be announced and unannounced which is often referred to as spot-weighing.

Table 1 provides an overview of methods of weight falsification and suggestions for possible countermeasures. However, some suggested approaches may not be appropriate for an individual patient as they might be perceived as too coercive. Examples of potentially inappropriately coercive measures are the use of metal detectors, patting a patient down, or letting them do jumping jacks. However, people with AN, like any other person, have an individual perception of shame, and the use of a metal detector might be less coercive for an individual patient than lifting their gowns.

3.3 Working collaboratively to prevent weight falsification

Transparency is a key aspect of communication around body weight. Clinicians should always maintain a therapeutic and supportive stance with the service user regarding their recovery and recognize that any weight falsification is a symptom attributable to the eating disorder. Direct questions should be asked with compassion, for example, "Many patients report that they have water loaded or tried to falsify their weight in any other way? Has this happened to you?"

The therapists should clarify the reasons for weight frailty-checking and should explain that the procedures are in place for every patient, out of concern for their well-being.

The expectation is that a gradual trajectory of change will be seen (occasional outliers can be ignored). Ongoing weight loss and weight falsification will have consequences, but the therapists and clinical staff will try to understand and support the patients with both.

Method of weight falsification	Measures to prevent it from happening
Water loading	• Limited access to water before weigh-ins. • Checking rooms for empty water bottles or weights. • Supervised toilet visits before weigh-in. • Blood drawing and measurement of sodium levels before or after weighing. • Mandatory toilet use before weigh-in. • Observing whether patients use the toilet shortly after weigh-in.
Consumption of salty foods	• Measurement of blood sodium levels.
Wearing weights and/or heavy clothing; hiding weights in hair or clothes	• Weighing in light gowns or underwear. • Shaking out the hair. • Letting the patient lift the gown to show that there are no weights hidden underneath. • Using metal detectors. • Patting down the patient.
Internal weights (e.g., anus, vagina, cheeks)	• Jumping jacks to dislodge any weights. • Checking the mouth.

The countermeasures should be explained to the service user and individually tailored to meet their needs and support therapy in the best way possible. Some measures are only feasible in an inpatient setting. Not all approaches are appropriate for all patients and might be perceived as too coercive. For further information, see [6, 10].

Table 1.
Methods of weight falsification and suggestions for possible countermeasures.

Communication goal	Examples	Rationale
Ask direct but compassionate questions before the weigh-in	• "Many patients have told me that they water loaded before being weighed. Have you water loaded today?" • "We know that the AN urges people to falsify their weight. Have you attempted weight falsification before this weigh-in?"	Encourage honesty, giving the option of talking about the weight falsifying.
Being transparent	• "We are noticing some ups and downs in your weight over the last few weigh-ins. I am concerned that some of the weights we are seeing may not be real. Is there anything that you would like to talk about regarding this?"	Giving the service user clarity and preparing them for what will come up, thus helping them to feel prepared and more comfortable and less overwhelmed.
Showing compassion	• "This must be really hard for you." • "You might feel very (emotion) right now and that's okay."	Making the patient feel heard and cared for. Improves communication between service users and staff.
Reassuring and comforting the service user	• "I know how hard this is for you, but I am here to help and if we do not know your real weight, it is not safe as we cannot accurately assess the risks to your physical safety." • "These are routine measures that we use for everyone." • "I am here to support you."	Reassuring the service user that the team is always here to support them and that they are not singled out for special treatment.

Table 2.
Questions and phrases to improve the communication regarding body weight and its measurement to prevent weight falsification.

Overall, it is important to be as transparent and reassuring as possible, to make the experience as minimally stressful as possible. A strong therapeutic relationship can help the service user to feel more comfortable, decreasing the need for them to falsify their weight, or be more open about this. **Table 2** provides examples of useful questions and phrases.

4. Conclusions and future perspectives

Even though weight falsification is a frequent clinical problem in the treatment of AN, little research has been done so far. Our chapter is only a first step which has been based on the scarce literature, and the experience and opinion of ED specialists and service user representatives. However, standardized approach to measure weight falsification and generally accepted methods to prevent weight falsification from happening are not available. Current treatment guidelines do not address this issue, even though some hospitals have local policies in place. Thus, research on weight falsification, its consequences and prevention is needed. It should take place in different settings, for example, outpatients, day care, and inpatients. Being weighed and seeing numbers on the scales can be a highly stressful and emotional experience for patients struggling with eating disorders, therefore it is highly important that empathy and compassion are at the forefront of further research and strategies to support service users in this area. A more open approach to encouraging discussion in this area would be appreciated. As weighing should become a collaborative process, methods to improve trust and the therapeutic relationship should be developed with the involvement of service users, their carers, and ED professionals.

Measuring the correct body weight might not only improve the assessment of physical health consequences of AN but could also lead to a better understanding of the emotional needs of people with EDs. For example, a recently published study has found that a higher BMI was associated with more severe ED psychopathology, more depressive symptoms, anxiety sensitivity, experiential avoidance, and lower mindfulness in patients across the whole spectrum of restrictive, binge-purge, and atypical AN [13]. Furthermore, recent research indicates that body weight at the start of inpatient treatment as well as weight gain kinetics during inpatient therapy for AN might help to predict treatment outcomes, improve clinical decision-making, and manage expectations of patients and clinicians [14]. Thus, a collaborative and more accurate way of measuring body weight might improve the clinical formulation and the decision-making process and lead to better treatment success and a more pleasant treatment experience in people with AN.

Acknowledgements

The authors would like to thank service users and staff members of the inpatient, day care, and enhanced treatment team ED services at the South London and Maudsley NHS Foundation Trust (SLaM), London. They would also like to thank their colleagues at the South London Partnership (SLP) for their helpful input and insights.

Conflict of interest

The authors declare no conflict of interest.

Author details

Marie Hehl[1], Gemma Peachey[2], Ivana Picek[2], Camilla Day[2], Georgia Faulkner[2], Alexandra Harvey[2], Janet Treasure[1,2] and Hubertus Himmerich[1,2]*

1 Department of Psychological Medicine, Institute of Psychiatry, Psychology and Neuroscience, Centre for Research in Eating and Weight Disorders (CREW), King's College London, London, UK

2 South London and Maudsley NHS Foundation Trust, London, UK

*Address all correspondence to: hubertus.himmerich@kcl.ac.uk

References

[1] American Psychiatric Association. Diagnostic and Statistical Manual of Mental Disorders. 5th ed. Arlington, VA, USA: APA Publishing; 2013

[2] World Health Organization. International Statistical Classification of Diseases and Related Health Problems. 11th ed. Geneva, Switzerland: World Health Organization; 2019. Available from: https://icd.who.int/

[3] Meczekalski B, Podfigurna-Stopa A, Katulski K. Long-term consequences of anorexia nervosa. Maturitas. 2013;**75**:215-220. DOI: 10.1016/j.maturitas.2013.04.014

[4] Treasure J, Duarte TA, Schmidt U. Eating disorders. Lancet. 2020;**395**:899-911. DOI: 10.1016/S0140-6736(20)30059-3

[5] National Institute for Health and Care Excellence (NICE). Eating Disorders: Recognition and Treatment. Manchester, UK: NICE; 2020. Available from: https://www.nice.org.uk/guidance/ng69

[6] Jaffa T, Davies S, Sardesai A. What patients with anorexia nervosa should wear when they are being weighed: Report of two pilot surveys. European Eating Disorders Review. 2011;**19**:368-370. DOI: 10.1002/erv.1093

[7] O'Regan E. Anorexic Patients 'sabotage weigh-ins' to Falsely Elevate What Is Shown on the Scales. Dublin, Ireland: Irish Independent; 2018. Available from: https://www.independent.ie/irish-news/anorexic-patients-sabotage-weigh-ins-to-falsely-elevate-what-is-shown-on-the-scales/37314966.html

[8] Quora. How Do I Fake Weight Gain before a Weigh-in if you Are Anorexic? Quora, Available from: https://www.quora.com/How-do-I-fake-weight-gain-before-a-weigh-in-if-you-are-anorexic [Accessed: April 24, 2024]

[9] ED Support Forum. Falsifying Weight. ED Support Forum, Available from: https://www.edsupportforum.com/threads/falsifying-weight.4160969/ [Accessed: April 24, 2024]

[10] Oden Akman A, Cak HT, Pehlivantürk-Kızılkan M, Balik Z, Akbulut O, Kanbur N. Sounds unrealistic: An adolescent girl with anorexia nervosa consumes 19 L of fluid in a few hours: What happens to the physiology? Eating and Weight Disorders. 2020;**25**:1487-1492. DOI: 10.1007/s40519-019-00777-7

[11] Shaw N, Duffield C. Surprising Health Conditions you Must Declare to DVLA from Diabetes to déjà vu. London, UK: Mirror Online; 2024

[12] Himmerich H, Treasure J. Anorexia nervosa: Diagnostic, therapeutic, and risk biomarkers in clinical practice. Trends in Molecular Medicine. 2024;**30**(4):350-360. DOI: 10.1016/j.molmed.2024.01.002

[13] Wong VZ, Lowe MR. Is there a basis for a weight cut-off point? A large-scale investigation of atypical anorexia and anorexia nervosa subtypes among patients at a residential treatment Centre. European Eating Disorders Review. 2024. DOI: 10.1002/erv.3077

[14] Di Lodovico L, Al Tabchi A, Clarke J, Mancusi RL, Messeca D, Duriez P, et al. Trajectories and predictive factors of weight recovery in patients with anorexia nervosa completing treatment. A latent class mixed model approach. European Eating Disorders Review. 2024. DOI: 10.1002/erv.3088

Chapter 12

Psychoeducation on Medication for People with Anorexia Nervosa: A Quality Improvement Project

Jessica McMahon, Ines Green, Titilope Omitogun, Ivana Picek, Gemma Peachey, Camilla Day, Janet Treasure and Hubertus Himmerich

Abstract

Whilst no medication has yet been approved for the treatment of anorexia nervosa (AN), clinicians often prescribe psychopharmacological and physical health medication to help with low mood, anxiety, obsessive-compulsive symptoms, sleep problems and pain. However, shared decision-making (SDM) requires an informed patient who feels confident to make the decision on their medication together with the medical doctor. We have therefore designed an intervention that consisted of a leaflet and two seminars, one on psychopharmacological agents and one on physical health medication, and we have measured the patients' own perception of their knowledge about medication before and after this intervention. A total of 11 patients with AN, 10 females and one gender-fluid person between 19 and 37 years of age who were currently treated in our inpatient or daycare service, agreed to participate in the quality improvement project. After the intervention, patients felt significantly better informed in four different domains: medications for eating disorders, mental health and physical health medication, and pro re nata (PRN) medication. The latter is medication that is given as required. Thus, a psychoeducational activity consisting of written information and seminars seems feasible to improve knowledge and SDM in people with AN. However, the small sample size limits the generalizability of our findings.

Keywords: eating disorder, anorexia nervosa, psychoeducation, medication, psychopharmacology

1. Introduction

1.1 Anorexia nervosa

Anorexia nervosa (AN) is a serious psychiatric disorder that can be associated with poor outcomes. The diagnostic criteria of the condition are characterized by the drive to achieve and maintain a low body mass index (BMI), an intense fear of weight gain and body image disturbance [1]. AN can take a chronic course and has a high mortality rate. Therefore, the standard mortality rate is ~5.9 [2] which is the highest mortality rate within psychiatric conditions. The high risk of dying is not only caused by the acute physical risks associated with AN but also due to the increased risk of suicide which is prevalent within this patient population [3, 4]. The lifetime risk for the development of AN is up to 4% in females and 0.3% in males with the peak incidence occurring within teenage years on average, aged 15.5 years old [5–7]. The course of AN can often be chronic with only 46% of patients managing to fully recover from the disorder and 20% of sufferers remaining chronically ill [3, 4]. The chronic course of the disorder compounds the significant impairment of the individual's physical health and psychosocial functionality [8]. The high mortality rate and significant debility caused by AN propagates the urgent need to optimize and explore psychopharmacological treatment options to improve both recovery rates and quality of life for current sufferers.

1.2 Psychopharmacological treatment for anorexia nervosa

Whilst psychopharmacological treatment options for other serious psychiatric conditions expanded exponentially through the 1950's with the development of new antipsychotics and antidepressants, the application of these medications within patients meeting the diagnostic criteria for AN was not successful [9]. At present, there is no medication approved to treat AN [3, 10] despite the correlation and overlap of symptoms with many other psychiatric diagnoses, namely, low mood, anxiety, and disrupted sleep [11].

The intense fear of weight gain, characteristic of the disorder, can often serve as a barrier to patients participating in trials of medication, where weight gain is a potential or known side effect. This barrier is both problematic for randomized controlled trials [RCTs] recruitment and for ongoing management by eating disorder teams [12]. Not only do some medications confront the fear of weight gain but other side effects such as metabolic changes, cardiac issues, sedation, and bone marrow suppression also may cause reluctance to commence such medication, without effective counseling of the risks presented. Even though medication has become an accepted means of self-management in many Western societies, patients with AN often see the refusal of recommended medication as a personally meaningful practice to resist their treatment [13].

The ambivalence of patients to engage in psychopharmacological treatment contributes to the lack of RCTs currently available in AN. The few published RCTs often have a small size [14], and the RCTs which have been published show only modest remission rates at the end of treatment varying between 13 and 43% [15]. The lack of RCTs with substantial sample sizes and with significant evidence of the benefits of psychotropic medications poses significant challenges to the medical management of this patient group.

Whilst there is no approved psychopharmacological treatment of AN, many medications are used by clinicians off-label to help improve specific symptoms patients may struggle with.

1.3 The patient's perspective

Self-starvation is a mechanism that serves people with AN to cope with difficulties such as acute stress, anxiety, and low mood. Within patients with acute AN, studies have demonstrated a positive correlation between low body weight and fewer emotional regulation difficulties, establishing that the maladaptive mechanism of caloric restriction is of benefit to the patient in managing aversive emotions [16]. Aiming at weight restoration could therefore be interpreted as a threat to the individual, forcing them to re-experience the underlying mood difficulties, whereas maintaining a low BMI mitigates experiencing their low mood; this mechanism impacts their motivation for recovery [17]. Thus, if the underlying psychological problem of low mood or anxiety could be treated, there would be a chance to mitigate the overall resistance to weight restoration.

Medication compliance and interest in commencing medication from a patient's perspective would be more acceptable if focused on emotional dysregulation as opposed to weight gain, due to the fears this elicits. Thus, psychological improvement of patients with AN should be pursued and interpreted as a separate important outcome measure independent of weight restoration [18]. Psychological improvement can be a tool to aid future recovery and reduce functional impairment.

With effective medication counseling and empowering patients' autonomy over their condition and treatment, medication compliance and psychological improvement could be seen.

1.4 Aim of the study

As explained above, no psychopharmacological medication has been approved for use in people with AN. Nonetheless, people with AN are prescribed various medications for off-label use. Off-label use, however, requires a shared decision based on sufficient information that should be given to the patients.

This study was designed to provide psychoeducation to people with AN on the use of medication to help with the AN and associated physical and mental health consequences. We hypothesized that patients would feel better informed about both physical health medication and psychotropic medications that may be used as part of the treatment of their eating disorder.

The intervention was added to treatment as usual (TAU). In our eating disorders service, TAU includes psychological therapy (Cognitive Remediation Therapy (CRT), Cognitive Remediation and Emotional Skills Training (CREST), Maudsley Model of Anorexia Nervosa Treatment for Adults (MANTRA), Cognitive Behavioral Therapy (CBT), Motivational Enhancement Therapy (MET), dietary advice, physical health monitoring, nursing and occupational therapy. A questionnaire was created to determine current knowledge of both physical health medications and psychopharmacological medications and how well-informed patients with AN felt about making decisions regarding medication they have been or may currently be prescribed. Following the collation of these data, two workshops were conducted to provide education on both physical health medications and psychopharmacological medications in relation to eating disorders. A leaflet with supplementary and supporting information was given to patients as a learning aid including the pharmacokinetics, pharmacodynamics of commonly prescribed physical health and psychotropic medications. The efficacy of these workshops was later assessed, and this information was collated to determine how useful these sessions and the leaflet were to the participants. Within this publication, we present the statistical analysis of the survey.

2. Methods

2.1 Patient sample

The psychoeducation was offered to all patients on the inpatient eating disorder unit and eating disorder day services within the South London and Maudsley NHS Foundation Trust. Thus, all the patients who were admitted to inpatients or day services were eligible to participate in the study. Our unit is specialized in the treatment of people with AN. No patients were excluded based on physical health conditions. No payments were made to participants included in the study.

A total of 11 patients with AN, according to the ICD-10 criteria, 10 females and one gender-fluid person, agreed to participate in the quality improvement (QI) project. Patients were between 19 and 37 years of age. The mean age (±standard deviation) was 27 (±6) years. Nine patients were treated in the South London and Maudsley NHS Foundation Trust eating disorders day service and two on the inpatient unit. The duration of current treatment in the named service ranged between 1 month and 9 months; the mean duration of treatment was 4.4 (±3.0) months. The duration of their AN was between 3 years and 28 years with a mean of 12 (±7.3) years.

The main psychiatric comorbidities were depressive disorder (46%), anxiety disorders (36%) and obsessive-compulsive disorder (18%). Some patients currently took or had regularly taken the antidepressants fluoxetine (18%), sertraline (36%), citalopram (9%), mirtazapine (9%) or venlafaxine (9%), the atypical antipsychotics olanzapine (36%) or quetiapine (18%), the anxiolytics diazepam (9%) or promethazine (18%), or melatonin as sleep aid (9%).

2.2 Questionnaires

The QI project team which consisted of patients and clinicians from the eating disorders inpatient ward and day service unit within the South London and Maudsley NHS Foundation Trust (SLaM) developed a questionnaire to measure the effectiveness of the psychoeducational intervention.

The questionnaire had four main sections. The first section provided personal information about the patient and their experience with prescribed medication, current or historical, relating to their eating disorder and general mental health. The second and third sections use a series of 4-point Likert scale questions, ranging from 0 to 4 (0 = strongly disagree, 2 = neutral, and 4 = strongly agree). The second and third sections focused on how well-informed patients feel about making decisions relating to medication before and after the workshop and leaflet being distributed, respectively. These questions had four domains: Medication for eating disorders, medication for other mental health disorders, pro-re-nata (PRN) medication, which means medication as required, and medications for physical health consequences.

The fourth section evaluated how helpful the participants found both the workshop and leaflet. The questionnaires were completed by 11 patients with AN between June and July 2023. The patient questionnaire used is depicted in the appendix of this article.

2.3 Workshops and leaflet

There were two separate workshops. One focused on physical health medications patients may have come across in the treatment of their eating disorder, and the other focused on psychopharmacological medication. A leaflet was also co-designed by patients and clinicians to provide concise information on pharmacokinetics and pharmacodynamics, physical health medication and psychopharmacological medication. Drawings, created by patients, were incorporated into the materials. The leaflet can be provided upon request to the corresponding author.

2.4 Data evaluation and statistics

The data collected were entered into an excel spreadsheet and fed into IBM SPSS Statistics Version 29. The differences between baseline and after the interventions were calculated using t-tests.

2.5 Ethical approval

The study was approved as a QI project by the QI committee of the South London and Maudsley NHS Foundation Trust in May 2023.

3. Results

3.1 Facilitation and acceptance

All (100%) QI project participants reported that they attended both workshops, the workshop on psychopharmacological medication and the workshop on physical health medication. All (100%) answered that they had been given written information on medications for physical health related to eating disorders. However, only 91% answered that they had been given the information on medications for eating disorders and on other mental health conditions. About 64% confirmed they had received written information on PRN medications for mental health, and 73% agreed they had received leaflet information on medications for physical health related to eating disorders.

3.2 Quantitative results

QI project participants rated their opinion regarding how well-informed they felt about making decisions on medication for eating disorders using a questionnaire that contained 47 questions. Questions 11 to 22 measured the feeling about being informed before the intervention on a 4-point Likert scale with values between 0 and 4, and questions 23 to 34 were corresponding questions which were asked after the intervention. **Table 1** depicts the mean scores ± standard deviations and the two-sided p-value of a t-test.

The patients who took part in the project felt significantly better informed about medications to make decisions for their own treatment. This applied to all questions asked in the four domains: Medication for eating disorders, medication for other mental health disorders, PRN medication and medications for physical health consequences.

Domain	Survey question before and after the intervention: I feel I have enough information ...	Mean ± SD before	Mean ± SD after	p-value
Medication for eating disorders	Regarding the intended effects of regular medications specifically for eating disorders.	1.6 ± 0.9	3.4 ± 0.5	< 0.001
	Regarding the side effects of regular medications specifically for eating disorders.	1.5 ± 1.0	3.4 ± 0.7	< 0.001
	To make decisions about medications specifically for eating disorders.	1.1 ± 0.8	3.4 ± 0.5	< 0.001
Medication for other mental health disorders	Regarding the intended effects of regular medications for other mental health conditions.	2.0 ± 1.1	3.3 ± 0.6	0.014
	Regarding the side effects of regular medications for other mental health conditions.	2.0 ± 1.1	3.0 ± 0.6	0.033
	To make decisions about regular medications for other mental health conditions.	1.9 ± 0.9	3.1 ± 0.5	0.007
PRN medication	Regarding the intended effects of PRN medications for mental health	1.6 ± 1.3	3.2 ± 0.8	0.009
	Regarding the side effects of PRN medications for mental health	1.5 ± 1.2	2.8 ± 0.8	0.026
	To make decisions about PRN medications for mental health	1.5 ± 1.2	2.9 ± 0.0	0.017
Medication for physical health consequences	Regarding the intended effects of medications for physical health related to eating disorders	2.1 ± 1.4	3.7 ± 0.5	0.004
	Regarding the side effects of medications for physical health related to eating disorders	2.1 ± 1.3	3.5 ± 0.7	0.013
	To make decisions about medications for physical health related to eating disorders	2.1 ± 1.2	3.5 ± 0.5	0.006

Abbreviations: Standard deviation (SD), pro-re-nata (PRN) medication.

Table 1.
Mean scores ± standard deviations before and after the intervention, and the 2-sided p-value of a t-test of corresponding questions measuring the feeling about being informed of all n = 11 study participants.

3.3 Qualitative results

In the free text, patients wrote that they want to be informed about how and where to bring up being prescribed the medication, when the medication should be reviewed and how to come off the medication. They also wanted to learn more about the statistics of effectiveness in patients. One patient wished to have more information on PRN medication for mental health during the workshops. While thanking the study team and the facilitators, one patient wrote "Thank you! It's not something that's relevant right now but was useful to think about past medication and hear about future research".

4. Discussion

4.1 Summary and interpretation of the results

In the reported QI project, we facilitated psychoeducational activity for people with AN in intensive care settings (inpatient and day service) to provide information on the use of medication to help with eating disorders. The psychoeducation consisted of three elements:

- A co-designed leaflet for people with eating disorders with information about psychopharmacological and physical health medication with a focus on eating disorders, their comorbidities and health consequences.
- An interactive seminar on psychopharmacological medications.
- An interactive seminar on medication for physical health medications.

The 11 patients who took part in the project felt significantly better informed about medications to make decisions for their own treatment. Thus, we achieved the aim of this intervention which therefore seems feasible to be tested in a larger group of patients.

However, areas that patients felt should have been covered better in the workshops and on the leaflets were as follows:

- How to approach clinicians to talk about medications and discuss prescriptions?
- When medications should be reviewed?
- How to come off medications?
- What makes a medication deemed effective in terms of the underlying statistics?
- PRN medication for mental health.

After the facilitation of the two workshops and handing out the leaflet on medication to help with eating disorders, patients felt significantly better informed about medications for eating disorders, psychopharmacological medication in general, PRN medication and medication for physical health conditions. They felt particularly better informed to make decisions about medication. This was the primary goal of our intervention. To make the best possible decision, a patient should be well informed about the realistic benefits and risks about medication to make the decision together with the clinician based on their own preferences and values, because this approach has been shown to be associated with higher adherence to and satisfaction with the treatment [19–22].

So far, no medication has been approved for the treatment of AN. However, the severity of the ED often requires supportive psychopharmacological treatment. The best possible recommendation for AN is olanzapine as there is strong evidence to suggest that it is an effective intervention for weight recovery. Despite this, effects on psychopathology are not clear. Weight gain was the primary outcome of most published studies. Therefore, olanzapine has not yet been authorized for use in eating disorders. Other medications that have been tested for AN include antiepileptics and mood stabilizers (e.g., lithium) and appetite stimulants (e.g., dronabinol), but the evidence for these medications is limited [23].

With the off-label use of these medications, a shared decision should be reached between patients and healthcare professionals about whether the medication is to be used to support treatment of their eating disorder. Patients require sufficient information about such medications before they can make an informed decision about whether they want to take the medication or not [24]. This QI project has demonstrated that, with psychoeducational activity, patients felt better informed to make decisions about medication.

There is a high percentage of co-morbid anxiety disorders within our sample which from our experience is representative of the wider eating disorder population. We hypothesize that co-morbid anxiety symptoms (presenting in different forms) often perpetuate inability to weight restore due to food restriction being a pathological safety behavior that reduces anxiety in general. Anxiolytic medications that reduce levels of felt anxiety but do not eradicate it could help patients to expose themselves to food intake and learn that food intake and weight restoration are not real threats to them (as in exposure therapy). Put in another way, anxiolytic medication could help food feel less scary, so one is willing to expose oneself to it and learn that you do not need to be scared.

4.2 Limitations

The reported psychoeducational QI project had only a small sample size of 11 patients. Thus, the statistical significance must be interpreted with caution. The patients who took part in the project were potentially more enthusiastic and motivated than patients who did not take part. We did not keep a record of patients who declined to come to the seminars and their reasons for this. Even though the information leaflet was co-designed with patients with AN and approved by the multidisciplinary ED team at the South London and Maudsley NHS Foundation Trust, it was not independently peer reviewed. Another limitation is that we did not assess the eating disorder psychopathology in a standardized way before and after the intervention.

4.3 Future directions

Our psychoeducational QI project mainly conveyed information on medication, pharmacodynamics, pharmacokinetics, pharmacological mechanisms and principles, efficacy, and side effects. Monitoring aspects and terminating pharmacological treatment were not covered extensively or comprehensively as the written feedback from patients revealed. Another area for improvement is the relational aspect of psychopharmacology, for example, when and how a patient with an ED should approach their clinician. In contrast to psychotherapy, there is not much research about the relationship between the prescriber and the patient in EDs available. From a practical experience, we are aware that a medication can remind the patient of the prescriber and is therefore a relational symbol, as such, it should be a source of productive cooperation, motivation, and mutual trust.

Acknowledgements

The authors would like to thank service users and staff members of the inpatient, day care and enhanced treatment team of the South London and Maudsley NHS Foundation Trust (SLaM), London, and the South London Partnership for their helpful input and insights.

Conflicts of interest

The authors declare no conflicts of interest.

A. Questionnaire

Quality Improvement Project – Shared decision-making regarding medications in treatment for eating disorders.

This questionnaire has been created to help improve shared decision-making around the use of medications in eating disorders as part of a quality improvement project. Please answer the questions according to your experience. Thank you for your participation.

To be completed BEFORE the leaflet has been distributed/the workshops have been facilitated:

Personal information.

1. My age.

2. My gender.

3. My current treatment: I am currently treated in the following service (e.g. FREED, Outpatients, Day Services, Inpatients):

   ____

4. Duration of my current treatment in the above-named service:

   ____

5. Diagnosis:

   ____

6. Duration of illness:

   ____

Are you currently taking/have you previously taken prescribed medication relating to eating disorder? Please specify which.

7. Regular medications specifically for eating disorders (e.g. for managing eating disorder thoughts or behaviors)

   ____

8. Regular medications for other mental health conditions (e.g. for managing mood, anxiety, OCD, etc.)

____

9. PRN (as and required) medications for mental health (e.g. sleep, acute anxiety)

____

10. For physical health associated with eating disorders (e.g. electrolyte supplements, vitamin supplements, constipation)

____

Opinion about how well-informed you feel about making decisions regarding medication for eating disorders

Strongly disagree Neutral Strongly agree

0 1 2 3 4

11. I feel I have enough information regarding the intended effects of regular medications specifically for eating disorders.

    0 1 2 3 4

12. I feel I have enough information regarding the side effects of regular medications specifically for eating disorders.

    0 1 2 3 4

13. I feel I have enough information to make decisions about medications specifically for eating disorders.

    0 1 2 3 4

14. I feel I have enough information regarding the intended effects of regular medications for other mental health conditions.

    0 1 2 3 4

15. I feel I have enough information regarding the side effects of regular medications for other mental health conditions.

    0 1 2 3 4

16. I feel I have enough information to make decisions about regular medications for other mental health conditions.

    0 1 2 3 4

17. I feel I have enough information regarding the intended effects of PRN medications for mental health.

    0 1 2 3 4

DOI: http://dx.doi.org/10.5772/intechopen.1006307

18. I feel I have enough information regarding the side effects of medications for PRN medications for mental health.

    0 1 2 3 4

19. I feel I have enough information to make decisions about medications for PRN medications for mental health.

    0 1 2 3 4

20. I feel I have enough information regarding the intended effects of medications for physical health related to eating disorders.

    0 1 2 3 4

21. I feel I have enough information regarding the side effects of medications for physical health related to eating disorders.

    0 1 2 3 4

22. I feel I have enough information to make decisions about medications for physical health related to eating disorders.

    0 1 2 3 4

To be completed AFTER the leaflet has been distributed/the workshop have been facilitated:
Opinion about how well-informed you feel about making decisions regarding medication for eating disorders
Strongly disagree Neutral Strongly agree
0 1 2 3 4

23. I feel I have enough information regarding the intended effects of regular medications specifically for eating disorders.

    0 1 2 3 4

24. I feel I have enough information regarding the side effects of regular medications specifically for eating disorders.

    0 1 2 3 4

25. I feel I have enough information to make decisions about medications specifically for eating disorders.

    0 1 2 3 4

26. I feel I have enough information regarding the intended effects of regular medications for other mental health conditions.

    0 1 2 3 4

27. I feel I have enough information regarding the side effects of regular medications for other mental health conditions.

0 1 2 3 4

28. I feel I have enough information to make decisions about regular medications for other mental health conditions.

0 1 2 3 4

29. I feel I have enough information regarding the intended effects of PRN medications for mental health.

0 1 2 3 4

30. I feel I have enough information regarding the side effects of medications for PRN medications for mental health.

0 1 2 3 4

31. I feel I have enough information to make decisions about medications for PRN medications for mental health.

0 1 2 3 4

32. I feel I have enough information regarding the intended effects of medications for physical health related to eating disorders.

0 1 2 3 4

33. I feel I have enough information regarding the side effects of medications for physical health related to eating disorders.

0 1 2 3 4

34. I feel I have enough information to make decisions about medications for physical health related to eating disorders.

0 1 2 3 4

Have you been given any information leaflets for:

35. Regular medication specifically for eating disorders?

Yes/no

36. If yes, how helpful is the leaflet?

Not helpful at all Somewhat helpful Very helpful

0 1 2 3 4

37. Regular medication for medications for other mental health conditions?

Yes/no

38. If yes, how helpful is the leaflet?

    Not helpful at all Somewhat helpful Very helpful

    0 1 2 3 4

39. PRN medications for mental health?

    Yes/no

40. If yes, how helpful is the leaflet?

    Not helpful at all Somewhat helpful Very helpful

    0 1 2 3 4

41. Medications for physical health related to eating disorders?

    Yes/no

42. If yes, how helpful is the leaflet?

    Not helpful at all Somewhat helpful Very helpful

    0 1 2 3 4

Have you attended the workshop for:

43. Medications for eating disorders and mental health conditions?

    Yes/no

44. If yes, how helpful is the workshop?

45. Medications for physical health problems related to eating disorders?

    Yes/no

46. If yes, how helpful is the workshop?

Any other suggestions/comments:

47. Is there anything else you feel would help you feel more informed to make decisions about medications? Or any other comments?

    ____

    ____

    ____

I agree that my data are used for service improvement and research. I am aware that my participation is voluntary and that my data will be anonymized and used for research purposes and service evaluation.
Signature or initials:

____

Thank you very much for your participation.

Author details

Jessica McMahon[1], Ines Green[1], Titilope Omitogun[1], Ivana Picek[1], Gemma Peachey[1], Camilla Day[2], Janet Treasure[1,2] and Hubertus Himmerich[1,2*]

1 South London and Maudsley NHS Foundation Trust, London, UK

2 Department of Psychological Medicine, Centre for Research in Eating and Weight Disorders (CREW), Institute of Psychiatry, Psychology and Neuroscience, King's College London, London, UK

*Address all correspondence to: hubertus.himmerich@kcl.ac.uk

References

[1] American Psychiatric Association. Diagnostic and Statistical Manual of Mental Disorders. 5th ed. Washington DC: APA Publishing; 2013

[2] Steinhausen HC. The outcome of anorexia nervosa in the 20th century. The American Journal of Psychiatry. 2002;**159**:1284-1293. DOI: 10.1176/appi.ajp.159.8.1284

[3] Cassioli E, Sensi C, Mannucci E, Ricca V, Rotella F. Pharmacological treatment of acute-phase anorexia nervosa: Evidence from randomized controlled trials. Journal of Psychopharmacology. 2020;**34**:864-873. DOI: 10.1177/0269881120920453

[4] Arcelus J, Mitchell AJ, Wales J, Nielsen S. Mortality rates in patients with anorexia nervosa and other eating disorders. A meta-analysis of 36 studies. Archives of General Psychiatry. 2011;**68**:724-731. DOI: 10.1001/archgenpsychiatry.2011.74

[5] van Eeden AE, van Hoeken D, Hoek HW. Incidence, prevalence and mortality of anorexia nervosa and bulimia nervosa. Current Opinion in Psychiatry. 2021;**34**:515-524. DOI: 10.1097/YCO.0000000000000739

[6] Momen NC, Petersen JD, Yilmaz Z, Semark BD, Petersen LV. Inpatient admissions and mortality of anorexia nervosa patients according to their preceding psychiatric and somatic diagnoses. Acta Psychiatrica Scandinavica. 2024;**149**(5):404-414. DOI: 10.1111/acps.13676

[7] Hebebrand J, Gradl-Dietsch G, Peters T, Correll CU, Haas V. The diagnosis and treatment of anorexia nervosa in childhood and adolescence. Deutsches Ärzteblatt International. 2024;**121**(5):164-174. DOI: 10.3238/arztebl.m2023.0248

[8] Zeeck A, Herpertz-Dahlmann B, Friederich HC, Brockmeyer T, Resmark G, Hagenah U, et al. Psychotherapeutic treatment for anorexia nervosa: A systematic review and network meta-analysis. Frontiers in Psychiatry. 2018;**9**:158. DOI: 10.3389/fpsyt.2018.00158

[9] Ten TJ. Years which changed psychiatry. In: Healy D, editor. The Psychopharmacologists. London: Arnold; 2000. pp. 543-559

[10] Himmerich H, Treasure J. Psychopharmacological advances in eating disorders. Expert Review of Clinical Pharmacology. 2018;**11**:95-108. DOI: 10.1080/17512433.2018.1383895

[11] Marucci S, Ragione LD, De Iaco G, Mococci T, Vicini M, Guastamacchia E, et al. Anorexia nervosa and comorbid psychopathology. Endocrine, Metabolic & Immune Disorders Drug Targets. 2018;**18**:316-324. DOI: 10.2174/1871530318666180213111637

[12] Miniati M, Mauri M, Ciberti A, Mariani MG, Marazziti D, Dell'Osso L. Psychopharmacological options for adult patients with anorexia nervosa. CNS Spectrums. 2016;**21**:134-142. DOI: 10.1017/S1092852914000790

[13] Lester R. Health as moral failing: Medication restriction among women with eating disorders. Anthropology & Medicine. 2014;**21**:241-250. DOI: 10.1080/13648470.2014.927824

[14] van den Berg E, Houtzager L, de Vos J, Daemen I, Katsaragaki G, Karyotaki E, et al. Meta-analysis on the

efficacy of psychological treatments for anorexia nervosa. European Eating Disorders Review. 2019;**27**:331-351. DOI: 10.1002/erv.2683

[15] Brockmeyer T, Friederich HC, Schmidt U. Advances in the treatment of anorexia nervosa: A review of established and emerging interventions. Psychological Medicine. 2018;**48**:1228-1256. DOI: 10.1017/S0033291717002604

[16] Brockmeyer T, Holtforth MG, Bents H, Kämmerer A, Herzog W, Friederich HC. Starvation and emotion regulation in anorexia nervosa. Comprehensive Psychiatry. 2012;**53**:496-501. DOI: 10.1016/j.comppsych.2011.09.003

[17] Pemberton K, Fox JR. The experience and management of emotions on an inpatient setting for people with anorexia nervosa: A qualitative study. Clinical Psychology & Psychotherapy. 2013;**20**:226-238. DOI: 10.1002/cpp.794

[18] Murray SB, Loeb KL, Le Grange D. Treatment outcome reporting in anorexia nervosa: Time for a paradigm shift? Journal of Eating Disorders. 2018; **6**:10. DOI: 10.1186/s40337-018-0195-1

[19] Lin GA, Fagerlin A. Shared decision making: State of the science. Circulation. Cardiovascular Quality and Outcomes. 2014;**7**:328-334. DOI: 10.1161/CIRCOUTCOMES.113.000322

[20] Stacey D, Légaré F, Col NF, Bennett CL, Barry MJ, Eden KB, et al. Decision aids for people facing health treatment or screening decisions. Cochrane Database of Systematic Reviews. 2014;**4**: CD001431. DOI: 10.1002/14651858.CD001431.pub4

[21] Greenfield S, Kaplan SH, Ware JE Jr, Yano EM, Frank HJ. Patients' participation in medical care: Effects on blood sugar control and quality of life in diabetes. Journal of General Internal Medicine. 1988;**3**:448-457. DOI: 10.1007/BF02595921

[22] Kaplan SH, Greenfield S, Ware JE Jr. Assessing the effects of physician-patient interactions on the outcomes of chronic disease. Medical Care. 1989;**27**: 110-127. DOI: 10.1097/00005650-198903001-00010

[23] Himmerich H, Lewis YD, Conti C, Mutwalli H, Karwautz A, Sjögren JM, et al. World Federation of Societies of biological psychiatry (WFSBP) guidelines update 2023 on the pharmacological treatment of eating disorders. The World Journal of Biological Psychiatry. 2023;**24**(8): 643-706. DOI: 10.1080/15622975.2023.2179663

[24] Himmerich H, Bentley J, Lichtblau N, Brennan C, Au K. Facets of shared decision-making on drug treatment for adults with an eating disorder. International Review of Psychiatry. 2019;**31**:332-346. DOI: 10.1080/09540261.2019.1571995

Chapter 13

Empowered by Hope: Insights from Lived Experience in Eating Disorder Recovery

Phoebe Saville

Abstract

This chapter will explore the transformative power of hope, drawing from both my personal battle with the eating disorder (ED) anorexia nervosa (AN) and the clinical insights I have gained since working on an ED inpatient unit during a placement as an MSc student. It was through fostering hope that I was able to support myself and promote recovery, a pattern I have observed frequently in practice. This chapter will explore how hope can be instilled through recovery-promoting strategies such as creativity and goal setting, alongside the value of relationships and lived experience support. Overall, I advocate for a more optimistic and empowering approach to mental health recovery, particularly in the context of EDs, which can be achieved through spreading hope and sharing stories of recovery.

Keywords: lived experience, eating disorders, anorexia nervosa, hope, creativity, goal setting, relationships

1. Introduction

Within the context of mental illness, hope emerges as an indispensable force, aptly defined by the late Desmond Tutu as 'being able to see that there is light despite all of the darkness' [1]. This chapter will explore the transformative power of hope, drawing from both my personal battle with the eating disorder (ED) anorexia nervosa (AN) and the clinical insights I have gained since working on an ED inpatient unit placement as an MSc student. I will share how hope can be fostered on the path to recovery through creativity, supportive relationships, goal-setting, and lived experience support.

1.1 My story

When I was 14 years old, I found myself entangled in a struggle with food and exercise. Initially, it was my enthusiasm for middle-distance running that contributed to my overexercising and focusing on 'clean' eating. Quickly, the foods I deemed healthy became less and less calorific, and the runs I went on longer and longer. Inevitably, my weight plummeted. Surprisingly, though my initial motivation was not driven by body image, I found myself besieged by body dysmorphia. I lost the ability to perceive myself accurately. Instead, I viewed my transformed body as a 'work in progress,' convinced that more weight needed shedding to achieve a prime athletic physique.

AN takes on two distinct forms: the restricting subtype and the binge-purge subtype [2]. It was when, in a desperate attempt to shed even more weight I engaged in the latter and could no longer deny the unhealthy path I was on. Despite this realization, I was terrified to even entertain the thought of the alternative—eating more and keeping it down. Indeed, AN cruelly operates on the paradoxical principle that the individual's worst fear, food, is their necessary medicine. Therefore, the preservation of destructive behaviors became my top priority, eclipsing everything else.

Fortunately, with intervention from my parents, who took me to a GP appointment, I was referred to Child and Adolescent Mental Health Services (CAHMS). On my initial visit, I was told I was grappling with AN (for formulation see **Table 1**). With a body mass index (BMI) of 14 kg/m2, I met the threshold for hospital admission [3]. However, I was granted a mere week to gain weight at home to avoid this. Outpatient treatments provide care in the least restrictive setting and thus are favored by current psychiatric practice [4]. So, for me, like many others, outpatient care was explored as the first-line treatment. I was subsequently placed on 'bed rest' at home for the following weeks to gain weight. The stringent measures imposed by the clinicians completely restricted my freedom and, in some ways, bore a resemblance to the sudden restrictions later imposed during the COVID-19 pandemic.

Poignantly, whilst I was away from school, a teacher cautioned my friends to not get their hopes up as I would 'never fully recover'. This prognosis instilled in me a profound sense of hopelessness. Not only was I physically confined to my home, but I also felt emotionally confined by the belief that any recovery efforts were futile. I felt trapped in a perpetual anorexic existence. My teacher was not alone in her concern, as many people question whether it is possible to ever fully recover from AN [5]. Indeed, even the statistics surrounding recovery seem poor, with less than half of people with AN fully recovering and a third relapsing after treatment, making it one of the most treatment-resistant psychological illnesses [6, 7].

Yet I did manage to find hope during this dark time, and against these odds, I find myself 9 years later typing this chapter as a testament to a fully recovered life. Although definitions of recovery do vary, I have met all definitions of complete recovery concerning physical, behavioral, and psychological indices for many years [8]. Therefore, I want to send the message that real, full, and lasting recovery is possible despite what we are so often told. Now, I am even working with individuals battling

Predisposing factors	**Perfectionism**
Precipitating factors	Loss of appetite and resulting weight loss
Perpetuating factors	Effects of starvation Parents not in charge of meals
Protective factors	Expresses a wish to gain weight Parental support and consistency Parental commitment
Phoebe meets the criteria for a DSM-5 diagnosis of Anorexia Nervosa. There are no current comorbidities.	

Table 1.
Table of formulation by my consultant child and adolescent psychiatrist.

DOI: http://dx.doi.org/10.5772/intechopen.1005460

with the same illness I overcame. My past has not hindered me but has actually enabled me to bring a deep experiential understanding and empathy to my clinical work. There was so much to be hopeful for.

2. Creativity

So, what enabled me to retain hope during this time?

During my time recovering at home, I created a self-guided scrapbook entitled 'Healthy Me'. To visualize what life could look like once I was healthy again, I sifted through magazines, selecting images and words to collage on each page. One page simply captured the essence of outdoor walks, emphasizing the sensations of being windswept, the scent of flowers in bloom, and the sights of the different seasons (see **Figure 1**). Other pages showcased my travel aspirations, one being Cornwall (see **Figure 2**) and another being South Africa, symbolizing faith that I would be well enough to explore these places for myself. In fact, the entire scrapbook echoed a theme of hope, envisioning my future beyond confinement. I have now witnessed everything I had scrapbooked come to fruition, having been on more walks than I can count, visited both Cornwall and South Africa, and even ventured further abroad. These experiences have been extraordinary, knowing how much I longed for each one, showing that my hope was not in vain.

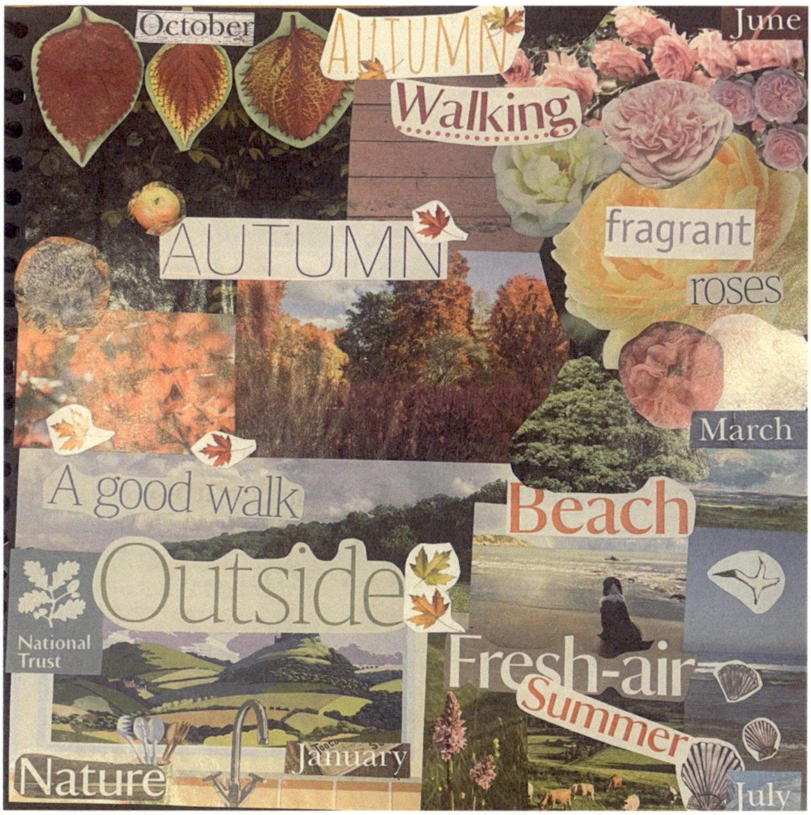

Figure 1.
The essence of outdoor walks.

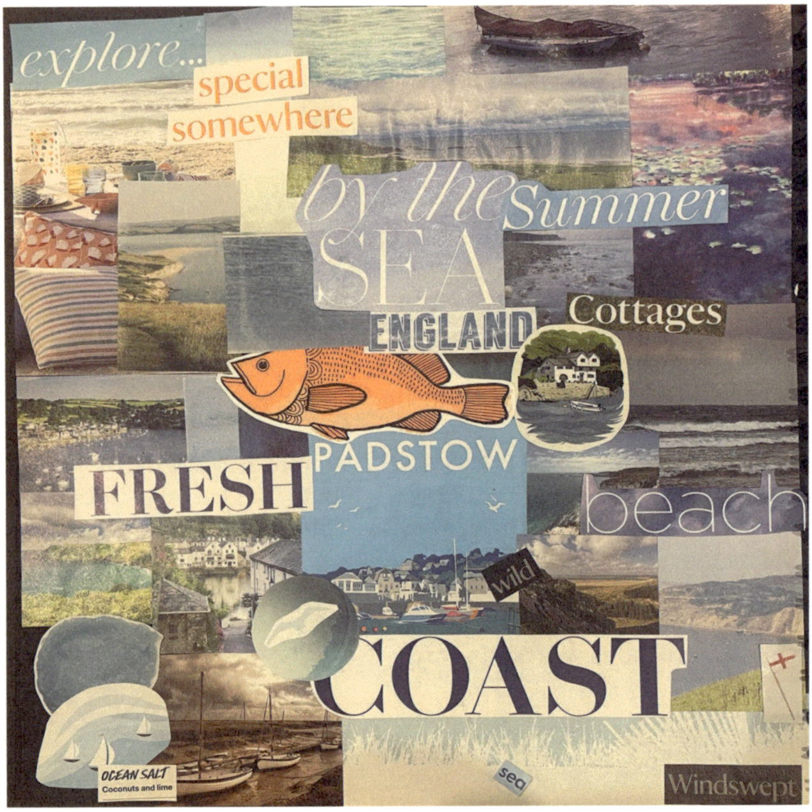

Figure 2.
My travel aspirations.

Although this was a self-led activity, scrapbooking is employed by creative arts therapy. The therapeutic and creative process of making art provides a non-verbal way to express thoughts and feelings [9]. This non-verbal process has been shown to reduce the use of defense mechanisms utilized by ED patients to protect themselves and provide a sense of control [10]. Indeed, I found this right-brain-engaging creative activity enabled me to shift from avoiding my feelings to actually feeling them. Furthermore, recent neuroscientific studies suggest that the brain reacts to mental images in the same manner as it does to reality [11]. Therefore, envisioning change through creativity is a very powerful tool. Thus, when I collaged images of going abroad, my mind pictured me there, providing me with a tangible vision of my future beyond AN.

Moreover, creativity in the form of scrapbooking provided me with temporary psychological relief as it served as a distraction from the negative thoughts and emotions that consumed me. Indeed, engaging in creative activities unrelated to disordered behaviors can be transformative for ED patients. I have witnessed this as part of my clinical placement, where I contributed to a weekly music therapy group in an ED inpatient unit. Staff and patients gather to sing and make music, creating a space where distinctions between residents and clinicians blur. Witnessing patients' faces light up and hearing remarks like 'We should go on X Factor!', highlights the escapism that they experienced during this time. The hour of immersive musical expression provides a mental sanctuary, pushing aside disordered thoughts. Therefore, it is no surprise that when used therapeutically, music has been shown to have a positive impact on ED symptomatology [12].

Despite creative arts therapy's efficacy in helping instil hope through envisionment and escapism, it was not a strategy utilized as part of my treatment. One reason for this may be that CAMHS treatment is mainly based on family interventions. By contrast, adult treatment is based on individual and group therapies and thus might allow more for the employment of techniques such as creative arts therapy [13]. However, I believe there is a need for creative arts therapy to be accessible to ED patients of all ages.

3. Relationships

Another aspect of my recovery that enabled me to retain hope was the presence of supportive relationships.

My parents played a fundamental role in my treatment: they prepared and oversaw all my meals and snacks, enforced the clinicians' guidelines regarding my freedom, took me to my weekly weigh-in sessions and provided unwavering emotional support. This very significant level of involvement in my recovery was helped by their ability to work from home. As indicated in my formulation (see **Table 1**), my parents' support, consistency, and commitment were identified as protective factors from the outset of my recovery journey. Their approach embodied tough love, necessitating difficult decisions on behalf of my well-being. Though I initially resented their firmness, I came to recognize it as a manifestation of their unwavering dedication to my recovery, which instilled in me a profound sense of determination. Their great efforts for my recovery gave me hope as it demonstrated that they believed recovery was possible. As I progressed through recovery and regained control of my life, our relationship evolved into a more balanced dynamic. Despite the extensive support they provided, the ultimate decision to embrace life and pursue recovery rested solely with me, but this was a journey on which they supported me unconditionally, for which I am immensely grateful.

Within the framework of CAMHS treatment, which is centred around family interventions, parents are recognized as pivotal in managing a young person's ED and bringing about change [13]. Parents are encouraged to take control of their child's eating until the child is deemed capable of regaining autonomy. Moreover, as parental involvement in the recovery process involves identification of early ED signs, seeking initial help, and navigating the many physical and psychological challenges faced by their child, this begins before commencing treatment [14]. Additionally, the central role of parents in treatment occurs amidst managing other responsibilities such as parenting siblings and maintaining relationships, work, and finances [14]. Optimal parental support has been shown to involve both parents and provide consistency, support, and affirmation [15]. Indeed, I am not alone in recognizing the pivotal role of familial relationships in recovery, as many individuals who have recovered describe their family's support as instrumental in their journey [16].

At 14, I was fortunate to have a supportive network of friends and in particular a best friend who I boarded with at school during the week. During my ED acquisition, I often appeared emotionally disconnected as I was preoccupied with internal struggles which consumed my thoughts and energy. Despite these challenges and then the additional hurdle of being separated for weeks, our friendship endured. Whilst recovering at home, she often sent me words of encouragement, shared songs that she thought I would like, and even came to visit. This further example of unwavering relational support gave me hope: both directly, through reassurance that I would get better, and indirectly, because it offered a lifeline to the rich friendships I longed to return to. Despite the damage an ED did to our friendship in the short term, it not only endured but ultimately grew stronger over time. Nine years later, we remain best friends. Like many others in recovery, a motivator to heal stemmed from the desire to return to normal, balanced friendships and reclaim my teenage experience. My friendships taught me that I was valued and loved regardless of my struggles, which gave me a strong foundation on which I found the strength to recover.

Friendship holds a central role in adolescent life, yet the onset of an ED can deeply affect these relationships. Developing an ED often leads to emotional and social distancing from friends, and a desire to heal damaged friendships can serve as a significant motivator for recovery [16, 17]. Individuals in recovery express increased hope when they strengthen emotional connections with supportive friends [16]. Additionally, patients with higher levels of social support, particularly from friends, show better outcomes in terms of recovery and reduction of symptoms. High-quality friendships, characterised by support, trust, and low conflict, promote the best outcomes for those in recovery.

In summary, support systems, such as family and friends, have the influence to significantly aid the ED recovery process. ED services must focus on providing support and guidance regarding fostering stable relationships for both parents and individuals in recovery. Due to the pivotal role parents play in child and adolescent ED recovery, it is vital to guide and support them throughout the recovery process. Offering parents training in skills to manage the illness can alleviate the distress of living with someone with AN and improve patient outcomes [18]. Furthermore, connecting parents with online support groups can be instrumental in offering them support, information, and empowerment throughout their child's recovery journey [19]. Similarly, individuals in recovery should be encouraged to seek and maintain supportive friendships, due to the positive impact this has on their recovery process [16]. Supporting young people in addressing any challenges that may have arisen in friendships due to their illness can help preserve these relationships and prevent long-term negative consequences for the individual.

4. Goal setting

A further strategy that enabled me to support myself and retain hope was goal setting.

Throughout my early adolescence, I battled with a paralyzing fear of underachievement and the pursuit of excessively high personal standards. Indeed, perfectionism has had longstanding implications in the pathogenesis of AN. Perfectionism often precedes ED onset, is implicated as a maintaining mechanism, and remains elevated after recovery [20]. Goal setting, closely linked to perfectionism, also emerges as a significant construct within EDs [21]. This involves making conditional associations between specific body shape and weight goals and the more abstract goal of attaining happiness as an outcome. The fixation on these conditional goals, irrespective of their appropriateness, organized my cognition and behavior whilst I was ill.

In my outpatient treatment plan, clinicians provided recovery goals which were staggered weight targets, each reinforced once achieved. The progression of reinforcement started with regaining the freedom to go on a walk, then returning to school gradually, reintegrating into sports sessions, and ultimately transitioning back to weekly boarding at school. As someone with high perfectionist tendencies, with goal setting ingrained in my illness attribution, I was used to thinking in a blinkered goal-centred way. My transition from prioritizing illness to prioritizing recovery began with these small weight gain goals, each achievement offering increased freedom and a return to aspects of my former life, ultimately shifting the focus of my perfectionism towards achieving full weight restoration. With each step, my hope of recovery was strengthened. Furthermore, within an inpatient setting, I have seen effective goals regarding the completion of nutrition and weight gain, rewarded by increased freedom. Literature supports the use of goals in recovery, as individuals who are provided with specific, challenging but attainable goals perform better than those given easy, nonspecific, or no goals at all [22].

However, my positive experience with goal-setting reinforcement was specific to the context of my care: As a minor at the time, my freedoms were restricted and subsequently reinstated by my parents in line with the goals set by clinicians. The dynamic becomes more complex upon reaching adulthood. In my clinical experience in an inpatient setting, where patients are sectioned, clinicians have the authority to revoke and reinstate freedoms as necessary. However, for adults undergoing outpatient treatment, the process of reinstating freedoms becomes less straightforward, as there are no mechanisms in place for their removal in the first instance.

Furthermore, Locke and Latham [23] outline, in the goal-setting theory of motivation, those goals must be accepted by the individual [23]. Simply assigning goals to someone is not indicative of their commitment to those goals, especially if the goal is difficult to accomplish, such as weight gain for ED patients. A powerful method of aiding acceptance is to allow patients to participate in the goal-setting process. Indeed, early on in Cognitive Behavior Therapy for Eating Disorders (CBT-E) treatment goals are set collaboratively, allowing the individual to then evaluate their progress throughout therapy [24]. However, concerning weight and food-related recovery goals, collaboration is more difficult as AN is defined by denial. Indeed, after my initial assessment, it was noted that I was not in total agreement with the clinician's plan for my care. However, as my goals were small increments and were reinforced by valued aspects of my former life, it was not long until I was in total agreement due to the motivation this strategy instilled in me.

5. Lived experience support

Finally, a strategy that I believe *would* have been instrumental in instilling hope during my treatment is the inclusion of lived experience support. Individuals with lived experience of EDs can play a crucial role in assisting those undergoing ED recovery, by offering treatment support, partaking in research, or even working as ED clinicians.

During my outpatient treatment at CAMHS, I expressed a strong desire for support from someone who had made a full recovery from an ED. Like all ED recoveries, my journey was marked by numerous challenges and triumphs, and I firmly believed that guidance from someone who had navigated a similar journey would have been invaluable. However, clinicians at CAMHS revealed a lack of contact with individuals willing to share their lived experience of ED recovery, highlighting a gap in available resources.

Stable ongoing support from individuals who are also in recovery or have recovered from an ED offers patients a connection with others who understand the complexities of the recovery process [16]. Indeed, patients with EDs express that support from individuals with lived experience alleviates feelings of isolation and poignantly provides tangible hope for recovery [16]. This perspective is echoed by both patients and caregivers alike [25]. Furthermore, adults post-recovery expressed that assistance and support had been the most forthcoming and helpful from other individuals who had recovered from an ED, in comparison to professional help which had generally been unhelpful and unempathetic [26]. Therefore, the resource of lived experience support for children in CAMHS could enhance treatment.

In ED research, studies should continue to venture beyond brief self-report questionnaires to capture the experiential perspective of individuals with lived experience of EDs [26]. Understanding the illness through the lens of lived experience offers a comprehensive picture that validates the experiences of those currently struggling with EDs. For example, Redenbach and Lawler's [27] study, revealed that none of the participants who had recovered from an ED had adopted dysfunctional eating habits to emulate the idealized body image perpetuated by the media [26]. If these findings had been accessible to me, they could have alleviated my perception of being misunderstood, particularly amidst a societal discourse of body image distortion as the primary driver of food refusal [27]. Additionally, gleaning insights from lived experience research would have offered me hope, knowing that others who had had a similar journey to mine had not only successfully attained full recovery but were able to share their narratives to help others.

Additionally, this research is invaluable in informing practice. If outpatient treatment programmes were informed by findings indicating that self-determination and self-acceptance significantly fuel recovery, rather than solely relying on treatment-focused interventions, individuals in recovery may feel more adequately supported and hopeful [26]. Integrating such insights into treatment modalities could empower individuals to take ownership of their recovery journey and foster a greater sense of agency, hope and resilience.

Being an ED clinician with lived experience can assist those undergoing ED recovery as the delivery of psychiatric services can be affected if clinicians have negative reactions to patients with EDs [28]. It is widely accepted that the lived experience of an ED deepens therapists' understanding of and empathy for clients [25]. A clinician's feelings towards patients directly impact the therapeutic alliance associated with patient outcomes. Patients stated that being treated by a recovered therapist had a positive effect on their recovery process as recovered therapists serve as positive role models and inspire hope for recovery [29]. This hope is not only due to the demonstration that recovery is possible but also that one can go on to lead a stable and productive life [30]. For me, always having had very high aspirations for myself, seeing clinicians occupying positions of status would have been very powerful. Furthermore, if I would been aided in recovery by someone who knows what ED recovery is like, I would have granted the clinician significant credibility.

However, there are particular challenges to this dual identity of clinician and lived experience expert in the field of EDs. Clinicians with lived experience may lack objectivity, be at risk of relapse, engage in comparison, and blur boundaries [25]. Nevertheless, these risks can be mitigated through therapists meeting specific conditions such as being fully recovered (though definitions of recovery vary widely), receiving additional training and supervision, having high levels of self-awareness, and engaging in therapy [25]. Furthermore, for clinicians, the longer the time since recovery and the more sophisticated the training, the less likely relapse will occur [30]. Personally, I would not have been equipped to handle working on an inpatient ward immediately after my recovery and it is only through the passage of time and the deliberate steps I have taken towards growth that I now feel confident in my ability to handle such responsibilities safely. Moreover, while sharing experiential knowledge can enhance empathy and understanding, it should be done thoughtfully, as it is not always necessary to disclose one's own experiences to be beneficial to those in care [29].

Furthermore, many clinicians hesitate to speak openly about their struggles due to the stigma surrounding mental health, even within their own field. Concerns about negative consequences for self and career and shame prevent some clinicians from disclosing and help-seeking [31]. Indeed, putting my name to this piece of work was something I thought through deeply, for this very reason. Additionally, while some employers actively seek out ED clinicians with personal experience, others may refuse to hire them, underscoring the diversity of opinions regarding this dual identity within the field [25].

6. Conclusion

Reflecting on my struggles in adolescence through the lens of this chapter has been a profound privilege, allowing me to discern more clearly what helped me 'see that there is light despite all of the darkness', and what might help others to see the same. Whilst I was recovering at home, I often sought reassurance from the fact that I could help others in the future with my experience. In ED recovery, the importance of spreading hope regarding recovery is crucial and may have broader implications for the wider field of mental health recovery. No one should ever be told they will never recover and instead sharing strategies and stories can aid recovery and help change this narrative.

After recovering from AN, I initially sought to avoid references to that chapter of my life, hesitant to revisit it in conversations with friends and family. One reason for this was I resisted the notion of being solely defined as a 'recovered anorexic', feeling that my identity extended far beyond that label. However, as time passed and I pursued my education, earning a bachelor's degree in Psychology and later studying for a master's in Mental Health Studies, I gained a profound appreciation for the power of lived experience insights and the value that comes with embracing a dual identity. Reclaiming the title of a survivor of one of the most challenging mental health disorders has been profoundly empowering for me. It is also a way of honoring the strength and resilience of individuals who have faced similar struggles. While that period of my life was significant, I have come to realize that it has not defined who I am nor confined my future; rather, it has opened doors to opportunities that have arisen directly from my experiences, like writing this chapter.

As more individuals with lived experiences bravely share their stories, the stigma surrounding mental health struggles diminishes, and we begin to see people for who they truly are—individuals with unique stories, strengths, and resilience. I am deeply grateful to everyone who supported me on my journey and told me that recovery was possible. My hope is that anyone facing similar struggles can find that same support and hope, in whatever form it may be. Additionally, the ultimate aim of this chapter is to serve as a testament to the transformative power of hope, illustrating how it can be found through various avenues. And while aspects of my experiences are unique, I hope they resonate with others, offering understanding and inspiration.

In summary, firstly, creativity was a powerful tool for promoting my recovery by fostering hope. Engaging in creative activities not only allowed me to envision life beyond my illness but also provided a means of expression whilst offering a break from disordered thoughts. Creative arts therapy, therefore, should be made available to individuals of all ages struggling with EDs.

Secondly, supportive relationships were instrumental not only in implementing my treatment plan but also in providing me with hope for recovery. The unwavering support from friends and family served as a constant reminder that recovery was possible and reinforced my determination to persevere. Services aimed at treating EDs must prioritize fostering stable relationships between parents, friends, and individuals in recovery, due to the significant role they play.

Thirdly, using small goals to focus my recovery, helped me to remain hopeful and thus support myself. Just one step at a time, achieving each milestone enabled freedom to be gained alongside a sense of accomplishment. While the nature of these goals may vary depending on the individual and their circumstances, the collaborative process of setting and working towards them should be encouraged to ensure optimal commitment and success.

Lastly, individuals with lived experience of eating disorders possess invaluable insights and the potential to contribute to the recovery of others. Whether through offering treatment support, sharing personal narratives in research, or even working as clinicians, their first-hand understanding can offer tangible hope to those undergoing recovery. The integration of support from individuals with lived experience into services, particularly within CAMHS, should be sought.

These are just a few strategies that I feel did or would have supported my recovery by providing me with hope for the future I am now living. I am proud to have joined the individuals who have bravely faced death and chosen life [32].

Notes/thanks/other declarations

I extend my heartfelt gratitude to Hubertus Himmerich for graciously reading my story and inviting me to write it in this book. His wisdom and encouragement have been invaluable, and it has been an absolute privilege to work with him. (This book chapter is a revised and extended version of an essay that I had written for my MSc Mental Health Studies programme).

I also want to express my deep appreciation to my wonderful parents. As highlighted in this chapter, their unwavering support was significant during my recovery; however, this has been a constant throughout my whole life. I hope this chapter can be a small token of my infinite thanks to them both.

Author details

Phoebe Saville
Mental Health Studies, King's College London, Institute of Psychiatry, Psychology and Neuroscience, London, UK

*Address all correspondence to: phoebe.saville@kcl.ac.uk

References

[1] SA News. A tribute to archbishop emeritus Desmond Mpilo Tutu. Available from: https://www.sanews.gov.za/special-features-archive/tribute-archbishop-emeritus-desmond-mpilo-tutu [Accessed: April 17, 2024]

[2] Peat C, Mitchell JE, Hoek HW, Wonderlich SA. Validity and utility of subtyping anorexia nervosa. The International Journal of Eating Disorders. 2009;**42**(7):590-594. DOI: 10.1002/eat.20717

[3] Le Grange D, Doyle PM, Swanson SA, Ludwig K, Glunz C, Kreipe RE. Calculation of expected body weight in adolescents with eating disorders. Pediatrics. 2012;**129**(2):e438-e446

[4] Madden S, Hay P, Touyz S. Systematic review of evidence for different treatment settings in anorexia nervosa. World Journal of Psychiatry. 2015;**5**(1):147

[5] Jenkins J, Ogden J. Becoming 'whole' Again: A qualitative study of women's views of recovering from anorexia nervosa. European Eating Disorders Review. 2012;**20**(1):e23-e31

[6] NICE. Eating Disorders. 2019. Available from: https://www.cks.nice.org.uk/topics/eating-disorders/background-information/prognosis/

[7] Touyz S, Le Grange D, Lacey H, Hay P, Smith R, Maguire S, et al. Treating severe and enduring anorexia nervosa: A randomized controlled trial. Psychological Medicine. 2013;**43**(12):2501-2511

[8] Bardone-Cone AM, Sturm K, Lawson MA, Robinson DP, Smith R. Perfectionism across stages of recovery from eating disorders. The International Journal of Eating Disorders. 2010;**43**(2):139-148. DOI: 10.1002/eat.20674

[9] Dokter D. Arts Therapies and Clients with Eating Disorders: Fragile Board. Jessica Kingsley; 2000

[10] Levens M. Eating Disorders and Magical Control of the Body: Treatment through Art Therapy. Routledge; 2002

[11] Nardone G, Balbi E. The Logic of Therapeutic Change: Fitting Strategies to Pathologies. Routledge; 2015

[12] Testa F, Arunachalam S, Heiderscheit A, Himmerich H. A systematic review of scientific studies on the effects of music in people with or at risk for eating disorders. Psychiatria Danubina. 2020;**32**(3-4):334-345

[13] Winston AP, Paul M, Juanola-Borrat Y. The same but different? Treatment of anorexia nervosa in adolescents and adults. European Eating Disorders Review: The Journal of the Eating Disorders Association. 2012;**20**(2):89-93. DOI: 10.1002/erv.1137

[14] Wilksch SM. Toward a more comprehensive understanding and support of parents with a child experiencing an eating disorder. International Journal of Eating Disorders. 2023;**56**(7):1275-1285

[15] Kyriacou O, Treasure J, Raenker S. The influence and importance of parents in care and treatment of an eating disorder. In: The Clinician's Guide to Collaborative Caring in Eating Disorders. The New Maudsley Method. 2010. pp. 241-249

[16] Linville D, Brown T, Sturm K, McDougal T. Eating disorders and social support: Perspectives of recovered individuals. Eating Disorders. 2012;**20**(3):216-231. DOI: 10.1080/10640266.2012.668480

[17] Galloway LL. Exploration of Friendship Experiences in Adolescent Eating Disorders. 2014

[18] Whitney J, Murray J, Gavan K, Todd G, Whitaker W, Treasure J. Experience of caring for someone with anorexia nervosa: Qualitative study. The British Journal of Psychiatry: the Journal of Mental Science. 2005;**187**:444-449. DOI: 10.1192/bjp.187.5.444

[19] Macdonald P, Hibbs R, Corfield F, Treasure J, Fuggle P. The use of the internet in the treatment of eating disorders. Current Psychiatry Reports. 2012;**14**(4):343-351

[20] Lethbridge J, Watson HJ, Egan SJ, Street H, Nathan PR. The role of perfectionism, dichotomous thinking, shape and weight overvaluation, and conditional goal setting in eating disorders. Eating Behaviors. 2011;**12**(3):200-206. DOI: 10.1016/j.eatbeh.2011.04.003

[21] Watson HJ, Street H, Raykos BC, Byrne SM, Fursland A, Nathan PR. Reliability and validity of the conditional goal setting in eating disorders scale (CGS-EDS) among adults with eating disorders. Eating Behaviors. 2010;**11**(2):113-118

[22] Lunenburg FC. Goal-setting theory of motivation. International Journal of Management, Business, and Administration. 2011;**15**(1):1-6

[23] Locke E, Latham G. Goal-setting theory. In: Organizational Behavior 1. Routledge; 2015. pp. 159-183

[24] Fairburn CG, Cooper Z, Shafran R. Enhanced cognitive behaviour therapy for eating disorders ("CBT-E"): An overview. Cognitive Behavior Therapy and Eating Disorders. 2008:23-34

[25] Bachner-Melman R, de Vos JA, Zohar AH, Shalom M, Mcgilley B, Oberlin K, et al. Attitudes towards eating disorders clinicians with personal experience of an eating disorder. Eating and Weight Disorders-Studies on Anorexia, Bulimia and Obesity. 2021;**26**:1881-1891

[26] Redenbach J, Lawler J. Recovery from disordered eating: What life histories reveal. Contemporary Nurse. 2003;**15**(1-2):148-156

[27] Katzman MA, Lee S. Beyond body image: The integration of feminist and transcultural theories in the understanding of self starvation. International Journal of Eating Disorders. 1997;**22**(4):385-394

[28] Thompson-Brenner H, Satir DA, Franko DL, Herzog DB. Clinician reactions to patients with eating disorders: A review of the literature. Psychiatric Services. 2012;**63**(1):73-78

[29] de Vos JA, Netten C, Noordenbos G. Recovered eating disorder therapists using their experiential knowledge in therapy: A qualitative examination of the therapists' and the patients' view. Eating Disorders. 2016;**24**(3):207-223. DOI: 10.1080/10640266.2015.1090869

[30] Costin C. Been there, done that: Clinicians' use of personal recovery in the treatment of eating disorders. Eating Disorders. 2002;**10**(4):293-303

[31] Tay S, Alcock K, Scior K. Mental health problems among clinical psychologists: Stigma and its impact on disclosure and help-seeking.

Journal of Clinical Psychology. 2018;**74**(9):1545-1555

[32] Garrett CJ. Sociological perspectives on recovery from anorexia nervosa. International Journal of Eating Disorders. 1997;**21**:261-272